COVID-19
Analysing the Threat

COVID-19
Analysing the Threat

Editors

Ajey Lele
Kritika Roy

PENTAGON PRESS LLP

COVID-19: Analysing the Threat

Editors: Ajey Lele and Kritika Roy

First Published in 2020

ISBN 978-93-90095-07-0

Published by

PENTAGON PRESS LLP
206, Peacock Lane, Shahpur Jat,
New Delhi-110049
Phones: 011-64706243, 26491568
Telefax: 011-26490600
email: rajan@pentagonpress.in
website: www.pentagonpress.in

Printed at Aegean Offset Printers, Greater Noida, U.P.

CONTENTS

North and South America

Europe and Russia

Africa

SECTION III: SCIENCE AND TECHNOLOGY

PREFACE

On 31 December 2019, the Wuhan Municipal Health Commission, China, reported a cluster of cases of pneumonia in Wuhan, Hubei Province. A novel coronavirus was eventually identified. Four days later on 04 January 2020, the World Health Organisation (WHO) corroborated the same information. Subsequently, this disease started spreading in some parts of the world. On 11 February 2020, the WHO gave the name for the new coronavirus disease as COVID-19. Finally, on 11 March 2020 taking note of the alarming levels of spread and severity, the WHO announced COVID-19 as a pandemic. This book presents some basic assessments of this pandemic during the first six months of its existence.

The editors are grateful to all contributors for taking out time for contributing to this volume. Amb Sujan R Chinoy, Director General, Manohar Parrikar Institute for Defence Studies and Analyses (MP-IDSA), New Delhi approved undertaking this work and the editors are deeply indebted to him. Acknowledgment is also due to Mr Vivek Kaushik for his assistance in providing editorial suggestions. The views presented in this volume are personal.

New Delhi
01 July 2020

Ajey Lele
Kritika Roy

ABBREVIATIONS

ACE2	Angiotensin-converting Enzyme 2
AI	Artificial Intelligence
AIDS	Acquired Immunodeficiency Syndrome
ALI	Acute Lung Injury
APEC	Asia-Pacific Economic Cooperation
ARDS	Acute Respiratory Distress Syndrome
BIMSTEC	The Bay of Bengal Initiative for Multi-Sectoral Technical and Economic Cooperation
BWC	Biological Weapons Convention
BTWC	Biological Weapons and Toxins Convention
CDC	Centers for Disease Control and Prevention
CNS	Centre for a New American Security
COBRA	Cabinet Office Briefing Room A
CRISPR	Clustered Regularly Interspaced Short Palindromic Repeats
CP	Convalescent Plasma
CT	Computed Tomography
DBT	Department of Biotechnology
HCQ	Hydroxychloroquine
HHS	U.S. Department of Health and Human Services
HIV	Human Immunodeficiency Virus
FDA	Food and Drug Administration
ECLAC	Economic Commission for Latin America and the Caribbean
IBV	Infectious Bronchitis Virus
ICMR	Indian Council of Medical Research
ICTV	International Committee on Taxonomy of Viruses

ICU	Intensive Care Units
IICT	Indian Institute of Chemical Technology
IMF	International Monetary Fund
INF	Intermediate Nuclear Forces
IRGC	Islamic Revolutionary Guards Corps
JAXA	Japan Aerospace Exploration Agency
LTTE	Liberation Tigers of Tamil Eelam
MERS	Middle East Respiratory Syndrome
NASA	National Aeronautics and Space Administration
NCVMC	National Corona Virus Management Committee
NHC	National Health Commission
NMPA	National Medical Products Administration
NSABB	National Science Advisory Board for Biosecurity
NSRA	National Security Risk Assessment
OECD	Organisation of Economic Cooperation and Development
OPEC	Organisation of Petroleum Exporting Countries
PAHO	Pan America Health Organization
PCR	Polymerase Chain Reaction
PPE	Personal Protective Equipment
RBD	Receptor Binding Domain
RT-PCR	Real-time Reverse Transcription-polymerase Chain Reaction
SARS-CoV-2	Severe Acute Respiratory Syndrome Coronavirus 2
SAARC	The South Asian Association for Regional Cooperation
STEP	Science and Technology Exchange Program
USAMRIID	United States Army Medical Research Institute of Infectious Diseases
WEF	World Economic Forum
WMD	Weapons of Mass Destruction
WHO	World Health Organisation

ABOUT THE CONTRIBUTORS

Dr Paulami Sanyal is a Research Analyst at the Manohar Parrikar Institute for Defence Studies and Analyses, New Delhi. She has a Ph.D. from the Centre for West Asian Studies, School of International Studies, Jawaharlal Nehru University, New Delhi and Master's in Politics with specialisation in International Relations.

Dr Anshu Joshi is an Assistant Professor in the School of International Studies, Jawaharlal Nehru University, New Delhi and has done her PhD on developing a comprehensive bio-defence mechanism. She has worked on diverse issues related to bioterrorism.

Mr A.Vinod Kumar is an Associate Fellow at the Manohar Parrikar Institute for Defence Studies and Analyses. His research interests include nuclear policy issues, missile defence and India's relations with the great powers. He is author of the book titled "India and the Nuclear Non-Proliferation Regime – The Perennial Outlier," Cambridge University Press, April 2014.

Dr Xie Chao is currently working as Assistant Professor at the Institute for International and Area Studies, Tsinghua University, and a visiting faculty scholar (2018-2020), Jindal School of International Affairs, O.P. Jindal Global University, India.

Dr Titli Basu is an Associate Fellow in the East Asia Centre at the Manohar Parrikar Institute for Defence Studies and Analyses, New Delhi. Her research interests include Japanese security, strategy and foreign policy; Japan and the Indo-Pacific; great power politics in East Asia; and India-Japan relations.

Professor (Dr) Ali Karami is currently working as a professor at Molecular Biology Research Center, Systems Biology and Poisonings Institute, Baqiyatallah University of Medical Sciences, Tehran, Iran. He is working and teaching in varied areas of Molecular Biotechnology and Rapid Molecular Detection of Infectious Diseases.

Dr Cherian Samuel is a Research Fellow in the Strategic Technologies Centre at the Manohar Parrikar Institute for Defence Studies and Analyses where he works on cyber security issues. His research interests have also covered Indo-US Relations, US Domestic issues, and the Indian Diaspora in the United States.

Mr Munish Sharma is a Consultant in the Strategic Technologies Centre at the Manohar Parrikar Institute for Defence Studies and Analyses, New Delhi. His research interests include cybersecurity, critical information infrastructure protection, space security and geopolitical aspects of emerging technologies. He is a Chevening Cyber Security Fellow (2018).

Mr Syed Ali works with the Embassy of Costa Rica in New Delhi. He is a regular contributor to newspapers sharing his observations on Latin American affairs. He worked with the RIS (Research and Information systems for Developing countries) under the Ministry of External Affairs. He did his M.A. from the United Nations-mandated University for Peace in Costa Rica.

Ms Elisande Nexon is a Senior Research Fellow at the Fondation pour la Recherche Stratégique, France. She focuses on biological and chemical non-proliferation, security threats arising from advances in life sciences, and major public health crisis response and governance. She holds a State Diploma of Doctor of Pharmacy and a master's degree in arms control and disarmament.

Mr Frédéric Coste is a Senior Research Fellow at the Fondation pour la Recherche Stratégique, Paris, France. He works on military sociology, crisis management and the integration of technologies in military organizations. He holds a master's degree in defence, geostrategy and industrial dynamics, as well as a research master's degree in political sociology.

Dr Maria J. Espona, Biologist, Master in Terrorism Studies and PhD in Criminology. She is the co-Director of the NGO ArgIQ (Argentina Information Quality), a nonprofit organization promoting information quality methodology in Spanish-speaking countries. She teaches postgraduate courses in Science and Technology and Disarmament, at Argentine universities.

Ms Chiara De Cuia is a terrorism and security analyst living in Rome and the deputy director of NextGen 5.0. She holds a master's degree in Security Studies from Georgetown University's School of Foreign Service.

Ms Kanchana Ramanujam holds a Bachelor's degree in Biotechnology (Goa University) and a Master's degree in Defence and Strategic Studies (University of

Madras). She has written extensively on matters pertaining to defence, warfare, China, Pakistan, and technology. She has also been associated with the Centre for Land Warfare Studies, New Delhi.

Professor Paul Rogers is Oxford Research Group's Senior Fellow in International Security, Emeritus Professor of Peace Studies at the University of Bradford and an Honorary Fellow of the UK Defence Academy. He is a frequent broadcaster on international networks and his most recent book is *Irregular War: The New Threat from the Margins,* I B Tauris, London, 2017.

Dr Nivedita Das Kundu, Ph.D, International Relations Expert and Foreign Policy Analyst. Teaches at York University, Toronto. She is also the President, Academic and International Cooperation Meadowvale College of Business Management and Technology, Brampton, Ontario. She has authored a few books.

Professor (Dr) Eucharia Kenya is a Professor of Biotechnology with expansive international experience and expertise on Biotechnology, Biosafety and Biosecurity issues. She holds a PhD in Applied Entomology and an Advance Master's degree in Business Administration. Currently, she is the Deputy Vice-Chancellor at the University of Embu in Kenya.

Dr Margaret Muturi is PhD holder in Immunology. She is a Senior Lecturer of Immunology, Biosafety and Biosecurity as well as a researcher in the area of Infectious Diseases in the Department of Medical Laboratory Science at Kenyatta University. She is also a resource person in several organizations and a member of several professional bodies.

Dr Mrinmayee Bhushan is a Bio-defence analyst, National Awards winning Technology Innovator & entrepreneur, Oxford University Chevening CRISP Fellow, PhD Medicine (Medical Pharmacology) & Microbiologist; Prospecting reforms of CWC and Biological and Toxin Weapons Convention (BTWC); CBRN preparedness, counter-terrorism and training.

Mr Ronnie Ninan is pursuing Post-Graduate Diploma at the Young India Fellowship (2020-21) from Ashoka University. He holds a Master's degree in International Studies from the Symbiosis School of International Studies, Pune.

Dr Namrata Goswami is an independent Senior Analyst and Author, and Subject Matter Expert, International Affairs, Futures Lab, USA. She was awarded the Minerva Research Initiative Grant for Social Sciences from the Office of the U.S. Secretary of Defense to study 'Great Power Competition'. Currently, she is working on a book 'Great Power Competition in Outer Space', Lexington Press, an imprint of Rowman and Littlefield.

Professor (Dr) Manish is currently Professor and Dean at the Centre for International Politics, School of International Studies, Central University of Gujarat. He has earlier served with Sikkim University. He is currently also an honorary Visiting Faculty at the Naval War College, Goa. His areas of research interest include foreign policy and strategic security aspects.

Mr Animesh Roul is the Executive Director of the Society for the Study of Peace and Conflict, New Delhi. He specializes in counterterrorism and armed conflict and issues relating to arms control and proliferation. He has written extensively on various aspects of national security. He has co-authored the book 'Indian Mujahideen: Computational Analysis and Public Policy', Springer, New York, 2013.

Dr Simon Whitby is Senior Lecturer at the Division of Peace Studies and International Development, Faculty of Management, Law and Social Sciences, University of Bradford. Dr Whitby graduated in 2000 with a PhD in Biological Security. Since 2009, Whitby has worked at the interface between life science and national security communities.

Mr Cheng Tang is an expert on Chemical demilitarization. He was also the Chairman of OPCW (Organisation for the Prohibition of Chemical Weapons) Scientific Advisory Board (SAB) and an advisor to the Chinese National Authority.

Professor (Dr) Lijun Shang holds a BSc and MSc in Mathematics and PhD in Physiology, London. His research is mainly focused on ion channels in health and disease. He also studies biomedical and clinical applications of biomaterials and nanomaterials. Recently, he expanded his research interests into biological and chemical weapons and science convergence.

Professor (Dr) Malcolm Dando trained originally as a biologist. After post-doctoral studies in the US he held the UK Ministry of Defence funded fellowships in Operational Research at the University of Sussex. He has worked on arms control and disarmament, particularly on chemical and biological issues. Currently, his work focusses on awareness raising and education of life scientists in regard to dual-use and biosecurity.

Dr David R. Franz served in the US Army Medical Research and Materiel Command during his 27 years on active duty and served as Commander of the US Army Medical Research Institute of Infectious Diseases (USAMRIID).

Mr Malinda Meegoda is a Research Associate working in the Global Governance program at the Lakshman Kadirgamar Institute of International Relations and Strategic Studies (LKI), Sri Lanka.

Mr Vikram Venkatram is a student at Georgetown University's School of Foreign Service and is pursuing graduate work through the accelerated BSFS/Security Studies M.A. programme. He is a scholar of the O'Neill-Pellegrino Programme in Science and Global Health Law and Policy of the Georgetown University Medical Centre, USA.

Dr Diane DiEuliis is a Senior Research fellow at National Defence University, USA. Her research areas focus on emerging biological technologies, biodefense, and preparedness for biothreats. Dr DiEuliis also lectures in a variety of foundational professional military education courses across the services.

Dr James Giordano is Professor in the Departments of Neurology and Biochemistry, Chief of the Neuro-ethics Studies Programme of the Pellegrino Centre for Clinical Bioethics, and Co-chair of the Program in Brain Science and Global Law and Policy at Georgetown University Medical Center, USA.

INTRODUCTION

Infectious disease outbreaks are a reality. These have happened many times in the past and are also likely to happen anytime in the future. But the case of coronavirus disease has caught most of the world unaware. Unfortunately, the scale and magnitude of the coronavirus epidemic has shocked one and all. Yet, humans are just not letting go of the world which they have 'shaped' with so much effort for centuries. The human race is a quick learner, hence today many states in the world are found facing this pandemic head-on and are trying to resolve the crisis in all earnestness. Unfortunately, the nature of the beast is so noxious that many are finding it extremely difficult to control the spread of the infection. The world is witnessing an unprecedented loss of life in a very short span of time.

The spread of infection owing to coronavirus had begun around November/ December 2019 in Wuhan, China. This infection has spread like wildfire in many parts of the world and within three to four months it has engulfed the entire world. For this type of coronavirus disease, as on date, no medicine or vaccine has been found. Obviously, various states are finding it extremely difficult to handle these crises. In some cases, there has been a very timely response by some states and they have implemented measures like social distancing, wearing of masks, quarantine, using Personal Protective Equipment (PPE), etc for individuals to follow and have ensured the complete lockdown of the state/cities.

Coronavirus disease is not something very new. During the mid-1930s, a severe respiratory infection in chickens was considered to be the earliest known form of coronaviruses, which is presently common avian infectious bronchitis, caused by avian infectious bronchitis virus (IBV).[1] In recent times, the recognition came during 1968 when an informal group of virologists claimed the arrival of a new group of viruses named coronaviruses.[2] Just a few years prior to that the era of human coronaviruses is said to have begun in 1965 when two scientists found that they could passage a virus named B814. It was found that this virus could be responsible for a substantial proportion of upper respiratory tract infections in children. Also, there was strong evidence that animal coronaviruses are life-threatening to multiple animal species, including rats, mice, chickens, turkeys, calves, dogs, cats, rabbits and pigs. Particularly, since 2003, few new human coronaviruses have been identified, including the severe acute respiratory syndrome (SARS) coronavirus, which caused significant morbidity and mortality. During 2002-2003, the SARS infection emerged from China and spread all over the world with quantifiable speed.[3] When the coronavirus is observed under an electron microscope it bears a resemblance to an optical phenomenon formed by the diffraction of sunlight or moonlight. In meteorology, this occurrence is known as 'corona' and hence the name to the virus.

During the 2019 pandemic, the World Health Organization (WHO) gave an official name for the new coronavirus disease as COVID-19. This is a short form of the coronavirus disease which began in the year 2019. In today's world, it is very important to name a disease appropriately. This is because, in the past, diseases were named based on the region for their origin or after considering a few other factors. Mostly, such names led to belittling a region or a city or a community. Also, naming was based on perceptions, like during 1918, the influenza pandemic was commonly known as the Spanish Flu, but actually, this infection had not originated in Spain. In general, the terminologies like the Middle East Respiratory Syndrome or Swine Flu should have been avoided. In the present case, there was a danger that the virus could 'earn' the name 'China virus' or 'Wuhan virus'. Hence, in order to avoid any such stigmatization, the name COVID-19 was decided.

So far, by the end of June 2020, more than four hundred thousand (>400, 000) deaths have taken place globally. This number is expected to increase significantly in the coming months. At the same time, the recovery rate of infected individuals is also reasonable. People with a mild form of the disease are normally recovering in about two weeks' time and for serious infection, it may take four to six weeks. The treatment for this disease involves the development of an appropriate vaccine and effective drug. It is expected that the vaccine may take 12 to 18 months for development. By May 2020 some agencies have already started testing the vaccine prototypes on animals/humans. There have been some efforts to check the effectiveness of existing drugs that have been used to cure Malaria, SARS, and Ebola. It appears that the medical community is focussing on antiviral drugs that are in use for various other diseases, particularly the drug Remdesivir, which was used during the Ebola crisis is known to have given good results in a few cases.

Also, a few drugs used for treating AIDS patients and people suffering from Hepatitis C are also known to have shown some encouraging results. The top-of-the-line drugs which are known to be consumed in many cases even by health workers including doctors as a preventive treatment include anti-malaria and chronic inflammatory disease drugs like chloroquine and hydroxychloroquine.

It is important to realise that globally there is a significant amount of dependence on global supply chains for critical pharmaceuticals and various equipment and instruments used in hospitals. There are a limited number of manufacturers for drugs and medical apparatus. Also, there are a limited number of suppliers for the raw material required for the pharmacy industry. To date states like China are known to be the major producers and suppliers for several industries in various countries. Since there are strict rules in place with regard to the issue of licenses and production and supply of medicines and medical equipment, it becomes difficult for the possible new entrants in this field to start immediate production to cater for an emergency situation like COVID-19. Hence, there is a possibility that globally there could be overdependence on a few states to handle the pandemic of this magnitude.

On the whole, the quest for effective medicine and vaccine development is currently work in progress. However, owing to the increase in the vast number of COVID-19 cases, there has been a significant impact on health services all over the world to the extent that has significantly impacted the global healthcare equilibrium. There is an acute shortage of doctors and nursing staff in many parts of the world. This is putting more pressure on the existing staff which is forced to put in additional hours of work. Also, there are shortages of medical equipment like ventilators. Obviously, the system could crumble at some point. On the other hand, people staying at home owing to lockdowns have generated tremendous financial pressure on the system, almost breaking the spine of the global economy. A significant increase in the number of jobless people, frustrated individuals and people not in a position to afford good medical facilities is leading to an increase in cases of depression and suicides. Eventually, all this is expected to increase lawlessness in society and severely impact the social fabric of the country in general and the safety and security of the individual and government assets in particular.

Now the question is, 'how is it that the human community, one of the smartest species ever to exist on earth was not able to anticipate such a threat'? How is it that in the 21st century, the century of Industry 4.0, humans are not able to find a permanent solution to address the challenge of COVID-19, even six months after the threat has become evident? The estimated loss of life owing to the atomic bombings of Hiroshima and Nagasaki (August 6 and 9, 1945) is more than 200,000. While a very moderate estimate indicates that loss of lives due to COVID-19 could be three to four times of this. This indicates that the situation of the day, is the result of major failures of various governments and other institutions on all counts. They failed to prepare the world to face an infectious disease outbreak in spite of having various warnings both in the near and distant past; for example, the 2003 outbreak of SARS and the 1918 flu pandemic.

There have been enough indications to realise the possibility of a threat like COVID-19. Unfortunately, society as such has been always reactive to the situation for all these years. Normally, humans are known to relate to a simultaneous large number of deaths (the meaning of large could be subjective and case-dependent) owing to wars, major terror attacks, natural disasters or pandemics. The problem is that the human community, as a whole, needs to get out of the 'syndrome' of reacting and preparing for yesterday's threats. The field of warfare tells us that humans draw lessons from past wars in order to prepare for future wars without realizing that the face of future wars may not be the same that they have experienced in the past. Techniques like scenario-building, net assessment and mathematical modelling have given limited relevance. There is a tendency of such techniques (in few cases) either to under-read or overread the possible threat. However, it appears that not much importance was given to the pandemic's modelling outputs as such by the policy makers in different parts of the world.

Broadly, there are two main categories of threats, called natural and human-induced.[4] Post-9/11, the world almost behaved in such a fashion as if terrorism is going to be the only threat in the future. Unfortunately, there has been a tendency for taking nature for granted, and as long as this tendency exists, the world would continue to face challenges like COVID-19 in the future too. At present, the process of obliteration is continuing and the need of the hour is to get the human population out of the woods first. By now, most of the political leadership across the globe have understood the severity of the situation and are found trying their best. The medical community which is bound by the Hippocratic Oath-the Oath written by Hippocrates, a Greek physician (460–370 BC), to treat the ill to the best of one's ability, is found abiding by this oath in true spirit. Kudos to them for their selfless service.

The frequency of natural disasters is not known and also, it is very difficult to predict in advance. There are some disasters, which possibly may not happen in the lifetime of a few generations. Obviously, the states are not prepared to handle such disasters. Take the case of the Tsunami. The Asian Tsunami, which occurred on 26 December 2004, is known to have taken more than 2,25,000 lives and had an impact on 14 countries. The deadliest Tsunami before this was Italy's 1908 Messina earthquake on the Mediterranean Sea and is known to have killed close to 1,23,000 people. The known Tsunami incident before 1908 and the science of seismology had made scientists conclude that the Indian and Pacific Ocean Region has very little probability of Tsunami occurrence. Possibly, the earlier Tsunami that happened in the region was around 400 years back. Obviously, Tsunami was not even considered to be a threat before 2004. Though, there was some indication two years before the Asian Tsunami. The 2002 Sumatra earthquake is believed to have been a "foreshock". The rupture area of the 2002 earthquake was very close to the rupture area of the 2004 earthquake. Such foreshocks are known to be the earthquakes that occur before a large seismic event. However, nothing much was 'read' from this quake.

The SARS (2002, 774 deaths), and MERS (2012, 858 deaths), incidents were possibly the "foreshocks" for the COVID-19 pandemic. Unfortunately, the world ignored them. There were few other diseases too, like Ebola and Zika, which did indicate that the destruction capability (in terms of human lives, economy, and impact on human physiology) of any 'virus' is much higher than the weapons created by the humans. Today, the spread of Coronavirus could be viewed as one of the biggest intelligence failures at the global level. Regrettably, the 'disease intelligence' was available, but we turned a blind-eye towards it. The history of pandemics and the forewarning given by the SARS and MERS diseases was the strategic intelligence available. Some risk assessment agencies indenting about the spread of some highly contagious virus over the Chinese region around December 2019 was the tactical intelligence available. But these visible signals were overlooked. More importantly, at a global level, we do not even have a structured Communicable Diseases Intelligence Gathering System which is functional.

During the year 2019, WHO had released a list of ten threats to global health. Apart from air pollution, non-communicable diseases, vaccine hesitancy, dengue and HIV (Human Immunodeficiency Virus) this list included threats like a global influenza pandemic, Ebola and high-threat pathogens and weak primary care.[5] This clearly shows that a correct assessment of the possible threats was done well in advance. However, it appears that all or most of the states in the world paid no heed to the warning. For more than a decade or so it was becoming evident that the next big threat could come from the influenza type of infection. In the past, the world had experienced what influenza can do. But sadly, no efforts were made even to strengthen the primary healthcare systems in most of the states.

The WHO has come under serious criticism for its ineptness as well as favouritism. But did the world ever seriously debate the challenges faced by the WHO? At a multilateral level, the focus always remained on the so-called organisations with glamour like World Bank, OPEC (Organisation of Petroleum Exporting Countries), OECD (Organisation of Economic Cooperation and Development), APEC (Asia-Pacific Economic Cooperation), IMF(International Monetary Fund), etc. Pandemics have never been an issue for focussed discussion when the Heads of State meet. Globally, health has got relegated more like a commercial issue than an issue for human survival. Hence, issues debated in the context of health were associated more with health insurance and medical tourism, but not pandemics.

Lately, the securitisation of a threat has become fashionable so as to attract the attention of the policy makers. This notion has given rise to terminologies like Environmental Security, Water Security, Food Security, and Cyber Security. Unfortunately, in order to 'secure' the interests of the pharmaceutical and biotechnology industry, the major world powers have never paid the required attention towards even strengthening the Biological Weapons Convention (BWC, 1975). Remaining prepared for any possible biological weapons attack or for any pandemic is almost one and the same. But for all these years, the world viewed both threats as almost zero-probability threats.

Pandemics are like health Tsunamis, they would never give any direct warning of their arrival but would definitely give a weak signal. For COVID-19, the world community collectively failed to effectively catch the correct signal in time. It is a failure of human intelligence.

Now, the world has realised that they would be required to co-exist with this virus for a few months or years. Normally, various known natural disasters and calamities are limited in geography and duration. Humans have no control of disasters like an earthquake. They can only plan for managing the disaster. Then there could be possible disasters like an asteroid strike on earth, where actually humans cannot do anything about such disasters. However, the case of pandemics is different and possibly much could have been done earlier to ensure that such a situation gets addressed properly.

For all these years, the human population as such was focusing their efforts towards gaining prosperity. They have followed various growth models to attain prosperity. At the same time, there was always power-dynamics associated with every act. As a society, people took positions based on religious, cultural, caste and social beliefs. Probably, while doing all this they forgot the basics – that for carrying forward any agenda the human race needs to exist first. Regrettably, for centuries, the global community has been passionate about every other thing except remaining prepared to address major health emergencies.

With regard to the spread of COVID-19, two conspiracy theories are doing the rounds.[6] There are some politicians in the United States (US) who had expressed a view that the Coronavirus was bio-engineered in a Chinese lab. To counter this view, some Chinese officials have mentioned that the US agencies' have bioengineered the virus. Generally, none of these conspiracy theories have found much of traction in the public mind.

In fact, COVID-19 is not the first disease suspected to be a bioweapon in recent times. Post-9/11 Anthrax attacks in the US ended up killing five people and was an act of intentional use of anthrax spores. Any subsequent disease spread gets normally suspected as a human creation. Particularly, since the coronavirus had its origins in a country like China, the 'conspiracy theory' that this virus is a bio-weapon has some takers. Probably, this is not based on any scientific facts but since the State of China has an 'image' issue for long, such stories would circulate.

Another view is that the main reason for the disease spread could be due to an accidental release from a laboratory in Wuhan province, where scientists were studying bat coronaviruses. Actually, at this point in time, it would be difficult to exactly claim what had led to the spread of this virus. Three options are being discussed: natural outbreak, accidental release from the laboratory and intentional biological attack (either by China or by the US). People are found mainly fixing their views based on personal opinions, political positions, and scientific understanding. Even for the scientific community to undertake a systematic and logical analysis at this point in time looks difficult owing to the data and assessment of location limitations.

It is a reality that the location of the virus origin was in China and the region of Wuhan is problematic even for the non-conspiracy theorists. As per some reports, the Wuhan Center for Disease Control and Prevention is located just 280 meters from the Hunan Seafood Market. Many claim this market as the source of the original outbreak. There is a bio-safety level four (BSL-4) laboratory situated in Wuhan. Presently, such a facility is the most high-ranking facility available globally. Only these facilities are permitted to undertake research on dangerous potentially life-threatening agents. Some coronaviruses related research was probably happening in this facility. However, there is no direct evidence to conclude that the virus could have leaked out from the laboratory. Scientists by comparing the available genome sequence data for known coronavirus strains have concluded, that the virus has originated through natural processes only.

The Spike Protein of coronavirus is found on the surface of the virus and allows the virus to bind to specific receptors on the surface of the human cell. This is considered as the first step towards infecting the cell. After the recent infections in Wuhan, scientists have found that the type of binding witnessed could happen only as the result of natural selection and not as the product of intentional genetic engineering. Also, the molecular structure of the virus is copybook and not bio-engineered. Hence, there is a general acceptance by many experts that the disease outbreak has happened naturally.

Currently, the focus of the entire world has been towards identifying a correct treatment for this disease and also towards the development of a vaccine. This is the need of the hour and any breakthrough in this regard would help to save many lives. However, it is also important to know about the exact origins of the pandemic, as the knowledge of virus transmission from animals to humans is important to understand, to avoid the risk of future re-emergence events.

Some pandemics have had a global impact in the past, while few were controlled within a limited geographical space. It was known that any major pandemic can alter lives, regionally or globally. But still, there was a general belief that this will not happen in our lifetime! Now, when this belief is challenged then obviously humans are getting restless. The COVID-19 crisis shows that the world is changing quickly and it is essential for the political leaders to recognize that in today's world almost everything is interlinked, from economy to environment to social aspects to geopolitics to security. Unfortunately, some states are found using this situation even to further their geo-economic and geo-strategic ambitions.

As of July 2020, more than six months have passed since the world has come under this threat. The world community together has suffered significantly. It was thought appropriate to take a view of how the world has responded to this ongoing crisis. This book is an attempt to look at a few important dimensions of the COVID-19 catastrophe. The chapters in this book have been written with hindsight. There are obvious pluses and minuses for analysing the issue with the advantage of hindsight. It is important for the readers to keep this in mind. Apart from the loss of human life, the other setback which the world is witnessing is the impact on the economy. Various states are trying to assess the impact on the economy based on various parameters. Also, states are taking various measures to improve their economies. The real economic picture would be clearer only after the situation gets totally under control. This book has not undertaken any major assessment of the economic aspects. The editors have tried to avoid any repetitions in the book. However, the nature of the debate is such that, at a few places it has been difficult to avoid repetitions.

The book has five parts. The first part takes a broad overview of the nature of the current crisis and how as such pandemics have impacted societies for all these years. The second part presents the condition of pandemics and responses by the states. Various technologies are at the forefront to address this disaster. The third section attempts to analyse this technology trajectory. Tragedy or joy, the human mind always tries to make good of any situation in their own interest. The fourth section looks at the geopolitics enacted at the backdrop of this misfortune. There has been some debate on biological weapons while analysing this calamity. The last section widens this debate by assessing the Biological Weapons Convention (BWC) and issues of biosecurity and biosafety.

Editors

NOTES

1. N.K. Jaiswal, and S.K. Saxena, 'Classical Coronaviruses,' *Coronavirus Disease 2019 (COVID-19): Epidemiology, Pathogenesis, Diagnosis, and Therapeutics*, 2020, pp. 141–150.
2. Virology: Coronaviruses, *Nature*, vol. 220, 1968, p. 650.
3. Kahn, Jeffrey, McIntosh and Kenneth, 'History and Recent Advances in Coronavirus Discovery,' *The Pediatric Infectious Disease Journal*, November 2005, Vol. 24, No. 11, pp. S223-S227.
4. Ajey Lele, 'COVID-19: Failure of Collective Human intelligence,' *SSPC Online,* 01 April 2020, available at https://sspconline.org/index.php/opinion-analysis/covid-19-failure-collective-human-intelligence-wed-04012020, accessed on 20 June 2020.
5. 'Ten Threats to Global Health in 2019,' *WHO*, available at https://www.who.int/news-room/feature-stories/ten-threats-to-global-health-in-2019, accessed on 14 June 2020.
6. Ajey Lele, 'Coronavirus: Assessing the Looming Threat,' *SSPC Online,* 27 March 2020, available at https://www.sspconline.org/opinion-analysis/coronavirus-assessing-looming-threat-fri-03272020, accessed on 20 June 2020.

SECTION I

THE GLOBAL OUTLOOK OF COVID-19

1

History and Politics of Pandemics

Paulami Sanyal

The World Health Organisation (WHO) during 2010, defined pandemic as the "world wide spread of a new disease". David M. Morens, Gregory K. Folkers, and Anthony S. Fauci (2009) define pandemic as a "disease of very different etiologies that exhibit a variety of epidemiologic features." Any pandemic will sure to possess one invariable common denominator: widespread geographic extension. In a Dictionary of Epidemiology (2008) Pandemic is defined as an "epidemic occurring worldwide or over a very wide area, crossing international boundaries, and usually affecting a large number of people."

The present pandemic has the world reeling under severe social economic and political pressure; not to mention the continuous surge in the loss of lives. As the spread of pandemic is now being shifted from developed countries to the developing world, the number of infected is rising and a basic change in the type of population infected are noticeable. Recently, it has even been reported that since the COVID-19 has been spreading to the developing world more middle-aged people are being infected and the number of deaths in that age group is also increasing. It should be noted here that previously many reports highlighted that majorly the elderly population was more prone to be infected from COVID-19.

This difference in the pattern of the spread of COVID-19 is nothing exceptional. The spread of any pandemic and the amount of population affected by it always depends on the respective countries' politics. How a country's government deals with a crisis and how it is in general prepared in situations such as these had a lot of influence in the country's handling a contagious disease.

Developing countries with their higher density of population and lack of a good education system and healthcare would have a larger number of the population prone to be affected by a contagious disease. However, sometimes a government's mismanagement of a crisis period can also stimulate the spread of a virus. For example, the way China handled COVID-SARS led to a rising number of infections and fatality rates. Thus, the politics of a country directly impacts the spread and influence of a pandemic.

On the other hand, highly contagious diseases with a higher fatality rate can influence and impact the way countries are governed. For example, the bubonic plague epidemic in the Middle Ages (discussed later) managed to change the economic and social conditions of the surviving labourers. In the last few decades, the infection rate and fatality rate of most pandemics were small in number. However, COVID-19 is different in terms of its infection rate. The disease possibly will seem more severe now with the developing countries being infected. From that perspective, this chapter attempts to have an understanding of previous major pandemics. The chapter is divided into two sections. The first section deals with political analyses of major pandemics throughout history and the second section briefly discusses how the present pandemic is shaping politics.

Political Analyses of Pandemics throughout History

A disease is considered a pandemic based on its reach and contagion. While selecting the diseases for the study of pandemics the definition of WHO is used as the primary source. However, it must be noted here that the WHO was only founded in 1948. Many of the diseases discussed in this section have occurred prior to WHO's formation. Moreover, due to a lack of documentation during the first few pandemics, it is almost impossible to specify what number of the infected population died. Lack of documentation, however, also appears in the Modern Ages due to governments' attitude to hide the numbers. This chapter has only selected diseases that were well-pervasive in its spread and had a large number of fatalities. Albeit malaria, smallpox, measles, or leprosy were highly contagious and had a huge death toll, their spread was limited compared to the ones discussed in this section. The only exception of that is SARS-COVID which had a limited reach. However, it was treated as a pandemic by the Centre for Disease Control and Prevention, the US within four months from the first infection and therefore it is included in this section. In cases of Zika and Ebola virus, both with less spread in the western world are not declared as pandemics by WHO or any of the international organisations. However, due to their maximum spread in the developing countries, it is argued that their potential is not given sufficient attention by institutions such as WHO while their true form might very well be equal to a pandemic (Adelaida Sarukhan 2016, David Morens and Anthoni Fauci 2017). In the case of Zika, the most disturbing phase is the secondary Zika-associated microcephaly and other birth defects and fetal losses which have affected a large but still unknown percentage of women infected with the Zika virus during pregnancy.[1]

Plague: "Plague of Justinian", "Black Death" and Plague in India

In the last two millennia, the plague has created several incidents of pandemics. The first recorded pandemic is known as Justinian's plague and it took place between 542 and 546 AD. It spread across Asia, Africa and Europe and claimed nearly 100,000,000 victims. The second plague pandemic is known as the "Black Death" which took place in the fourteenth century from 1347 to 1350. It caused the death of approximately 50,000,000, half of which was from Asia and Africa and the other half from Europe. One-fourth of the European population succumbed to this disease. The third phase of the plague-pandemic began in Canton and Hong Kong, China in 1894 and spread by rats to 77 ports in five continents within 10 years from 1894 to 1903. Plague entered India in the third phase when it caused nearly 13,000,000 deaths. The cause of this disease was only understood in the late 19th century to be a bacterium called *Yersinia Pestis*. This strain of *Yersinia* infects the oriental rat fleas or *Xenopsyllacheopis* forcing them to regurgitate concentrated bacteria into the host. Such infected hosts then transmit the disease to humans. Humans can transmit the disease by droplets, leading to pneumonic plague.[2]

The spread, source and severity of the first plague-pandemic are disputed due to lack of documentation. Plague of Justinian, the first of three human plague pandemics, either spread from central Asia or Africa across the Mediterranean basin into Europe through the ships loaded with grain which also carried rats. This plague killed an estimated 100 million people. According to the contemporary scholar Procopius, this is approximately 50 to 60 percent of the population of these regions contributing to the end of the Roman Empire.[3]

People died of starvation along with the disease as staple foods were scarce. The tax base reduced and the economic revenue decreased resulting in the Empire forcing the survivors to share the tax burden. The Byzantine army suffered as well, being unable to carry out military campaigns as it has fewer serving soldiers in its rank. As a result, the army failed to retake Rome for the Empire. By 600 AD the population of the Empire probably was reduced by 40 percent. Moreover, due to the lack of understanding of the events, it was during this time Christian tradition began to enter the realm of interpreting nature and calamity. Plague and other such misfortunes were explained as a punishment for sins or retribution from God. As the Byzantine Empire began to experience challenges during this outbreak the Arabs who were a nomad tribe moving through deserts and practicing a natural form of isolation, prepared to expand its territory in the name of Islam.[4]

Religious interpretation of a certain event was more prominent during the next plague pandemic in the 14th Century. Owing to the absence of medicinal progress during this century many people turned to religion. Catholic Europe sought to identify sinners against God and in the process frequently singling out minorities, women, Jews or Non-Catholic Christians. During this phase, young doctors from any ranks were contacted to perform the duty of the plague doctor and address the shortage of specialized physicians. Venice was among the first city-states to establish such practice during 1348. These doctors' principal task was to care for plague-infected people and to put in public records the cases of deaths. In cities such as Florence and Perugia, plague doctors were the only ones allowed to perform autopsies to help determine the cause of death. This period also understood the significance of quarantine or isolating the infected population. They noted that, after a period of isolation, individuals who had not developed symptoms of illness would likely not spread the disease any longer. Thus, the rule of mandatory isolation was initiated. The first known instance of quarantine was found in 1377 in Ragusa, the city-state of Dubrovnik where all new arrivals went into self-isolation for 30 days before entering the city.[5]

The social effects of the plague were immediately understood after the worst outbreaks were mitigated. There was an extreme labor shortage making the servants, once tied to the land, benefit. They began to have a choice of whom to work for. Landowners were compelled to make conditions better lest leaving their lands untended. This immediately led to wage increases across Europe. The poorer section of the population began to grow more confident about the importance of their service. Therefore, when landowners tried to revert to the old social and economic system there were peasant revolts throughout Europe. On the other hand, the Catholic Church and Jewish populations in Europe faced trouble as a long-term consequence of the 14th Century plague epidemic. Both among the poor and the propertied sections distrust in God and the church increased. People began to realise that religion could not prevent the spread of the disease and their family's suffering. So churches and religion, in general, lost their popularity and influence and church services in many areas ceased.[6]

The third wave of plague began in China's Yunnan province in 1894 and then spread through the shipping routes to the United States (US). A ship with infected rodents from Hong Kong came to Hawaii in December 1899, and then San Francisco, where the pandemic began in March 1900.[7] However, except for China and India, its spread was limited.[8] In India as well the spread was contained to selected zones. It arrived in India in 1896. During the first three years, almost fifteen percent of the total number of deaths in India was from Bombay. In the year 1903 Bombay witnessed 20,788 plague deaths, and in 1907 total death toll of India was 1,315,892. Till 1921, an estimated twelve million Indians lost their lives, in comparison with three million in the rest of the world. Punjab had the second-largest number in plague mortality.[9]

India, then a British colony witnessed severe actions from the rulers. People were forced into hospitals, bodies were searched without any sensitivity, houses were torn down, and streets and sewers were overflowing with disinfectants. For many people, being admitted to a hospital meant a death sentence. The occasion was also used to forbid festivals organised by the nationalist movement. The British government's control and legitimacy were already being questioned by the rise of nationalist movements in different parts of the country. Moreover, Indians were not considered for advice at the outbreak of the plague. All these situations together created conditions for violent confrontations. Hospitals were attacked in Bombay and Pune (Poona). One of these confrontations claimed the life of a plague commissioner Walter Charles Rand and his escort Lieutenant Ayerst, both assassinated by Damodar Chapekar, Balkrishna Chapekar, Vasudev Chapekar and Mahadev Ranade.[10]

Due to the increasing riots, the British government changed its strategy by emphasising more on voluntary initiatives to stop the plague and began collaborating with the leaders of the Indian nationalist movement. With the altered British policy, while the confrontations were averted the plague pandemic remained ineffective. The outbreak of the plague continued to spread in India till 1907 when the fatality reached more than a million. The plague outbreak in Indian cities and the citizen's responses against the British government have later been considered significant milestones in Indian national movements.[11]

Another British colony in South Africa, Cape Town too witnessed significant political developments due to the Plague pandemic during this time. Based on the notion that Africans were dirty and disease-infested, an idea of physical segregation of the coloured population from the white elite section was being formed. As a result, in 1902, the 'Native Reserve Location Act' was passed, making the temporary forced segregation permanent.[12]

Influenza Virus: "Spanish Flu" or H1N1, and "Swine Flu" or H1N1/09

There are two bouts of influenza virus that had reached a level of the pandemic. One took place from 1918 to 1919 and another in 2009. Both influenza viruses have similar flu-like symptoms such as fever or feeling feverish/chills, cough, sore throat, runny nose, muscle or body aches, headaches, fatigue, and diarrhea.[13] However, one distinctive trait of both these viruses was their ability to affect the younger healthier population whereas common flu tends to impact children and elder generation more.

An estimated one-third of the world's population was infected during the 1918–1919 influenza pandemic. The fatality rate was more than 2.5 percent, compared to other influenza viruses with less than 0.1 percent fatality rate. The first wave of influenza pandemic appeared in March 1918, followed by two much more fatal second and third waves in September to October of 1918 and January of 1919 respectively.[14]

Despite advances in epidemiology and public health, the true origin of Spanish flu remains unknown. The pandemic took place in the middle of World War I in a time of uncertainty, press censorship and advanced modes of transportation, including intercontinental travel. Within months, it spread from Europe, where military movements contributed to larger spread, to the US, Asia, Africa, and the Pacific Islands. Spain was one of only a few major European countries to remain neutral during the First World War. Therefore, the Spanish media was free to report all the details and developments of the War. This is why news of this particular illness was first published in Madrid in May 1918. The coverage of this influenza increased after the Spanish King Alfonso XIII was infected a week later. The rest of the nations were going through a media blackout because of their alliance with any one of the parties of World War I. The only way other nations could read about the flu was from Spanish news sources. Thus, they assumed that the country was where the pandemic began. Spain, however, believed that the virus had begun to spread from France, so they called it the French Flu.[15] The mortality rate of Spanish flu ranged from 10 percent to 20 percent. This influenza virus had the highest fatality rate among the H1N1 strains, approximately 100 million. This virus affected mostly younger and healthier populations. By August 1918, the virus had mutated to another form which was supposedly even deadlier than the first wave.[16]

Spanish flu to some extent also determined the outcome of the First World War because it affected armies of Germany and the Austrian–Hungarian Empire more virulently than their Allied opponents. Many notable politicians, artists, and scientists were either affected by the flu or succumbed to it. Its distinguished survivors include Walt Disney, Greta Garbo, Raymond Chandler, Franz Kafka, Edward Munch, Franklin Delano Roosevelt, and Woodrow Wilson; whereas painters such as Gustav Klimt and Egon Schiele, and poets like Guillaume Apollinaire were among the fatalities of this virus.[17]

The influenza virus of 1918 had differently influenced politics in different parts of the world. In the United States, the then President Woodrow Wilson probably had contracted Spanish flu while en route to the Paris peace conference in 1919. As a result, he may also have suffered from a stroke a few months later. This probably was the reason President Wilson was unable to persuade Congress and the Senate to back the League of Nations. Spanish flu in the Indian subcontinent exposed the British as incapable of handling a crisis of this scale. Mohandas Karamchand Gandhi too contracted the flu and was temporarily unable to act. The pandemic, meanwhile, aggravated a drought-related famine all over India. During this deeply vulnerable situation, a number of grassroot level local and caste organisations mobilised themselves for relief efforts laying the groundwork for future liberation movements. When Gandhi recovered, he was too weak to respond to a bill initiated by the British government that continued the rule of martial law and eventually led to the Amritsar massacre in April 1919.[18]

The 2009 H1N1 pandemic started in Mexico in April 2009. By the end of April, cases were reported in several states in the US, and in countries such as Canada, Spain, the United Kingdom (UK), New Zealand, Israel, and Germany. On 25 April 2009, the WHO declared the situation a public health emergency of international concern.[19] It continued to spread for over a year and on 10 August 2010, the Director-General of WHO, Dr Margaret Chan declared the end of this pandemic. The first doses of the H1N1 pandemic vaccine were administered on 5 October 2009. The virus infected over 10 percent of the global population and had a death toll approximately from 20,000 to over 500,000. The largest of these fatalities may have occurred in countries in the African and Southeast Asian regions as per a report published by the Centers for Disease Control and Prevention (2012), where more than half of all 2009 H1N1-related deaths occurred. This study estimated that 80 percent of H1N1 fatalities were younger than 65 years of age. It is different from seasonal influenza epidemics which usually kills 80 to 90 percent of the population that is 65 years of age and older. It was estimated that 0.001–0.007 percent of the world's population died of respiratory complications caused by the 2009 H1N1 virus infection during the first 12 months.[20] Although its death rate was lower than the regular influenza death rates, at its peak it was perceived as threatening because it primarily affected healthy young adults. This pandemic was the first disease where mental health was considered an important aspect of preparedness and mitigation of policy efforts.[21]

As per the media reports, there were approximately 2,400 Mexicans infected by H1N1. Only 10 states (Arizona, California, Indiana, Kansas, Massachusetts, Michigan, Nevada, New York, Ohio and Texas) of the US were affected by the disease. New York City was most affected according to the data of the Centers for Disease Control and Prevention, US. Swine flu epidemic exposed the risk of unemployment, poverty and undernourishment due to the spread and severity of a contagious disease.[22] The WHO faced criticism due to its systemic difficulties. It lacked a consistent, understanding of the severity of a pandemic. Throughout the pandemic period, the WHO failed to procure a cohesive set of procedures and priorities for timely guidance. From the time of defining the disease as pandemic to the disease's progression from one phase to another, WHO failed to make a simple and all-pervasive strategy for the affected countries. The WHO also discontinued routine press conferences thus giving birth to a lot of speculation and misunderstanding among the affected countries. The most serious operational shortcoming was the failure to distribute vaccines for influenza timely. In total, 78 million doses of vaccine were delivered to 77 countries long after they could have helped in controlling the spread. This delay happened due to a shortfall in global vaccine-production capacity, technical complications, and distributional problems.[23]

HIV Virus

The first cases of Acquired Immuno-Deficiency Syndrome (AIDS) were reported in 1981, and very quickly infection with the virus (HIV) has grown to pandemic proportions. At present treatment of HIV infection with antiretroviral therapy (ART) are available.

From 1981 till the end of 2018, 74.9 million people have become infected with HIV and 32 million have died.[24] It causes about one million deaths a year worldwide. This virus's spread is especially alarming in some Sub-Saharan African countries such as Botswana, Lesotho, and Swaziland, where it has infected more than 25 percent of the population. As per the WHO report of 2018, 67.99 percent of the total HIV positive patients are from Africa, 10.5 percent from South East Asia, 9.26 percent from both the continents of America, 6.61 percent from Europe and 5.03 percent from Western Pacific.[25] In the US, approximately 1.2 million people are HIV positive and the death toll is 12,000 per year. It used to be over

40,000 per year in the late 1990s. Additionally, HIV has disproportionately affected the gay population, transgender women, and African-Americans both in terms of the number of infected and social discrimination in the country.[26]

Despite spreading slowly than any other pandemic, HIV has received significant public health attention from national and international administrations and pharmaceuticals. It is also a disease that has managed to focus on the mental health of the patients so as to make others comprehend some of the challenges generally associated with infectious diseases.[27]

AIDS has always been highly political, more because of the stigma associated with sexual intercourse and intravenous drugs that is the cause for most of the patients. Initially, the identification of the disease and its containment was much politically motivated due to the 1980s gay activism and community mobilization. When a particular type of disease began to increase among the gay community it was associated with a much larger anti-gay stigma of the society. Later with the gradual understanding of the disease, the stigma saw a gradual decline. However, it is not completely done away with. Now, this disease is handled with more political support. In a United Nations Security Council debate and a special session in the United Nations General Assembly both in 2000, it was confirmed that AIDS was a political issue requiring global action.[28]

Corona Virus: SARS

Severe Acute Respiratory Syndrome (SARS) was caused by the SARS Coronavirus (SARS-CoV) and first appeared in China in 2002 where it had infected almost 10,000 individuals, mainly in China and Hong Kong.[29] By the end of 2002, the disease spread to 26 other countries, such as Canada with 251 cases. The outbreak was contained by mid-2003. Although there are disputed theories regarding its inception, SARS-CoV is thought to come from an animal probably bats, which spreads to other animals (civet cats).[30]

Symptoms of SARS-CoV are primarily similar to influenza and include fever, malaise, myalgia, headache, diarrhea, and shivering. However, the disease has no proven specific symptoms so far. For example, fever, one of the most frequently reported symptoms, is sometimes absent at the beginning of the infection, especially in elderly and immune-suppressed patients. From the perspective of severity and mortality rate of about 10 percent, SARS-CoV created a global health concern. The outbreak of SARS also witnessed an increase in the study of patient's mental health both among the active patients and survivors of the disease.[31]

Following the habit of bureaucratic secrecy, initially, information about the disease was not made available to the public in China. On 27 January a report was first presented from Guangdong health officials where the disease first began to spread. However, standard measures were applied so that the news of the outbreak does not reach the public. Gradually the disease reached Hong Kong, and under its increasing pressure and criticism, the Chinese government on 26 March admitted that the number of patients with a similar disease is much higher (305 to 792). From November 2002 to March 2003, Jiang Zemin and Zhu Rongji were stepping down and Hu Jintao and Wen Jiabao were taking their places as General Secretary and Premier on Communist Party of China respectively. It was a time to avoid any trouble and maintain calm and stability. But the new leadership had to endure a lot of pressure. China at the time was witnessing international hostility and loss of business confidence. Furthermore, rumours were spreading among the local population. Thus, as a strategic measurement, on 17 April's Politburo meeting called for complete openness. On 20 April, the health minister and Mayor of Beijing were replaced. Under the new Mayor, strict quarantine provisions were announced, and daily updates were announced. Hong Kong's response to SARS was, on the other hand very different than Beijing. It had a free press making the cover-up entirely impossible. But the leadership was indecisive to take strict measurements. The government's indecisive measurements were a response to the Chinese stand on the disease. Chief Executive of Hong Kong Tung Chee-Hwa had Chinese support and, in an attempt, to continue with the support, he could not take a strong stand.[32]

Ebola Virus Disease

Ebola Virus Disease (EVD) first appeared in 1976 in two simultaneous outbreaks, one in the present Nzara in South Sudan, and the other a village near the Ebola River in Yambuku, Democratic Republic of Congo.[33] The 2014 to 2016 outbreak in West Africa was the largest EVD outbreak since the virus was first discovered in 1976. Most likely it was first spread through fruit bats in a village in Guinea in December 2013. From Guinea, it reached Sierra Leone and Liberia, where it infected over 28,000 and the fatality rate was approximately 11,000. Cases were registered in Nigeria and Mali as well, albeit small in number and quickly contained. In September 2014, a passenger from Liberia died in Texas simultaneously infecting two nurses caring for him which led to a significant public concern over possible Ebola outbreak in the US.[34] This again led to the US Department of Defense deploying military personnel for training Liberians to manage the disease and build hospitals. This mission was called Operation United Assistance.[35]

As per WHO guidelines 2020, EVD is introduced into the human body through contact with the blood, secretions, organs or other bodily fluids of infected animals such as fruit bats, chimpanzees, gorillas, monkeys, forest antelope or porcupines. After it enters a human-body, EVD spreads through human-to-human transmission via direct contact through blood or body fluids or objects that have been contaminated with body fluids from a sick person. The symptoms of EVD include fever, fatigue, muscle pain, headache, sore throat vomiting, diarrhea, rash, impaired kidney and liver function, internal and external bleeding.[36]

The political structure of Sierra Leone was severely affected by the outbreak of EVD. The government's day-to-day service began to deteriorate when it stopped spending money on services not directly related to battling the virus. As a result, citizens of Sierra Leone started questioning President Dr Ernest Bai Koroma regarding his capacity to handle the challenges. President Koroma also faced disapproval for supporting the Minister for Health and Sanitation Miatta Kargbo. She was severely criticized for suggesting that infection and deaths could have been minimised if victims had appropriately responded. She was removed from the office on 29 August 2014. Similarly, in Liberia, the pandemic sheds light on people's lack of trust for their government. Because of the uncertainties due to the EVD spread, several investors, aid workers, and skilled employees started to leave the country despite urges from the government to stay. Government of the United States, even without any true concern regarding infection had to face criticism for the Center for Disease Controls deficient efforts. The Republicans criticised the Obama government for not providing a realistic assessment of the situation. A demand was also raised to enforce new travel constraints for those countries in Africa where the outbreak began.[37]

Zika Virus

Zika virus is found in rhesus monkeys in Uganda in 1947.[38] The only known outbreaks of this virus were recorded in Micronesia in 2007 and South America and the US from 2015 to 2016. It was identified in Brazil in 2015. Symptoms of the Zika virus are flat pink rashes, bloodshot eyes, joint pains, fever, and headaches. It is a mosquito-borne disease, typically borne by the species *Aedes Aegypti* but it also can be sexually transmitted. Initially, its mild symptoms made it rather insignificant form the public health perspective. However, as later infections showed that Zika can cause Guillain-Barre syndrome in adults and cause microcephalia (a condition in which the brain does not develop or has stopped growing thus making the circumference of the head smaller than normal[39]) in unborn children of infected mothers (a risk of about 1%).[40] Guillain-Barre syndrome is a neurological disorder for which the body's immune system attacks part of its nervous system located outside of the brain and spinal cord. GBS can cause mild weakness to paralysis.[41]

For example, in the year 2015 Brazil witnessed 2400 birth defects and 29 infant deaths due to suspected Zika infection. Zika transferred from Micronesia, across the Pacific, to Brazil, where it continued to spread. Since 2016, Zika has spread throughout South America, Central America, the Caribbean, and several states within the USA. It remains a significant public health concern, as there is no vaccine available so far.[42]

Zika brought out the socio-economic factor that plays an important role during any disease. This pandemic spread more to the poorer regions with a lack of public health infrastructure that allows illnesses to spread without significant resistance. These poor communities also did not have access to health hygiene. Brazil is the country most affected by the virus and provides a clear example of the importance of social and economic aspects that the government did not take into consideration. In 2016 at the initiation of its spread Brazil government had announced a war against Zika.[43] By 2018 data from the Brazilian Ministry of Health shows that majority of cases of babies with congenital malformations (which could be caused by Zika, but also could be caused by infections like syphilis and rubella) are concentrated in the north-east of Brazil, especially in the states of Pernambuco, Bahia, Paraíba and Maranhão. The average family income in these four states is 180 percent lower than the rest of the country. These are also the states with a higher level of young pregnancy, lower levels of education, fewer women with jobs. It should also be mentioned here that in general in Brazil as well as in most regions of Southern America, women have limited access to contraception; abortion is illegal and are prone to a higher rate of sexual violence.[44]

In Colombia and El Salvador women were cautioned by the Health Ministers to avoid being pregnant creating a paradoxical situation as approximately 50 percent of pregnancies in Colombia are unplanned. Moreover, El Salvador in the South America region has one of the highest rates of adolescent and teenage pregnancy. Zika virus thus gave prominence to the demands for the right to reproduction. Some of the countries in this region have strict anti-abortion rules which led many women infected by the virus to go for clandestine and illegal abortions. In 2016 a group of Brazilian activists demanded from the Supreme Court to allow abortions due to Zika infection. However, most of these countries continue to have restrictions against abortion.[45]

COVID-19

The virus causing a respiratory infection was first detected in the city of Wuhan, China, in late 2019. In the second week of December, doctors in Wuhan of Hubei Province china began to find cases that indicated the virus was spreading from one human to another. Wuhan Municipal Health Commission reported a cluster of cases of pneumonia on 31 December. Even though the official statement still does not agree to the human-to-human transmission factor of the disease a novel coronavirus was identified. By 6 January 2020 as many as 59 cases of the "pneumonia-like illness" were reported in Wuhan already. China reported its first death of a 60-year old man associated with this virus on 11 January. On 13 January 2020, a case was confirmed in Thailand, the first recorded case outside of China. On 22 January WHO mission to China issued a statement on the evidence of human-to-human transmission in Wuhan. By the end of January, Japan, South Korea, the US and France all issued its first cases of the virus, France being the first country to catch the virus outside south Asia on 24 January.[46]

By the month of February china went into complete lockdown; travel ban on china was issued from the US, Singapore, Russia and Australia; Italy sealed off its most hit Lombardy and Vento region and the virus already managed to spread into Europe and the Middle East with Italy and Iran becoming the new epicenter of the virus. By 6 March the number of infected people globally was more than 100,000 with a death toll of approximately 3,400. On 14 March and 24 March, France and Spain and India respectively went into complete lockdown. By the end of March South Africa, the Democratic Republic of Congo and Kenya went into lockdown. By 1 April with almost half of the world under lockdown, global infected cases rose to more than one million and death toll reached 100,000 by 10 April.[47]

Due to lockdown, many companies went bankrupt creating an economic crisis worldwide. For example, J. Crew Group Inc filed for bankruptcy protection after temporary store closures cost it almost 900 million USD on 4 May. In the following weeks, Neiman Marcus Group and J.C. Penney Co Inc also went bankrupt. On 26 May Latin America's second-largest airline Avianca Holdings and LATAM Airlines Group, the continent's largest carrier filed for bankruptcy. It was followed by Hertz Global Holdings Inc filing for bankruptcy protection on 22 May. The US economy lost around 20.5 million jobs in April which is the steepest plunge since the Great Depression. The unemployment rate in the country increased to 14.7 percent by the end of April.[48]

From the month of May countries such as China, the UK, Italy, Germany partially lifted the lockdown. On 8 June New Zealand became one of the first countries to lift all social and economic restrictions except border controls and return to pre-pandemic normality. However, the virus began to reappear as countries such as South Korea, Germany, Iran, Saudi Arabia, Switzerland, New Zealand and China were hit by further infections. As of 30 June, the total number of COVID-19 infected cases worldwide were 10,590,724 and the death toll was 514,020. The US has the maximum number of cases (2,727,853) with Brazil, Russia and India being the second, third and fourth highest number of infected cases.[49]

Potential Political Changes due to COVID-19

The measures taken by many governments to prevent the spread of the virus have created pressure on its population. The people living in slum areas or economically poorer parts of a city often live in a cramped condition. It is implausible for them to self-isolate. Their minimal and inconsistent income makes it impossible to stay home for weeks without working. Citizens of the poorer countries, who make up around 25 percent of the world's population, innovated several coping mechanisms to manage financial security for a long time. But these mechanisms which were built and followed for generations are now being undermined due to many constraints imposed by the government. In India, a lockdown was imposed for three weeks without taking into account the millions of internally migrated populations mostly residing in the metro cities such as Mumbai and Delhi. This triggered a mass exodus from these cities along with panic, confusion and clashes as migrant workers attempted to return without transport. Cases were reported where several migrant workers died due to exhaustion in their attempt to walk. Similarly, in Zimbabwe, where the staple foods were already expensive due to inflation, citizens protested against a lockdown fearing that they may have to starve to death. Many countries have tried to introduce relief packages in terms of providing necessary amenities to the poor and help revive economic activities. For example, governments of Nigeria and Rwanda have initiated relief measures to feed vulnerable families. There is a probability that when the governments are unable to meet these needs people will breach lockdown, resulting in clashes with the security forces.[50]

Clashes have been reported from areas such as Chilean capital Santiago in May[51]; in the suburbs of Paris in April[52]; and in Uttar Pradesh[53], West Bengal[54], and Maharashtra[55] of India. The governments' efforts to heavy-handedly enforce the curfew further reduced public confidence in the government and the security forces. In countries such as Kenya and South Africa lockdown has been enforced with blatant human rights abuses.[56] Such growing tensions between the hungry population and the governments can undermine efforts to contain the spread of the virus in the short run. As the long term impact the present situation that many poorer economies will soon be engulfed by possible debt crises. Moreover, some of the foreign-aid providers have their own financial crises now. Therefore, politically and economically weak states can face a risk of debt, mass unemployment, and social unrest.

President Trump announced on 20 April that he would temporarily suspend immigration into the US as a response to the COVID-19 crisis. Subsequently, he issued an executive order which only paused green cards from being issued for at least 60 days. It did not, for example, affect green card applicants who are already in the country. The situation has also led to a re-evaluation of a social safety net for the US's citizens. Questions have arisen regarding introducing universal basic income, paid sick leave, unemployment benefits and so on.[57]

Millions of Americans have lost their jobs and the benefits such as health insurance associated with it within a month. Government assistance is slow to reach them due to partisan politics. The class inequality among the citizens of the US is more prominent now and experts believe that this might lead to demands for better protection.[58]

Not only has the virus increased class rift among citizens, but data from the government of New York City shows that the virus is also disproportionately affecting the ethnic minorities and the black community of the US. The following figure sums up the understanding of the ratio in which the white community and coloured community in the US are affected.

Figure 1: Age Adjusted Rate of Fatal Lab Confirmed COVID-19 Cases per 100,000 by Race/Ethnicity Group
as of 6 April 2020

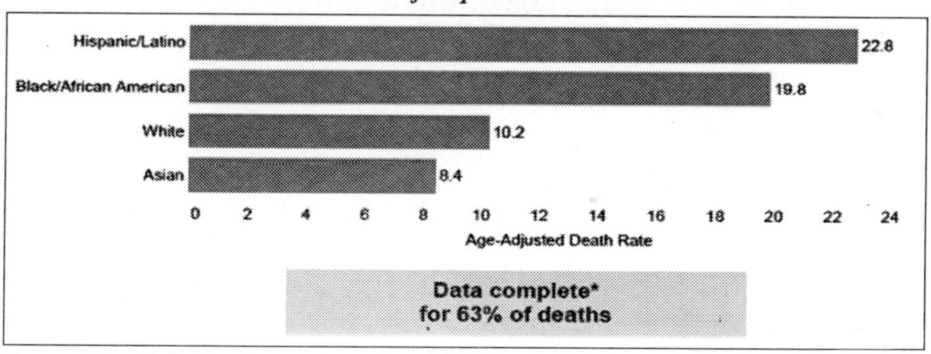

Source: New York City Department of Health and Mental Hygiene, available at https://www1.nyc.gov/assets/doh/downloads/pdf/imm/covid-19-deaths-race-ethnicity-04082020-1.pdf, accessed on 27 June 2020.

The COVID-19 crisis has also provided an opportunity for countries such as France and Germany to showcase their venture at humanitarian diplomacy. French humanitarian organizations such as Médecins Sans Frontières (MSF) have set up hospitals across the EU to strengthen health infrastructure. France has also announced a 1.4 billion USD relief package to assist African countries during the corona pandemic. Germany has been treating ICU patients from Italy, France, and the Netherlands and has supplied food aid to the Sahel region in Africa.[59]

Conclusion

COVID-19 has created an uncertain environment to an extreme that was not witnessed for almost a century. This is a situation where people are forced to incorporate different personal, social, and communitarian habits. As seen from the examples discussed in this chapter, such rapid changes in the societal structure have significant impacts on international trade, economics and politics. The states with a weaker economy and a high number of the illiterate population tend to suffer more from such crisis situations as its citizens are unable to cope up with required changing habits in a short time span. Thus, it can be assumed that developing countries will bear most of the brunt of this pandemic.

The politics have a causal relationship with society and in a crisis period, such relations become more apparent. From that perspective, there is a possibility that the developing countries will face some major changes in their present political scenario. Developed countries going through an immediate economic crisis may continue to witness the same for some time. Moreover, in the immediate future, there might be an antagonism towards globalization and free trade even though such an attitude cannot be continued in the long run. Therefore, the presence of COVID-19 for the next three to four years unvaccinated may not create radical changes in world politics but there will be some structural adjustments among the governments.

* * *

A shorter version of the essay was published in the CBW Magazine, Vol. 13, No. 1, Jan-June 2020.

NOTES

1. Morens David, Anthoni Fauci, 'Pandemic Zika: A formidable challenge to medicine and public health', *The Journal of Infectious Disease*, Vol. 216, 15 December 2017, pp. 857-859.
2. David T. Dennis, and Kenneth L. Gage, 'Plague Manual: Epidemiology, Distribution, Surveillance and Control', *World Health Organisation*, available at https://www.who.int/csr/

resources/publications/plague/whocdscsredc992a.pdf, accessed on 10 May 2020.

3. Wagner David M et al, "Yersinia pestis and the Plague of Justinian 541–543 AD: A Genomic Analysis", *The Lancet Infectious Diseases*, 28 January 2014, available at https://cpb-us-e1.wpmucdn.com/blogs.cornell.edu/dist/c/2716/files/2012/12/Wagner-1te9if4.pdf, accessed on 13 May 2020.
4. Damir Huremović, 'Brief History of Pandemics (Pandemics throughout the history)', *Psychiatry of Pandemics*, vol. 16, May 2019, pp. 7-35.
5. Ibid.
6. Heather Whipps, 'How the Black Death Changed the World', *Livescience*, 28 April 2008, available athttps://www.livescience.com/2497-black-death-changed-world.html, accessed on 13 June 2020.
7. Nicholas Wade, 'Europe's Plagues Came From China, Study Finds', *The New York Times*, 10 October 2010, available at https://www.nytimes.com/2010/11/01/health/01plague.html?auth=login-email&login=email, accessed on 11 June 2020.
8. Samuel K Cohn Jr., '4 Epidemiology of the Black Death and Successive Waves of Plague', *Cambridge Journals Medical History*, vol. 27, 2008, pp. 74-100, available at https://www.ncbi.nlm.nih.gov/pmc/articles/PMC2630035/,accessed on 10 June 2020.
9. Natasha Sarkar, *Fleas, Faith and Politics: Anatomy of an Indian Epidemic, 1890-1925*, National University of Singapore, Department of History, 2011, available at https://core.ac.uk/download/pdf/48655733.pdf, accessed on 10 June 2020.
10. Niels Brimnes, 'When Epidemics Change the World: Can we Learn Anything from the Third Plague Pandemic?', *ScienceNordic*, 25 May 2020, available at https://sciencenordic.com/denmark-epidemic-history/when-epidemics-change-the-world-can-we-learn-anything-from-the-third-plague-pandemic/1685595, accessed on 16 June 2020.
11. Ibid.
12. See note 9.
13. Centers for Disease Control and Prevention, "H1N1 Flu: Know the symptoms of the flu", 5 December 2009, available at https://www.cdc.gov/h1n1flu/homecare/symptoms.htm, accessed on 9 May 2020.
14. Jeffery K. Taubenberger and David M. Morens, "1918 Influenza: The Mother of all Pandemics", *Emerging Infectious Diseases*, vol. 12, January 2006, pp. 15-22.
15. Anton Erkoreka, 'Origins of the Spanish Influenza Pandemic (1918-1920) and its Relation to the First World War', *Journal of Molecular and Genetic Medicine*, vol. 3, December 2009, pp. 190-194.
16. See note 3.
17. See note 3.
18. Crawford Killian, 'Pandemics, Politics and the Spanish Flu', *The Tyee*, 15 September 2017, available at https://thetyee.ca/Culture/2017/09/15/Pandemics-Politics-Spanish-Flu/, accessed on 12 June 2020.
19. Harvey V. Fineberg, 'Pandemic Preparedness and Response: Lessons from H1N1 Influenza of 2009', *The New England Journal of Medicine*, Vol. 370, April 2014, pp. 1335-1342.
20. Centers for Disease Control and Prevention, 'First Global Estimates of 2009 H1N1 Pandemic Mortality Released by CDC-led Collaboration', 25 June 2012, available at https://www.cdc.gov/flu/spotlights/pandemic-global-estimates.htm accessed on 27 May 2020.
21. See note 3.
22. David Walsh and Sean South, 'Politics and Economics Dominate Response to Swine Flu

Epidemic', *World Socialist Web Site*, 30 April 2009, available at https://www.wsws.org/en/articles/2009/04/sflu-a30.html, accessed on 29 May 2020.

23. Harvey V. Fineberg, 'Pandemic Preparedness and Response: Lessons from H1N1 Influenza of 2009', *The New England Journal of Medicine*, vol. 370, April 2014, pp. 1335-1342.
24. UNAIDS, 'Global HIV & AIDS Statistics – 2019 Fact Sheet', 2019, available at https://www.unaids.org/en/resources/fact-sheet, accessed on 14 June 2020.
25. World Health Organisation, 'HIV/AIDS: Data and Statistics', available at https://www.who.int/hiv/data/en/, accessed on 23 May 2020.
26. See note 3.
27. See note 3.
28. Peter Piot, Sarah Russell and Heidi Larson, 'Good politics, Bad politics: The Experience of AIDS', *Am J Public Health*, vol. 7, November 2007, pp. 1934-1936.
29. See note 3.
30. World Health Organisation, 'SARS (Severe Acute Respiratory Syndrome)', 2020, available at https://www.who.int/ith/diseases/sars/en/, accessed on 20 May 2020.
31. Ibid.
32. Tom Christensen and martin painter, 'The Politics of SARS- Rational Responses or Ambiguity, Symbols and Chaos', *Policy and Society*, vol. 23, 2014, pp. 18-48.
33. World Health Organisation, 'Ebola Virus Disease', 10 February 2020, available at https://www.who.int/news-room/fact-sheets/detail/ebola-virus-disease, accessed on 20 May 2020.
34. See note 3.
35. Clinton K. Murray et al, 'Operation United Assistance: Infectious Disease Threats to Deployed Military Personnel', *Military Medicine*, vol. 180, pp. 626-651, 1 June 2015.
36. World Health Organisation, 'Ebola Virus Disease', 10 February 2020, available athttps://www.who.int/news-room/fact-sheets/detail/ebola-virus-disease, accessed on 20 May 2020.
37. Al Qureshi, 'Economic and Political impact of Ebola Virus Disease', *Elsevier Public Health Emergency Collection*, 19 February 2016, available at https://www.ncbi.nlm.nih.gov/pmc/articles/PMC7150125/,accessed on 17 May 2020.
38. John Cohen, 'Zika's Long, Strange Trip into Limelight', *American Association for Advancement of Science*, 8 February 2016, available at https://www.sciencemag.org/news/2016/02/zika-s-long-strange-trip-limelight#, accessed on 17 May 2020.
39. National Institute of Neurological Disorders and Stroke, NINDS Microcephaly Information Page, 30 June 2015, available at https://web.archive.org/web/20160311132503/http://www.ninds.nih.gov/disorders/Microcephaly/microcephaly.htm, accessed on 17 May 2020.
40. See note 3.
41. National Institute of Neurological Disorders and Stroke, Guillain-Barre syndrome Fact Sheet, 16 March 2020, available at https://www.ninds.nih.gov/Disorders/Patient-Caregiver-Education/Fact-Sheets/Guillain-Barr%C3%A9-Syndrome-Fact-Sheet#3139_1, accessed on 17 May 2020.
42. See note 3.
43. Kruskal Joshua, 'Zika Virus: How Poverty and Politics will Determine its Social Cost', *International Policy Digest*, 19 February 2016, available at https://intpolicydigest.org/2016/02/19/zika-virus-poverty-politics-will-determine-social-costs/, accessed on 15 June 2020.
44. Barbara Ribeiro and Sarah Hartley, 'Why Brazil's Zika Virus Requires a Political Treatment', *The Conversation*, 17 February 2018, available at https://theconversation.com/why-brazils-zika-virus-requires-a-political-treatment-91955, accessed on 15 June 2020.
45. Kimberly Gressick, Adriane Gelpi and Toni Chanroo, 'Zika and Abortion in Brazilian

Newspapers: How a New Outbreak Revived an Old Debate on Reproductive Rights', *Sexual and Reproductive Health Matters*, vol. 27, 2019, pp. 20-23.

46. World Health Organisation, 'Archived: WHO Timeline" COVID-19', 27 April 2020, available at https://www.who.int/news-room/detail/27-04-2020-who-timeline--covid-19, accessed on 30 June 2020.
47. Hindustan Times, Timeline: How the Global Coronavirus Pandemic Unfolded', 29 June 2020, available at https://www.hindustantimes.com/world-news/timeline-how-the-global-coronavirus-pandemic-unfolded/story-IEe31EwqvuEwnE6DKIC5EN.html, accessed on 30 June 2020.
48. Ibid.
49. BBC News,' Coronavirus Pandemic: tracking the global outbreak', 30 June 2020, available at https://www.bbc.com/news/world-51235105, accessed on 30 June 2020.
50. Nic Cheeseman, 'The Coronavirus could Topple Governments around the World', *Foreign Policy*, 31 March 2020, available athttps://foreignpolicy.com/2020/03/31/coronavirus-regime-change-could-topple-governments-around-the-world/, accessed on 10 June 2020.
51. BBC News, 'Coronavirus: Chile Protesters Clash with Police over lockdown', 19 May 2020, available at https://www.bbc.com/news/world-latin-america-52717402, accessed on 1 June 2020.
52. Financial Times, 'Clashes Breakdown in Locked-down Paris Suburbs as Tensions Rise', 24 April 2020, available at https://www.ft.com/content/85014164-601d-439a-b434-44fcc0d4ed98, accessed on 1 June 2020.
53. DNA India, 'Uttar Pradesh: Clashes break out between Police and Locals amidst lockdown in Aligarh', 22 April 2020, available at https://www.dnaindia.com/india/report-uttar-pradesh-clashes-break-out-between-police-and-locals-amidst-lockdown-in-aligarh-2822044, accessed on 10 June 2020.
54. Hindustan Times, 'Coronavirus: 10 Injured as Clashes Break out in Kolkata over Distribution of Relief Material', 30 March 2020, available at https://www.hindustantimes.com/india-news/kolkata-10-injured-as-clashes-break-out-over-distribution-of-relief-material/story-qxURwEVJadZ3R7l97yH40J.html, accessed on 20 May 2020.
55. Rajiv Singh, 'Clashes break out between Locals and Police amid lack of essential items in Malegaon', *India TV*, 23 April 2020, available at https://www.indiatvnews.com/news/india/coronavirus-lockdown-maharashtra-containment-zone-malegaon-clashes-locals-police-610454, accessed on 20 May 2020.
56. Jason Burke, 'South African Police Fires Rubber Bullets at Shoppers Amid Lockdown', *The Guardian*, 20 March 2020, available at https://www.theguardian.com/world/2020/mar/28/south-africa-police-rubber-bullets-shoppers-covid-19-lockdown, accessed on 1 June 2020.
57. Stanage, Niall, 'Five ways the coronavirus could change American politics', *The Hill, 2 may 2020*, available at https://thehill.com/homenews/campaign/495761-five-ways-the-coronavirus-could-change-american-politics, accessed on 28 June 2020.
58. Ibid.
59. Pant, Harsh V., 'COVID-19 and the Middle Power Moment in Global Politics', *Observer Research Foundation*, 6 May 2020, available at https://www.orfonline.org/research/covid-19-and-the-middle-power-moment-in-global-politics-65726/, accessed on 29 June 2020.

2

Mapping the Global Outbreak of COVID-19

Anshu Joshi

For the past couple of years, the world has been witnessing changes that have impacted global politics, world order, economies, and societies at an inconceivable scale. On the one hand, many countries have still been struggling with the challenge of providing basic facilities and infrastructure to their people. On the other hand, advances in Information Technology (IT), Artificial Intelligence (AI) and Robotics are on the verge of dominating the world. Additionally, the world has seen the emergence of new challenges, such as cyber warfare and the use of new chemical and biological agents by the terrorist organisations and rogue states to create a state of panic among people and the governments.

Today, we are living in a world of highly advanced technologies where drones can deliver pizzas, robots can serve food in restaurants, chatbots can help us online and more. In this world of IT-enabled lifestyle, things seemed to be perfect until a virus, without any alarming symptoms, entered our lives, created havoc, and brought everything to an unexpected halt. How this virus, known as Corona, spread across the world? Is it natural or artificial? How can it be contained? Is there any medication available for this deadly virus? What will be the future of the world? There are many unanswered questions. However, one thing is crystal clear, biological agents, whether leaked accidentally or deliberately, whether natural or laboratory-made, have the power to bring the entire world to a standstill. Apart from the immediate life-threatening effect, they also instigate long-term political, social, economic, and psychological consequences that can change the world forever.

To date, more than eight million cases of COVID-19 have been reported across the world with over 440 thousand deaths. Despite having the best technologies, modern workforce, and world-class infrastructure, even the most developed nations like the US (United States of America) seem to be helpless in fighting against this lethal virus outbreak. With no medication and vaccine available for COVID-19 so far, the most significant question remains how can a comprehensive civil defence system be prepared against such outbreaks?

COVID-19 Around the World

Beginning in China, the deadly virus created an unimaginable mayhem in other parts of the world. There are confirmed cases in at least 200 countries and territories across the globe. The US has reported the highest number of cases with over 2 million confirmed infections and over 1 lakh deaths till June 2020.

In Europe, the UK (United Kingdom) has been the worst impacted country due to Coronavirus. The UK Prime Minister, Boris Johnson struggled for his life after getting infected from Coronavirus. After the UK, Italy has recorded the highest number of deaths in Europe, with over 34,000 people while over 240 thousand infected people. Spain has over 296 thousand confirmed infections and over 28,346 deaths. Germany has comparatively lower numbers than other European countries with over 9,000 deaths. Latin America has been a late entrant in the list of COVID-19 affected regions. However, now the Latin American countries like Brazil, Argentina, Ecuador, Chile, Columbia and more are registering new cases of COVID-19 every day. Initially, Brazil did not endorse any lockdown mentioning economic reasons. Now, the number of infected people in Brazil has crossed Germany and France growing at a daily pace second only to the US. In this critical situation, its second health minister has resigned within a month time indicating the internal political issues during such testing times.[1] India, being the world's second largest populated country has registered over 5 lakh cases so far with over 17,000 deaths. It had followed the step-by-step lockdown mechanism that helped containing the virus to certain extent. Otherwise, the projections made in April 2020 by the reputed institutions like Jawaharlal Nehru Centre for Advanced Scientific Research (JNCASR), Indian Institute of Science, Bangalore, Indian Institute of Technology (IIT), Bombay and Armed Forces Medical College, Pune through a joint study anticipated over 500 thousand cases and 38,000 deaths by mid-May in India.[2]

In the Middle East, where the countries are already struggling to establish peace over cross-border conflicts and political instability, COVID-19 has created a big-time challenge. Additionally, the healthcare facilities are not adequate in most of these countries and are controlled by external factors other than the government. Iran alone has registered over 227 thousand cases and over 10,000 deaths. Amid the global smouldering of COVID-19, there was a fear of a viral spread of the virus in Africa. However, so far, less than two percent of the total number of global cases have been reported from Africa that has around 17 percent of the global population.[3]

Almost all major countries in the world are facing the fatal challenge of COVID-19, Italy, and the US have become the case studies for the experts for being the worst-hit countries despite having cutting-edge technology and the healthcare system.

China and the Curious Case of COVID-19

By the end of December, Wuhan Municipal Health Commission, China, reported mysterious cases of spread of an unknown virus that had flu-like symptoms in Wuhan, Hubei Province. Eventually, this novel virus was identified as Corona by the Chinese experts, later classified as COVID-19. On 4 January 2020, the World Health Organisation (WHO) reported the cases in Wuhan on social media, with no deaths.[4]

Soon the cases started rising exponentially with reports of death of few patients. As per the timeline maintained by the John Hopkins University and reported in *Hindustan Times*, by 23 January, China registered over 500 cases and 20 deaths due to COVID-19. By this time, Wuhan was in a complete lockdown. By 3 February, China registered over 13,000 cases with nearly 500 deaths. By mid-February, this number crossed 60,000 with over 2000 deaths. China banned trade, consumption of wild animals, and postponed its annual parliamentary meeting.[5] Though, by this time, the virus had reached other parts of the world through the travellers. Even at this stage, the world did not wake up to the alarming call of Coronavirus. Only if China would have sealed its borders at this stage and stopped both incoming and outgoing flights the world might not have had to suffer from a dreadful pandemic.

The first recorded case outside China was registered in Thailand on 13 January 2020. Post this, the WHO experts from its China and Western Pacific regional offices visited Wuhan to analyse the related facts and situation. At this juncture, the experts acknowledged the risk of a wider spread. By 30 January, the WHO Director-General reconvened the Emergency Committee (EC), which was constituted to analyse various aspects related to COVID-19. The EC advised the Director-General that the outbreak constituted a Public Health Emergency of

International Concern (PHEIC). The Director-General accepted the recommendation and declared the novel coronavirus outbreak (2019-nCoV) a PHEIC. Still, the WHO remained reluctant to call it a pandemic. After registering the cases reported in 18 countries outside China, several visits to Wuhan and alarmingly growing levels of spread and severity of COVID-19 worldwide, finally WHO announced COVID-19 as a pandemic on 11 March 2020.[6] By this time, the virus had already spread to the rest of the world and the experts were questioning the origin of the virus and the role of China in this whole situation.

The role of China in the global outbreak of COVID-19 is currently under question by many governments, institutions and experts. Many news articles, news channels and reports suggest that China not only provided wrong numbers about the infected people but also concealed the facts related to COVID-19 from the world, which resulted in a global outbreak. China did later admit that it made mistakes in the calculation of the death toll and recording the infected cases. Many reports claim that China was busy hiding the facts instead of sharing them with the world. In fact, the whistle-blowers were chided, who tried to raise the alarm for COVID-19 online, by the Chinese government.

The following was reported and shared by WHO officials:[7]

> "Wuhan, the COVID-19 epicentre, admitted gaffes in tallying its death toll, abruptly raising the city's count by 50 percent-following growing world doubts about Chinese transparency over the outbreak. The WHO further said Wuhan had been overwhelmed by the virus, which emerged in the city in December, and the authorities had been too swamped to ensure every death and infection was properly recorded. Authorities in Wuhan initially tried to cover up the outbreak, punishing doctors who had raised the alarm online, and there have been questions about the government's recording of infections as it repeatedly changed its counting criteria at the peak of the crisis. Later, China added many more cases to its earlier reported numbers of infected people and the death toll."

Also, there are media reports on the unpublished data of the Chinese government that suggest that the first case of COVID-19 was reported in China in November 2019. However, the official statements by the Chinese government to WHO stated that the first confirmed case had been diagnosed on 8 December. "Authorities did not publicly concede there was human-to-human transmission until 21 January. Jonathan Mayer, professor emeritus at the University of Washington's department of epidemiology, said it was 'entirely conceivable' there were cases as early as mid-November. He said there were three possibilities: first, the cases were not detected at the time, second, they were detected but not recognised as a new disease and last, they were detected and recognised but reporting was suppressed."[8]

Then, the reason provided by the Chinese experts for the spread of COVID-19 is also under the radar of suspicion by many scientists and experts. The Chinese authorities believe that COVID-19 spread from the local seafood market of Wuhan. It was stated that the local seafood market of Wuhan sold wild animals like bats, rabbits and snakes, and from here the transmission of the fatal virus started from animals to humans. Although a study by the scientists of Wuhan Institute of Virology claimed 96 percent similarities between the genetic makeup of the new Corona virus and the ones found in bats. However, later studies by many experts questioned this claim as many of the initially infected people had no link to this market.[9] To date, the exact reason behind the spread of Coronavirus is under question and is a matter of study. Many experts also believe that Coronavirus is a laboratory-made virus. French Nobel prize-winning scientist, Luc Montagnier, claimed that the SARS-CoV-2 virus was an outcome of the Chinese attempt to develop a vaccine against the AIDS virus. In his interview with a French news channel, he explained that the Wuhan city laboratory has been working on Coronaviruses since the early 2000s. Montagnier, who co-discovered Human Immunodeficiency Virus (HIV), claimed the presence of elements of HIV in the genome of the Coronavirus and the probability of elements of the Malaria too. Although his claim has been discarded and criticised by many of his colleagues, still many experts are not denying the possibility of Coronavirus being laboratory-made.[10]

Due to these reports, China is now under question by many countries and experts who believe the virus has been accidentally or deliberately leaked by China as a part of its ambitious biowarfare programme. In recent days, US President Donald Trump and Secretary of State Mike Pompeo also claimed that COVID-19 has originated from the Wuhan Institute of Virology in Wuhan. The two leaders also stated that China must explain why it declined to provide international scientists access to understand what happened. On the other hand, China has responded wrathfully to these allegations and has demanded proof for making such claims.[11] Thus, due to the lack of transparency, the origin of the virus has become a reason for a concerted US-China diplomatic conflict, fuelled by US officials calling the disease 'Chinese Coronavirus' or 'Wuhan virus'.[12]

Also, it has been alleged by Donald Trump that China stopped all incoming flights to its provinces however did not stop any outgoing flights that resulted in the global spread of COVID-19. It is also a matter of study how Coronavirus reached the rest of the world from China and spread rapidly, however, the neighbouring regions of Wuhan remained comparatively less affected.

Although China put Wuhan under lockdown in February, yet it was late for the people who travelled across the globe and became the reason for the transmission of this deadly virus in various countries. After declaring itself almost COVID-19 free, wherein very few cases were getting reported post quarantine period, China itself has reported 14 new COVID-19 cases on 10 May. This includes one new case from Wuhan where no new COVID-19 case was reported in over a month, as per the reports from Reuters.[13] This indicates the dangerous recurring tendency of the virus, wherein it may reoccur despite it's spread being controlled.

COVID-19 in Europe

Within Europe, Italy has been the hardest hit country, with the death toll passing 10,000 in late March. Spain, France, and the United Kingdom also have rapidly growing death tallies. Germany has recorded a large number of cases, but its fatalities are relatively low.[14]

The first case in Italy was reported on 30 January when the virus was found in two Chinese tourists visiting Italy.[15] By 21 February, 16 people were found to be Corona positive in Lombardy and Veneto. This was the time when the WHO was still insisting the virus was 'containable' and not nearly as infectious as the flu. Soon, the cases started increasing exponentially.[16]

Although Italy announced the first lockdown on 21 February itself, the virus kept spreading across the country. Epidemiologists believe that what went wrong in Italy is a matter of study and research for years, as the healthcare system of Italy is one of the best in Europe. The situation became so critical in Italy, that the country was forced to ask the patients to stay in-home care because of its low Intensive Care Unit (ICU) capacity. Due to COVID 19, Italy was left with 8.6 ICU beds per 1,00,000 people, below the average of 15.9 within the developed countries of the Organisation for Economic Cooperation and Development (OECD).[17]

It seems that initially, Italy was confident about its well-equipped medical care system. Italy has 3.2 hospital beds per 1000 people (as compared with 2.8 in the US). However, when the situation went out of control, all non-critical surgeries were cancelled, and operating rooms were turned into makeshift ICUs. With all beds occupied, corridors and administrative areas too filled with patients, the preparedness eventually turned into panic.[18]

Although, there is another set of studies, where experts state that Italy has the most elderly population in Europe and the second most elderly population in the world after Japan. According to an analysis, the average age of people infected with COVID-19, who died in Italy, has been 80 years, and the average age of patients requiring critical care support has been 67 years. On the other hand, Italy has a high proportion of patients with heart diseases. Since COVID-19 mortality is strongly dependent on the age group and the presence of associated serious diseases, the researchers believe Italy had to face the worst effect of the outbreak.[19]

Some experts suggest that when the entire world started following social distancing and other precautions to check the spread of COVID-19, Dario Nardella, Mayor of Florence, Italy, initiated a 'Hug a Chinese' campaign on Twitter on 1 February. Many Italians followed the mayor and posted their pictures hugging Chinese people. Although no study proves that COVID-19 spread in Italy due to this particular act, the probability of rapid and wide transfer of infection due to such acts cannot be denied.

After rounds of lockdown across the country, now Italy has started providing gradual relaxations. Apart from the immediate effect of COVID-19, that is, the health crisis across the country, Italy is also facing severe economic challenges. To cope up with the situation and start rolling up its economy again, Italy's government has allowed the café, restaurants and other outlets to open. It would gradually be opening the travel and other facilities too. However, this may prove to be a perilous step as there is still no treatment or vaccine available for COVID-19 and Coronavirus has a tendency to reoccur.

As reported by many news agencies, Coronavirus reached the UK in mid-March 2020. With its Prime Minister himself suffering from COVID-19, the country announced a lockdown on 23 March 2020. Since then, the country struggled to cope with the numbers of infected people every day in terms of providing them with adequate healthcare facilities and containing the virus. The situation in the UK became worse so much so that the prime minister of the UK has been facing criticism for being overconfident and underestimating the frightful impact of COVID-19. However, after implementing social distancing and lockdown to check the massive spread of the virus, the UK announced a decrease in the number of COVID-19 impacted people. Since June 2020, fewer cases are being reported in the UK, Scotland and Ireland, however, the authorities and experts are now anticipating the second wave of COVID-19 and planning to prepare against the same.[20] Also, the country now seems to be under a political and economic crisis where the government has to make a way out for both anticipated and unexpected economic challenges that may occur due to issues such as unemployment. Amid this grave socio-politico-economic situation and challenge of containing COVID-19, scientists at Imperial College, London have recently come up with the plan of starting vaccine trials on selected people shortly as the developed vaccine candidate against COVID-19 has shown some great results.[21]

France is the first country in Europe that reported the first case of COVID-19 on 24 January 2020 in Bordeaux.[22] Soon more cases were reported, and the first COVID-19 death of a Chinese tourist was reported on 14 February 2020 in France.[23] It was later revealed that the first case of COVID-19 had already been reported in December. At that point in time, the patient was treated for flu-like symptoms. However, the swab taken from the recovered patient was tested later for COVID-19, as cases were reported in France.[24]

France was also initially reluctant towards lockdown, cancellation of assemblies and mass gatherings which resulted in rapid transmission of the virus. It was only in March that the President, Emmanuel Macron, announced the shutdown of all schools and universities. A day later, the Prime Minister, Édouard Philippe announced a ban on meetings of more than 100 people. The next day, immediate closure of all non-essential public places, restaurants, cafés, cinemas and nightclubs was announced.[25]

After a considerable reduction in the number of COVID-19 cases, and readiness in terms of healthcare and other infrastructure facilities, the country has been easing the lockdown since May 2020. Now, it is preparing to open the schools and theatres from 22 June 2020, by laying down essential guidelines related to COVID-19, in its third phase of lockdown. Restaurants and café, shopping malls and transportation have already opened in France depending on the zone of virus infection. As the country is also following red, orange and green zones to imply the level of infection and the stage of easing lockdown.[26]

France, the second biggest economy of Europe, is also facing the challenge of a great economic slump due to the COVID-19 situation and is trying to come up with various solutions. In fact, most of the European countries now seem to be in a mode of reviving their economies by lifting the restrictions imposed during the lockdown periods. Additionally, President Macron is looking forward to 'relaunch' the economy of France and be self-reliant instead of relying on other countries in terms of supply of goods.[27]

Signs are slowly emerging that Europe may have turned a corner on the virus as infection rates begin to fall and parts of Europe are starting to relax restrictions.

But social distancing guidelines remain in place, as leaders attempt to balance a return to normal life with protecting populations from new spikes in infections.

Why the US Failed to Contain COVID-19?

Amidst the global toll of COVID-19, what is happening in the US is indeed shocking. With over 2 million cases and over 1 lakh deaths, the US is another case study to understand why and how the so called 'superpower' failed against a virus outbreak. This sounds more dreadful as the US has been working for years on preparing a comprehensive civil defence mechanism against the usage of biological agents or an outbreak through various programs. It has a strong normative framework, agencies, healthcare system, proficient workforce, very advanced technologies and most importantly, enough funds to invest in the required facilities to fight such outbreaks. However, what is happening in the US can be considered as an alarming bell for those who are working on preparing holistic and efficient responses against any biological agent outbreak. When other countries were announcing total lockdown, the US preferred to keep its economic interests above social distancing. The US kept itself engaged in a blame game with China instead of paying attention to its measures to contain the virus. Despite huge numbers of infected people every day, the US continued to remain reluctant to announce nation-wide lockdown. It appeared that the country was overconfident about its healthcare preparedness and vaccine development program. Later, even when lockdowns were announced in several states, both government and people did not support it wholeheartedly, which resulted in a failed response against COVID-19.

Korean Peninsula: Treatment, Recovery and Relapse

Although a political predicament emerged due to the deadlock in the denuclearisation process of North Korea due to COVID-19, both North and South Korea seemed to be fortunate enough of not being adversely impacted due to COVID-19 as compared to other countries like Italy, France and the US. Compared to the western part of the globe, both North and South Korea have been successful in containing the virus effectively.

For many days after COVID-19 hit the world, the infection and eventual death of the North Korean dictator Kim Jong-un kept making headlines. However, his public appearance cleared all rumours. North Korea has been claiming that it is COVID-19 free and has not reported any case so far. However, given the secretive nature of the North Korean government and that absence of any international institution in the country, the same cannot be verified.

South Korea has reported more than 12,000 COVID-19 infected people with 282 deaths so far. The WHO has recognised South Korea as an example for the countries that could contain COVID-19 effectively with their comprehensive measures. South Korea noted the second largest number of COVID-19 cases after China in March 2020. However, it followed a strict lockdown mechanism complemented with mass testing, contact tracing and similar means to contain further spread of the virus and it succeeded.[28]

Despite its success in fully containing the virus, South Korea is again witnessing another spike in the numbers of COVID-19 positive people. The country started lifting its lockdown in April 2020, and the government officials of Korea did not consider re-imposing stronger social distancing guidelines mentioning a weak economy as the reason. On the contrary, many health experts, including the director of the Korean Centre for Disease Control, Jung Eun-kyeong, warned that the country may have to face another wave of COVID-19, and this time in its most populated regions.[29]

The Spread of the Deadly Virus in Latin America

Although a late entrant in the list of COVID-19 affected regions, currently Latin America has become the epicentre of COVID-19 as noted by WHO. The virus has infected more than 1 million people in Brazil, leading to more than 50 thousand deaths. Peru has also registered more than 282,000 cases, while nearly 275,999 have been infected in Chile.[30] Brazil, Peru, Chile, Colombia and Ecuador tops the list of the worst impacted countries in the region. However, there is no country left in the region, which has not recorded COVID-19 positive cases. The news reports also cover how these countries are facing tough times due to their ill-prepared public and community health and government systems. For instance, many reports mentioned abandoned dead bodies on the streets and completely collapsed the public health system in Ecuador.[31]

Latin American countries have already been facing many political, social and economic challenges. Amid politically unstable environments and economically fragile conditions, it has been challenging to fully prepare against an outbreak of this scale. Inadequate healthcare facilities, unavailability of PPEs (Personal Protection Equipment) and masks, poor testing and surveillance capabilities and lack of coordination among departments are the major reasons behind such massive spread in the Latin American region. Currently, the situation seems to be deteriorating as few countries of Latin America never implemented lockdown while others are getting ready to lift the restrictions. This, coupled with the fact that no vaccine or treatment is available for COVID-19 yet, makes the situation more challenging as social distancing seems to be the only measure to check the viral containment.

Impact of COVID-19 in South Asia

South Asia has almost 25 percent of the world population and in that comparison the impact of COVID-19 has been considerably low. Most people dwell in the densely settled areas and many have limited access to quality infrastructure and healthcare. The COVID-19 pandemic was expected to be a "perfect storm" for the region. However, as of 30 June, South Asia had reported a total of only 966,920 confirmed cases and 23,761 deaths, which is way less compared to total world fatalities – even as the numbers in some South Asian countries have spiked drastically in the past few weeks.[32] A very puzzling situation that was noticed in this region by the experts. As compared to North America, Western Europe and East Asia, the number of infections and deaths in this region has been comparatively low. Obviously, it is still early to come down to a definitive conclusion in this respect as many believe that many countries are still in the early stages where community transmission has not gathered momentum. An exponential growth in infection numbers could yet surface later, or in a second phase.[33] Many hypotheses have been offered over the past few months as to why South Asia might be an outlier in the pandemic: "its tropical climate, the protection offered by a tuberculosis vaccine called Bacillus Calmette-Guérin (BCG), exposure to malaria, and a weaker strain of the virus in the Indian subcontinent."[34] However, a more acceptable explanation regarding this phenomenon states that the lack of testing capability and the massive size of the population in these regions could actually be shadowing the reality. Additionally, the strict lockdown measures imposed by India, Bangladesh, Pakistan, Sri Lanka and Nepal by the last week of March may have helped in curbing the rapid spread of transmission to some extent.[35]

In South Asia, the coronavirus pandemic is simultaneously a health, economic and humanitarian crisis. A UNICEF report noted that an estimated 120 million children living in South Asian countries could slip into poverty within the next six months due to the COVID-19 crisis. The reports also flag the negative impact of the COVID-related disruption to vaccination, nutrition and other vital health services.[36]

Pandemic has also heavily dented the economy of this region. Especially countries like Maldives, Sri Lanka, Nepal, and Bhutan that are dependent on tourism, for fuelling their economies are seeing huge losses. Many states are also seeing losses in remittances from workers in the Middle East that contribute to their national economies.

The pandemic has also been exacerbating the existing political and security challenges from the civil war in Afghanistan and the civil-military seesaw in Pakistan to the Rohingya refugee crisis on Bangladesh's southern border, to the stand-off between India-China.[37]

India's Measures to Contain COVID-19

India, which has a huge population and limited resources comparatively, adopted the lockdown way of containing COVID-19. After facing the initial hiccups and challenges, India successfully created a comprehensive response against COVID-19. First of all, India announced a day's Junta Curfew or lockdown on 22 March 2020. After a supportive response from its system and the people, it then announced the first phase of nation-wide lockdown on 24 March 2020. Except for essential services like healthcare, banks, sanitation, administrative and security facilities, all other services were suspended. The state borders were sealed, and the government banned on all non-essential travel except in cases of inevitability. The government also announced the closure of teaching in schools and universities. This led to the adoption of online modes of teaching and assessments. The country also followed under-surveillance quarantine of infected persons. This way, India delayed the spread period of the virus so that it does not face a situation like Italy. These lockdowns also provided enough time for the government to prepare against the dreadful outbreak with required measures, infrastructure and policies. This also created a well-planned awareness and preparedness among the masses. Currently, India is gradually easing the lockdown with strict measures in place.

In its report based on data from 73 countries, the Oxford COVID-19 Government Response Tracker (OxCGRT), appreciated India's Government that has responded more stringently than other countries in managing COVID-19. It also acknowledged the government's emergency policy making, instant investment in healthcare, financial measures, investment in vaccine research and active response to the situation and scored India with a '100' for its strictness.[38]

It is important to note that most of the developed countries with enough funds, good infrastructure and advanced public and community health systems have failed in tackling the pandemic effectively. Generally, the availability of good infrastructure and advanced public and community health systems are considered as one of the most significant components for building a strong and holistic civil defence against biological agents or outbreaks. Then what went wrong? Here the scale of the outbreak and unavailability of accurate medications or vaccines against the virus played the most important role in causing the obliteration of a global scale. None of the countries were prepared for an outbreak of such a scale. Moreover, the human-to-human spread created another challenge as the medical staff too started getting infected. Most of the countries had made make-shift arrangements for new hospitals overnight for accommodating COVID-19 infected people. This is the reason the countries that followed a complete lockdown could relatively contain the virus more effectively.

World Order Post-COVID-19

How will the world look post-COVID-19? First of all, it is very important to note that COVID-19 is not going to vanish all of a sudden. It will exist and would again hit the world in its second wave, as predicted by many scientists. Hence, it is critical at this stage to be more vigilant and cautious with all measures in place to mitigate its infection. Then, it is also significant to accept that the world has entered into a stage of acceptance where biological outbreaks through the novel agents are no more a fallacy. Also, such novel agents may be used by terrorist organisations or the rouge states to disrupt the global system and challenge the international security and create a state of panic. At the same time, it is no more a secret for masses that such outbreaks, natural or deliberate, may disrupt their lives.

Although it is too early to comment on the future world order, a debate is going on about shift in the power centres, upcoming challenges and the status of regional and global alliances. The nature of the global system post-COVID-19 would depend on the emerging leaders and countries based on their response to COVID-19. Experts believe that even in the era of globalisation, counties would prefer to keep their priorities at the top and hence COVID-19 would certainly change the world forever where multi-realities could be the new realities. Multilateralism would continue, in fact, may get more strengthened.

Then, we are learning to live in a new way where social distancing, face masks and remote work environments could become the new normal. The power centres will shift too as the world is living in a shadow of the threat of economic slump due to COVID-19. Be the elements of conventional or hard power such as military capabilities and funding or the factors associated with soft power such as culture, diaspora and tourism, all have been impacted due to COVID-19, and it would be interesting to see how countries would get over the associated challenges caused due to COVID-19. Basically, COVID-19 seems to be working as a catalyst for prevailing political, social and economic problems in different countries. It seems that the prevailing problems may reach their peaks during or post COVID-19 and hence would change the existing global system in both scenarios if they get solved or they get worst.

Conclusion: What is Needed?

Natural or laboratory made, we cannot deny the fact that COVID-19 has changed our lives forever. Today, the world is facing a war without any missiles or guns. The enemy is right in front of us and not visible. A comprehensive civil defence is the need of the hour. A strong global mechanism is required to combat the plausible threat of usage of biological agents for outbreaks along with belligerent use of technology. However, at present, the most critical requirement to defeat COVID-19 is the right treatment and vaccine. Although many countries are working on it, so far, no verified medication or vaccine is available to treat COVID-19. Many countries have reported about the successful outcomes of using plasma of the recovered people to treat infected people, however it cannot be considered as the exact treatment for the disease. On the other hand, the normative procedure for development, verification and production of vaccine for COVID-19 needs to be expediated so that the containment and reoccurrence of the outbreak can be checked. However, one more significant point has to be considered here. The possibility of use of more novel biological agents cannot be denied, and we cannot vaccinate ourselves every time for a novel agent. Hence, in terms of vaccination, a well-planned global vaccination strategy needs to be developed based on the experts' advices.

From futuristic perspective, strong normative framework for both, the tactical challenges as well as the strategic roadmap keeping outbreaks like COVID-19 in mind, usage of advanced technologies for developing easy and fast detection systems, promoting vaccination programs to develop broad-spectrum vaccines, mass production of PPEs, creating general awareness among public so that they can learn to respond to such outbreaks without panic and most significantly, collaboration are the key steps in solving this global issue.

Collaboration and connectedness seem to be the most critical key for combating COVID-19 efficiently. First of all, countries need to form a web of networks from local to global levels either directly or through International Organisations. Sharing information immediately holds the most critical solution for COVID-19 like outbreaks. Imagine if China would have shared the information related to COVID-19 immediately with the world and had quarantined itself? Then, there is a need to prepare the public and community health systems to act effectively.

Underdeveloped and developing countries' health infrastructure should be aided by economically stronger countries to prepare themselves for such outbreaks. Multi-spectrum vaccination programs should also be discussed and run at a global level.

COVID-19 opens a new world of challenges coming from the unseen and novel biological agents. Whatever the source be, the world needs to respond effectively and collectively based on scientific remedies. Biosecurity and biodefence seem to be and need to be 'the' priority for the world to ensure the existence of the human race.

* * *

A shorter version of the essay was published in the CBW Magazine, Vol. 13, No. 1, Jan-June 2020.

NOTES

1. 'Brazil's New Health Minister Quits as Prez Bolsonaro Grabs Reins in Coronavirus Crisis,' *Reuters, India Today.com*, available at https://www.indiatoday.in/world/story/brazil-new-health-minister-teich-quits-prez-bolsonaro-grabs-reins-coronavirus-crisis-1678607-2020-05-16, accessed on 15 May 2020.
2. Richa Sharma, 'Projection: 38,220 deaths, 5.35 lakh COVID-19 Cases in India by mid-May,' Indian Express, 23 April 2020, available at https://www.newindianexpress.com/nation/2020/apr/23/projection-38220-deaths-535-lakh-covid-19-cases-in-india-by-mid-may-2134087.html, accessed on 29 April 2020.
3. 'Why COVID-19 Seems to Spread more Slowly in Africa,' *The Economist*, 16 May 2020, available at https://www.economist.com/middle-east-and-africa/2020/05/16/why-covid-19-seems-to-spread-more-slowly-in-africa, accessed on 16 May 2020.
4. 'WHO Timeline-COVID-19', *WHO Website*, 12 May 2020, available at https://www.who.int/news-room/detail/27-04-2020-who-timeline--covid-19, accessed on 14 May 2020.
5. Sparshita Saxena, 'Revisiting Hubei: How did COVID-19 events unfold in China?,' *Hindustan Times*, 10 May 2020, available at https://www.hindustantimes.com/world-news/revisiting-hubei-how-did-covid-19-events-unfold-in-china/story-VWslylVgiFWJ9gebDEEgrO.html, accesses on 12 May 2020.
6. See note 1.
7. 'WHO says All Countries will Face This' After China Revises COVID-19 Death Tally', *Livemint*, 18 April 2020, available at https://www.livemint.com/news/world/who-says-all-countries-will-face-this-after-china-revises-covid-19-death-tally-11587180452852.html, accessed on 30 April 2020.
8. 'First COVID-19 Case Happened in November, China Government Records Show-Report,' *The Guardian*, 13 March 2020, available at https://www.theguardian.com/world/2020/mar/13/first-covid-19-case-happened-in-november-china-government-records-show-report, accessed on 15 April 2020.
9. Matt Reynolds and Sabrina Weiss, 'How Coronavirus Started and What Happens Next, Explained,' *The Wire*, 12 May 2020, available at https://www.wired.co.uk/article/china-coronavirus, accessed on 14 May 2020.

10. 'Nobel Winning Scientist Claims COVID-19 Virus was Man-made in Wuhan Lab,' *LiveMint.com*, 19 April 2020, available at https://www.livemint.com/news/world/nobel-winning-scientist-claims-covid-19-virus-was-man-made-in-wuhan-lab-11587303649821.html, accessed on 29 April 2020.
11. China Asks US to Show 'Enormous Evidence' of COVID-19 Originating From Wuhan Lab, *India.com*, 6 May 2020, available at https://www.india.com/news/world/china-asks-us-to-show-enormous-evidence-of-covid-19-originating-from-wuhan-lab-4021893/, accessed on 10 May 2020.
12. See note 5.
13. See note 2.
14. Mapping the Global Spread of the Coronavirus, *National Geographic*, 28 June 2020, available at https://www.nationalgeographic.com/science/2020/03/mapping-coronavirus-infections-across-the-globe/,acessed on 29 June 2020.
15. Angelo Amante and Elvira Pollina, 'Two First Coronavirus Cases Confirmed in Italy: Prime Minister,' *Reuters*, 31 January 2020, available at https://www.reuters.com/article/us-china-health-italy/two-first-coronavirus-cases-confirmed-in-italy-prime-minister-idUSKBN1ZT31H, accessed on 15 March 2020.
16. 'Italy's Daily COVID-19 Death Toll Lowest Since mid-March,' *Hindustan Times*, 27 April 2020, available at https://www.hindustantimes.com/world-news/italy-s-daily-covid-19-death-toll-lowest-since-mid-march/story-LWIjKmrNvUOy4MEGDRlsBI.html, accessed on 30 April 2020.
17. Ibid.
18. Lisa Rosenbaum, 'Facing COVID-19 in Italy-Ethics, Logistics, and Therapeutics on the Epidemic's Front Line,' *The New England Journal of Medicine*, vol. 382, 18 March 2020, pp. 1873-1875, available at https://www.nejm.org/doi/full/10.1056/NEJMp2005492, accessed on 25 April 2020.
19. 'Lessons Countries can Learn from COVID-19 in Italy decoded,' *Economic Times*, 12 April 2020, available at https://economictimes.indiatimes.com/news/international/world-news/lessons-countries-can-learn-from-covid-19-in-italy-decoded/articleshow/75105308.cms?from=mdr, accessed on 29 April 2020.
20. UK sees Fewest COVID-19 Deaths Since Lockdown, but Threat of Second Wave Looms, *Livemint.com*, available at https://www.livemint.com/news/world/uk-has-fewest-covid-19-deaths-since-lockdown-but-threat-of-second-wave-looms-11591543097175.html, accessed on 12 June 2020.
21. UK Begins Trial of Latest COVID-19 Vaccine Candidate this Week, *PTI*, 16 June 2020, available at https://www.timesnownews.com/health/article/uk-begins-trial-of-latest-covid19-vaccine-candidate-this-week/607036, accessed on 20 June 2020.
22. S. Bernard-Stoecklin, 'First Cases of Coronavirus Disease 2019 (COVID-19) in France: Surveillance, Investigations and Control Measures,' *Eurosurveillance*, 13 February 2020; vol. 25, no. 6, available at https://www.ncbi.nlm.nih.gov/pmc/articles/PMC7029452/, accessed on 19 June 2020.
23. 'Chinese Tourist in France dies of COVID-19, First Death in Europe,' *Reuters*, 15 February 2020, available at https://www.thehindu.com/news/international/chinese-tourist-in-france-dies-of-covid-19-first-death-in-europe/article30829346.ece, accessed on 18 June 2020.
24. 'Coronavirus: France's First Known Case 'was in December', *BBC News*, 5 May 2020, available at https://www.bbc.com/news/world-europe-52526554, accessed on 18 June 2020.

25. 'Coronavirus: Spain and France Announce Sweeping Restrictions,' *BBC News*, 15 March 2020, available at https://www.bbc.com/news/world-europe-51892477, accessed on 18 June 2020.
26. 'What Changes as France Enters 'phase 3' of lockdown on Monday?,' *The Local*, 18 June 2020, available at https://www.thelocal.fr/20200618/what-changes-as-france-enters-phase-3-of-lockdown, accessed on 19 June 2020.
27. 'France to Accelerate Easing of Coronavirus Lockdown Restrictions,' *NBC News*, 15 June 2020, available at https://www.nbcnews.com/news/world/france-accelerate-easing-coronavirus-lockdown-restrictions-n1231039, accessed on 19 June 2020.
28. Kyungji Cho and Jihye Lee, 'Coronavirus: South Korea Faces 2nd Wave of COVID-19, Bars & Clubs closed,' *Bloomberg*, 10 May 2020, available at https://www.livemint.com/news/world/coronavirus-south-korea-faces-2nd-wave-of-covid-19-bars-clubs-closed-11589094342314.html, accessed on 19 June 2020.
29. Kim Tong-Hyung, 'COVID-19 Resurgence Threatens South Korea's Success Story,' *The Diplomat*, 12 June 2020, available at https://thediplomat.com/2020/06/covid-19-resurgence-threatens-south-koreas-success-story/, accessed on 19 June 2020.
30. 'WHO Declares that South America is the New Coronavirus Epicenter,' *Washington Post*, 23 May 2020, available at https://www.washingtonpost.com/nation/2020/05/22/coronavirus-update-us/, accessed on 19 June 2020.
31. 'Anthony Faiola and Ana Vanessa Herrero, 'Uncollected Bodies Lie for Days in the Streets of Ecuador: The Emerging Epicenter of the Coronavirus in Latin America,' *Stuff*, 13 April 2020, available at https://www.stuff.co.nz/national/health/coronavirus/120818001/uncollected-bodies-lie-for-days-in-the-streets-of-ecuador-the-emerging-epicenter-of-the-coronavirus-in-latin-america, accessed on 20 June 2020
32. Puja Changoiwala, 'Why South Asia's COVID-19 Numbers Are So Low (For Now),' *Quanta Magazine*, 23 June 2020, available at https://www.quantamagazine.org/why-south-asias-covid-19-numbers-are-so-low-for-now-20200623/, accessed on 24 June 2020.
33. Deepak Nayyar, 'The COVID-19 paradox in South Asia,' *The Hindu*, available at https://www.thehindu.com/opinion/lead/the-covid-19-paradox-in-south-asia/article31417806.ece, accessed on 22 June 2020.
34. See note 32.
35. Ibid.
36. 'COVID-19 Might Push 120mn Children into Poverty in South Asia, including India: UNICEF,' 24 June 2020, available at https://www.hindustantimes.com/health/coronavirus-covid-19-might-push-120-mn-children-into-poverty-in-south-asia-including-india-unicef/story-37mxXGFGghFOO5UubKtSoJ.html, accessed on 22 June 2020.
37. Srinath Raghavan, 'South Asia's Battle with the Coronavirus,' *Carnegie India*, 21 May 2020, available at https://carnegieindia.org/2020/05/21/south-asia-s-battle-with-coronavirus-pub-81850, accessed on 22 June 2020.
38. India Scores High on COVID-19 Response Tracker Made by Oxford University,' *India Today*, 10 April 2020, available at https://www.indiatoday.in/india/story/india-scores-high-on-covid-19-response-tracker-made-by-oxford-university-1665573-2020-04-10, accessed on 14 May 2020.

SECTION II
ASSESSMENT AND RESPONSES

Asia

3

Saving a Billion: How India Confronted COVID-19

A. Vinod Kumar

The outbreak of the Coronavirus Disease (COVID-19) in the final months of 2019 in China had led to a global pandemic with the disease-causing pathogen, the SARS-CoV-2 (Severe Acute Respiratory Syndrome-Coronavirus-2), spreading virulently to almost all habitable land on Earth within a matter of 2-3 months. Even over seven months after its first imprint in Wuhan, the pathogen remains unconquerable with close to 9 million being infected and more than 4.5 lakh dead. Most nations had largely responded uniformly by locking down economies and halting all ways of outdoor lives to break the chain of contagion. Yet, most of the heavily affected countries, particularly the populous ones, have had their own distinct operational experiences and institutional challenges in the dual effort of halting the spread of the virus and effectively curing the infected populace.

Unlike the high-casualty rates in the Western world, known for their superlative healthcare systems and practices, the developing world, particularly China and India, which together accounts for close to one-third of world population, has had comparatively much lesser infection and mortality rates from the pandemic. While the Chinese experience has been mired in secrecy despite being the source of the outbreak, India's COVID-19 campaign, with its extensive population imprint and transparent disease control measures, provides significant insights for global public health systems and pandemic management strategies.

Protecting 1.37 billion people from an epidemic, for that matter, involves a colossal political and policy challenge. There are some key attributes to the strategies that India adopted in dealing with the spread of CoV-2, which has ensured that the country's infection rate remained below 0.0072 percent of its total population and deaths even a further minuscule percent of that at a lockdown peak during mid-May and rising to 0.015 percent by the time of unlocking by early June (and stretching to 0.021 percent by end-June when total infections crossed 5 lakhs).[1] Assuming, at the current spiralling rate of the first wave,[2] the infection may peak to over 10-20 lakhs before stabilizing, subsiding or triggering herd immunity (in high-impact pockets),[3] it will still account for only around 0.10 percent of the population, and thus mark an effective pandemic management strategy for the world's second-largest populace. Notwithstanding the peculiar epidemical curve (of a late nation-wide surge and regional pockets with community spread despite effective mitigation measures) that India has experienced, the country's COVID-19 campaign needs a cursory assessment to know its intrinsic features and key contours.

First, despite being of third-world standards, India's public health systems responded and functioned robustly to tackle the COVID-19 challenge in contrast to what was seen as world-class health-systems collapsing under the weight of the rapid contagion in western nations. India's public health infrastructure was instantly prepared to provide free and dedicated trauma care and treatment to the affected communities, whereas it was widely reported that the healthcare system in western nations was not easily accessible and costly.[4] Public healthcare institutions in many of the western countries had reportedly turned into critical care systems that resulted in large segments of infected patients having to confine to home-isolation and over-the-counter drugs thus aggravating the risk of those with co-morbidities. This was in sharp contrast to the scenario in India where COVID-positive patients were subjected to instant clinical exposure in highly sanitized public health premises and provided with dedicated treatment and highest possible recovery opportunities. However, as the cases rapidly increase in India, various states are planning to ramp up critical care facilities by going beyond public health systems and harnessing infrastructure from the hospitality industry in order to ensure the widest possible availability of clinical and critical care exposure.

Second, India managed to inhibit rapid initial virus contagion by early restriction of flights from affected countries (especially in the first wave of global CoV-2 imprint), enforcing access control at border points, initially, and thereafter (by early March) closing borders and terminating all international traffic from and to the country. This was in sharp contrast to the situation in many Western capitals where international air traffic and free movement of people, particularly in transit hubs like London, were happening uninhibited despite virulent spread in the region. By implementing early access control and opportunity denial, India was highly effective in delaying the swift surge of virus transmission in the country though many early infected carriers had already entered the country by the time these measures were initiated.

Third, India has had a distinct experience with the phenomenon of community spread. In fact, the core of India's contagion mitigation strategy was to ensure that community spread does not occur rapidly or could be effectively controlled in as best ways possible in a country with thousands of urban areas that have a high intensity of populations. Unlike the rampant community spread that was witnessed in many of the Western hotspots, India was effective in mitigating rapid contagion beyond initially-formed clusters through mitigation exercises including nationwide lockdown, active contact tracing and containment thus ensuring that even the bulging of clusters does not result in a community spill-over that could permeate to a national scale. Nonetheless, as is consequent for virulent pathogens, there were mild trends of community spreads subsequently visible in various localized hotspots in some parts of the country even during the peak lockdown period and resulting in a cumulative increase of newer clusters across the country matching the national spiral. For example, infection spirals in Dharavi in Mumbai,[5] Jehangirpuri in Delhi and Koyembedu Market in Chennai were instances of localized community spreads with clusters rapidly bulging and spilling over towards newer cluster formations despite being sealed off through rigorous containment measures.

The mutative intensity of the pathogen apart, such virulent contagion trajectories are a testament to the fact that any extent of mitigation measures may fall short when dealing with an epidemical spread in dense urban centres. With the intense infection spiral coinciding with the phased easing of lockdown and initiation of unlocking process in early June, there have been instances of rapid community spreads in states like Delhi and across numerous districts in Maharashtra, Gujarat and Tamil Nadu, among others, though a nation-wide community spread was not visible even 135-150 days after the first COVID-19 case was reported in the country in late January, thus underlining the relative efficacy of the conglomeration of measures taken to protect 1.37 billion from the pandemic. In fact, the Indian epidemical map of the CoV-2 spread is largely about primary to secondary permeation in the initial phase and tertiary spread in the later phases expanding many of the infected clusters in the highly populous urban centres and their eventual spill-over causing community spread to contiguous communities and beyond.[6]

Having identified these significant divergences from how the rest of the world dealt with the CoV-2, India's response strategies could be described through two key elements:

(a) Contagion Mitigation

Since 30 January 2020, when the first COVID-19 case in the country was identified in Kerala, the country's contagion course has been akin to a roller-coaster ride. With its experience of containing an outbreak of Nipah virus in 2018,[7] Kerala managed to control the spread of the initial CoV-2 cases through immaculate mitigation measures including patient isolation, contact tracing and clinical improvisation, an exercise it pursued on a sustained basis to come up with the most efficient response methods in India.[8] The significant gap between patient zero in January and the sudden spiral through fresh cases in Delhi and Telangana in the first week of March could be attributed to the decision to enforce surveillance at airports with an initial focus only on East Asian hotspots like China and South Korea and later expanded to other affected regions like the Middle East and Europe. While the first case was a direct Wuhan import, the slow but certain surge in the rest of India since early March can be attributed to the cases from the Middle East and Europe who either evaded entry-point monitoring or were asymptomatic.

The decision to follow the Chinese model of lockdown for contagion mitigation was intended to contain infection within the then-existing clusters and deny the scope for a community spread through an extended mutation period of around 21 days, assuming the extent of spread could have been evident and mapped by then. These calculations went awry as spontaneous new clusters formed by undetected external inducers – cases like the Tablighi Jamaat spreading across the country, arrivals from the Middle East causing clusters in Maharashtra, pilgrim- and traveller-driven spirals in Punjab, among others causing primary-to-secondary spiral in the 21-day mutation period. This was followed by swift secondary and tertiary spread leading to the expansion of clusters and creation of new ones (as in West Bengal), and the migrant exodus from cities to states like Bihar and UP (Uttar Pradesh) being later cases.

While the initially infected states like Kerala, Rajasthan, Karnataka and UP had used effective tools of mitigation including rigorous containment of hotspots, contact tracing and clinical exposure to stem the spread, there are later cases like Gujarat, Tamil Nadu, West Bengal and Punjab (besides Maharashtra) where the dynamics of community spread and cluster bulges are beyond easy explanations. With the socio-economic costs of the nation-wide lockdown becoming overbearing, particularly over the mass exodus of migrant workers, who were also aggravating the contagion risk in their cross-country movement, the Indian government was forced to adopt a phased relaxation of rigorous mitigation exercises like the nation-wide lockdown and instead adopt a bottom-up approach of identifying containment zones and containing infection and inhibiting cluster bulges within the designated hotspots.

Notwithstanding arguments that this approach if adopted initially could have offset the socio-economic costs of a national closure, the rapid spiral seen during the easing phases could also be seen as an indicator of how the march of the virus was delayed, and its potency negated, through the nation-wide lockdown. Thus, with its own distinct epidemical curve, the Indian experience in contagion mitigation through different approaches (lock-down and phased unlocking) covering over 80 days (at the time of writing) and destined to stretch into another 30-45 days, could still be seen in terms of its relative efficacy in ensuring that not more than 0.025 percent is likely to be infected by the virus even at its estimated peak of around 10-20 lakhs. Thus, the outcome of India's contagion mitigation seen in five months of the campaign has been the creation of an elongated epidemical curve that had ensured that a high-consequence national contagion impact could be averted and the intensity of infections and moralities had been restricted to a significantly lower benchmark in contrast to the mass deaths expected to have occurred when the highly-virulent passed through the world's second-largest population.

(b) Disease Control

Clinical Remedies: COVID-19 being a disease caused by a new pathogen, notwithstanding its other Coronavirus familial links,[9] is yet to be confronted with a potent treatment remedy. The domineering clinical methods adopted across India have been to use generic medications for symptoms associated with the virus infection particularly on mild and moderately-affected patients. At the same time, various anti-viral drugs that have been developed for other viral strains like HIV, Ebola and Influence, among others, have been repurposed to be being tried out individually or in combinations on the severely-affected and those with a risk of co-morbidities as placebo formula.

Of the over 25 drugs that were proposed for repurposing for COVID-19 treatment, some have found greater acceptance among public health authorities across the globe and accordingly have also been allowed for usages at various stages of COVID-19 treatment in India. Notable among the preferred anti-virals is remdesivir, a drug originally developed for the treatment of Ebola by US-based Gilead Sciences in 2014, and subsequently tried out on SARS and MERS patients, though not without much success in the latter cases. Notwithstanding, this drug is now being positioned as the most promising prospect for COVID-19 treatment following encouraging results seen in various stages of treatment of severe and moderate COVID-19 patients during the Gilead conducted clinical trials, besides favourable results in the Solidarity Trials of the World Health Organisation (WHO).[10]

Remdesivir's emergence as the frontline CoV-2 medication, in the absence of suitable alternatives, did not find easy acceptance going by its supposed limited impact during on SARS and MERS. Initial studies published in journals like *Lancet* had dismissed any significant clinical benefits from remdesivir to speed up recovery time,[11] though many national medical authorities including the US Food and Drug Administration (FDA) approved emergency-use authorization based on Gilead's claim of improved recovery time seen during patient trials.[12] By early June, Gilead had shared results of clinical trials that showed the drug as being effective in reducing recovery to as low as five days for moderately-ill COVID-19 patients.[13]

In fact, India had by then already started clinical trials at nine designated hospitals and had received over a thousand doses of remdesivir as part of the Solidarity Trials.[14] Accordingly, the Indian Institute of Chemical Technology (IICT) has initiated the key starting materials (KSM) to develop the pharmaceutical ingredient of the drug and conducted technology demonstrations for drug manufacturers to begin commercial production of remdesivir in India.[15] In fact, contrary to concerns of commercial exploitation, Gilead issued royalty-free licenses to four Indian pharmaceutical companies – Cipla, Jubliant Life Sciences, Hetero and Mylan – for generic production of the drug and its supply to over 127 countries, and later expanding the list to include Dr Reddy Laboratories, Zydus Cadila and Syngene, besides announcing its own brand likely to be unveiled in India by July.[16] Accordingly, it is assumed that the drug will be widely available in the Indian market in the coming months, including, possibly as an over-the-counter drug which will lessen the load considerably on the public health system and enabled home-based remedies. On the other hand, despite the nodal regulator, the Drug Controller of India, granting emergency use approval to Gilead and the licensees known to be ready with the generic versions, the Central Drugs Standard Control Organisation (CDSCO) was reportedly undertaking quality checks based on inputs given by the manufacturers before granting approval for production.[17] Furthermore, the Health Ministry revised on 13 June the clinical management protocol for COVID-19 to include the use of remdesivir (along with tocilizumab and convalescent plasma therapy).

Hydroxychloroquine (HCQ), a drug used to treat autoimmune diseases such as rheumatoid arthritis and lupus, widely used for anti-malaria treatment, after initial usage as a placebo pivot is now preferred as a precautionary dose for health workers and is a key element in the Solidarity Trials amid contestations about its efficacy.[18] It was US President Donald Trump who initially championed the efficacy of HCQ by claiming in March that HCQ taken together with Azithromycin is an effective cure and preventive cure against COVID-19, and continuing to use the medicine himself as a preventive despite caution sounded by the US health authorities. Amid concerns expressed that the HCQ might be detrimental for those with heart problems, many countries including India, and others where chloroquine remains an effective remedy, continue to use HCQ in high numbers on patients and health workers.

The WHO, however, temporarily halted use of HCQ in its Solidarity Trials in May after a study in Lancet concluded limited or no efficacy of the drug in COVID-19 treatment based on research by an American health group, whose findings, though, were heavily contested and later red-flagged by the *Lancet* itself for insufficient data.[19] The study by the Chicago-based Surgisphere registry based on health records of supposedly over 96,000 patients had concluded that treatment with HCQ showed no benefit, and in turn, increased likelihood of mortality.[20] While Lancet decided to retract this study based on concerns of transparency and methodology raised by an independent audit, an earlier study published by the same group in the *New England Journal of Medicine* was also retracted for a similar reason. Notwithstanding the fact that the credibility of organisations including the WHO and the Lancet was severely eroded over this and many similar episodes of inaccurate prognosis and recommendations, the Indian medical establishment, having termed the WHO reaction as 'knee-jerk', continued to repose faith on the limited use of HCQ, and stood out as an example of how individual national health systems have instilled best practices that were often more effective and reliable than the globally-induced standards by agencies like WHO. Nonetheless, with the WHO maintaining its position on the limited efficacy of HCQ in reducing mortality of hospitalized COVID-19 patients, India had decided to withdraw the 22 HCQ trial sites that were involved in the Solidarity Trials of this drug. [21]

The other anti-viral medications that have found greater acceptance in India is the Lopinavir/ritonavir, which is a combination of medicine for HIV and used earlier also for SARS and MERS.[22] Even for HIV patients, this combination has been used in limited terms as second-line drugs and is largely manufactured in India for export to African countries. An integral part of the Solidarity Trials, there were mixed results from various studies with some suggesting reduction of mortality risk and a few others finding no significant impact. Following instances of successful usage in China, there were initial unconfirmed reports that Kerala had tried out the combination, on its first three COVID-19 patients. Thereafter, both Kerala and Rajasthan were given regulatory clearance to try out this combination dose on patients.[23] Following these experiences, the Indian Council of Medical Research (ICMR) had approved extensive usage of this combination even while subjected to clinical trials.[24]

Other drugs under consideration of Indian health authorities on a case-to-case basis include the mycobacterium W, an anti-leprosy drug; tocilizumab, an immunomodulator used to treat Arthritis; favipiravir which was anti-viral treatment for Influenza, etc.[25] In fact, a governmental task force had found favipiravir and tocilizumab as among the most promising drugs for potential use against COVID-19, notwithstanding their high-pricing and relatively unaffordability for the Indian market, albeit results from clinical trials had encouraged the health authorities to include them in the clinical management protocols.[26] Besides these remedies, Indian health authorities have also tried out limited use of plasma therapy on critical patients with low oxygen saturation levels, and seen to have derived marginal efficacy through numerous recovery cases.[27] This is done when patients who have recovered from severe infections donate their plasma which is then injected into other critical patients to boost their immunity. While the Indian government has included plasma therapy in its 'clinical management protocol' of early June, it continues to be only recommended for critically-ill patients, and in select moderate cases, as there remain concerns that wrong usage methods could cause fatalities or other complications.

Testing: The other key aspect of India's disease control strategy has been the efforts to set up a dependable nation-wide testing and surveillance infrastructure. Identifying a COVID-19 infected person or a CoV-2 carrier is a complex and uncertain endeavour if one considers the fact that over 60-70 percent of India's COVID-19 patients, on an average, are reported to have been asymptomatic in various assessments.[28] The initial efforts at pre-emption in the initial epidemical months of February-March were centred on heightened monitoring of international arrivals at airports which revolved on one simple benchmark – whether an in-bound traveller showed COVID-19 symptoms. That a thermal scanning of body temperature or assessment of visible symptoms was not good enough to detect an infected person was amply proven by how CoV-2 managed to enter the country and caused the subsequent contagion.

Accordingly, the actual detection of COVID-19 cases in the country effectively started only after people who were subjected to compulsory isolation tested positive, which led to a whole series of tracking and hospitalization protocols including contact tracing (states like Kerala used to publish route maps of the positive cases to prompt social reporting from impact zones), quarantine measures and clinical exposure. For a considerable part of the initial contagion period (March-April), testing was confined to quarantine zones and of symptomatic or suspected cases. The grave shortage of RT-PCR (Real-time reverse transcription-polymerase chain reaction) kits and absence of production facilities in the country seriously curtailed the ability to measure community spread and intensity of anti-bodies presence, besides limiting detection of infections in asymptomatic and immune communities. While the rejection of China-origin RT-PCR kits came as a further setback, the swift breakthrough attained by the National Institute of Virology, which developed an indigenous anti-body test kit, enabled the government to rapidly scale up to over 1 lakh daily tests nationwide by the end of April.[29]

The enhanced testing ability, in fact, allowed the government to ramp up diagnostic and clinical infrastructure with a realistic picture of the CoV-2 spread, including the instances and imprint of community spread that was visible in various pockets around the country. With the rapid availability of RT-PCR kits, the Indian public health authorities were able to conduct around 1 lakh tests per day by the beginning of May to around 1.5 lakh tests daily by early June. With an extended network of 907 laboratories (659 in the government sector), Indian authorities aim to enhance the testing capability to 3 lakh samples per day by end of June, and over 5 lakhs by July.[30] This rapid expansion of testing capacity on a national scale was enabled by the deployment of additional testing tools and technology including TrueNat machines, new ELISA kits, rapid antibody test and antigen-based test kits.

The active participation of the private sector accrued benefits which enabled the deployment of technologies like TrueNat, a system used earlier for tuberculosis and HIV detection, but being similar to RT-PCR technology and available as smaller kits allow for faster results.[31] While TrueNat complements the active infection detection process, there has been rapid progress in parallel measures for the detection of both active cases and community spread through a whole set of systems available to identify antibody development. The Indian government facilitated this by assigning mass production of COVID-specific ELISA (enzyme-linked immunosorbent assay) kits by prominent pharmaceutical companies.[32] Besides efforts to fast-track the production of rapid antibody test kits, the ICMR, in June, approved a new kind of diagnostic test for COVID-19 through rapid antigen test kits, which will function on similar lines as RT-PCR, implying a major breakthrough for national testing capability.[33]

The key outcome of this ramped-up national testing capability could reflect in the high detection rates and rapid rise in caseloads. The daily highs recorded in the national infection rate during the May-June period could easily be attributed to the high testing rate, which, in turn, also indicates the large-scale exposure to the virus among the population, in other words, the likelihood of community transmission in various parts of the country with high infection presence. For instance, the first serosurvey to assess the spread of the transmission and infection conducted by ICMR till April end had found that about 0.73 percent of the 28,500 people surveyed in the survey in 83 districts across the country.[34] Some reports that appeared earlier of an ICMR serological survey in 69 districts (unknown if both surveys are part of the same exercise) had indicated that an estimated 7 lakh people could have been indicated, making experts wonder whether the data was under-reported or tailored towards specific informational goals.[35]

While it is known whether the variegated efforts were meant to impress upon the fact that community spread has not massively happened across the country, other than in a few pockets, the government had actually revised its original target of conducting serosurveys in all 733 districts of the country as declared in end April by deferring to plan to focus the survey only on the hot-spot districts. While serosurvey could have largely generated data about the extent of antibodies produced in a given community, the massive expansion of RT-PCR testing has enabled a realistic understanding of the spread across the country.

The Way Forward

As of 21 June, over five months after the first infection was reported in the country and over 85 days after the country implemented complete lockdown, India's COVID-19 cases have surged beyond the four lakhs mark. As in the case of other populous countries, two variables will determine the future course of this campaign: (a) the progress towards vaccine development and availability, and (b) the creation of herd immunity in communities and regions across the country.

Vaccine development: While some reports indicate that at least three dozen ventures or more are ongoing across the world to develop a vaccine against the CoV-2, the troubling question is about the actual time needed to develop a reliable vaccine and ensure its global reach, and whether commercial and political interests will make accessibility to the vaccine(s) a costly affair. Even as the WHO considers 5-7 of the ongoing initiatives as promising,[36] declarations by organisations in Italy, Israel and China of vaccine and anti-body breakthroughs have not, surprisingly, found much endorsement. This could be because a credible vaccine process could take between 2-5 years to be proven as effective after many rounds of trials on animals and humans.[37] While the efforts of the global initiatives are to develop a vaccine in 12-18 months, it is noteworthy that over 14 projects have been commissioned by various bio-research institutes in India to develop a vaccine in the shortest possible time.[38] Notwithstanding such substantial push by the Indian government to gain an indigenous vaccine breakthrough, India has also partnered with some of the global projects, notably the Serum Institute's tie-up with the Oxford University Vaccine Group.[39]

Such enthusiasm apart, the arrival of a first-comer or multiple vaccines should not be seen as a magic potion as vaccines inherently come with limited timelines of efficacy when having to match the genetic stability or mutative attributes of the pathogen, which might drastically make them redundant as proven in earlier microbial experiences like the HIV.[40] Furthermore, vaccination endeavours constantly run the risk of creating medical complications for the immunized population particularly when the injected agent may turn out to be incompatible with the physiological status of many vaccinated people or could detrimentally affect existing morbidities, thus reducing its effect or complicating the presence of a microbial in a particular segment of the population.

Herd immunity/effect: Even if the vaccine projects may not come in time to resolve the current waves of contagion, there is now greater acceptance of the need for communities to develop herd immunity to halt the further spread of CoV-2. Herd immunity or protection presupposes that the healthier members of a community with their strong immune systems will break the contagion chain of the pathogen, or, in other words, a form of community protection from infectious diseases which occurs when the majority of the population becomes immune to the disease, either by earlier infection or immunization.[41] According to one definition, herd immunity is "the proportion of subjects with immunity in a given population," which implies only a large portion of the population which is immunized, as opposed to the unimmunized segment for whom the indirect protection observed is termed as the "herd effect," or the reduction of infection in the unimmunized segment as a result of immunizing a proportion of the population.[42]

Thus, herd immunity remains a complicated phenomenon on which faith cannot be irrefutably placed as it involves subjecting huge segments of the population to the virus exposure, assuming their physiological integrity will remain unaffected and that anti-bodies will be generated in sufficient terms to develop immunity against the pathogen, and above all, that will shield against further transmission of the virus in the community. Besides the fact that countries like the United Kingdom and Sweden which attempted herd immunity initially saw massive death spirals, especially among vulnerable age groups, the assumption that immune people could stymie its further spread seems too costly a gamble considering a prevailing belief that healthy carriers of the virus can transmit it on to vulnerable sections even while remaining immune to the morbid impact of the virus.[43] Consequently, not many countries were willing to subject their populace to herd immunity experimentations though in cases like Italy and Spain there are indications that communities that survived the virus onslaught might have developed natural herd protection.

The decisions taken by respective governments to lift lockdowns, open economies and restore normal life in countries like the US, UK and India, despite intense epidemical trends, seems to be driven by the belief that beyond a threshold of contagion spike, herd immunity will naturally set in. As India moves towards phased unlocking of its economy and daily life, the huge spike in caseload might prompt many to surmise the possibility of herd immunity beginning to form in India. However, this amounts to a difficult and risky proposition owing to the numbers that determine the chances of herd protection forming in a community. Though previous cases of measles and chickenpox have been cited in public health literature of effective instances of this phenomenon, the fact that at least 70-90 percent has to be immunized either by previous infection or vaccination in order for herd immunity to be formed in itself makes it a highly risky endeavour to be tested in the world's second-largest populous nation.

Albeit herd protection might naturally be formed in pockets where community transmission has happened with higher intensity, considering that this syndrome is restricted to various clusters across the country, attempting herd immunity on a national scale is an improbable and avoidable strategy that should not be consciously attempted even at an epidemical peak. Instead, the actual emphasis should be on augmenting the public health infrastructure, and developing and implementing precautionary protocols in a manner that will enable India to effectively tackle future waves of the contagion as well imbibing lessons from this pandemic to instill new community health cultures and practices.

* * *

A shorter version of this essay was published with the same title in CBW Magazine, Vol. 13, No. 1, Jan-June 2020.

NOTES

1. As of May 15, 2020, which happens to be 105 days after the first Covid-19 case was reported in Kerala, and 52 days after a nationwide lockdown was enforced on March 24, 2020, the total cases of infection in the country were 85,761 with 2752 deaths and 53, 219 cases of patients under treatment. In the subsequent two fortnights, however, the numbers rapidly crossed 1 lakh total infections and another swift spiral to the 2 lakh. On 75th day (7 June 2020) since the lockdown was implemented, India's total numbers stood at 2, 46,628 total cases and 6,929 deaths, with daily new cases of 10,000 beginning to be reported from 6 June 2020. While it took 109 days for the total toll to reach the one lakh mark, it took just 9 nine days to cross 1.5 lakh and less than a fortnight to cross 2 lakh, thus indicating the rapid infection growth rate after easing of lockdown restrictions and augmented testing rate. By June 13, the caseload had cross the 3 lakh mark with over 11,000 infections detected per day. The daily cases touched 14,052 on June 18, with overall infections crossing 3.81 lakhs and 12,602 deaths, with a revised data set in the previous week causing a swift jump in number of total deaths to past 12,000. By June 20, the daily cases had crossed the 15,000 mark which took the total case load past 4 lakhs with deaths touching 13,500.
2. The question of contagion wave had different connotations as governments are yet to conclusively determine between phases of spikes, surges and spreads. In India, for example, it is widely assumed that the first wave that started from early March is peaking at the moment. Public health groups have warned that the second wave might be in coming months, probably followed by subsequent waves. On the other hand, some states that had successfully contained the first bout of infections have seen recurrences that raise the question whether they amounted to new contagion waves. In fact, Wuhan, the original epicenter, and countries like South Korea have reported new waves.
3. Various estimates through statistical model undertaken by some organizations have projected wide-ranging estimates ranging from 23 lakhs to 70 lakhs cases that were claimed to have been averted by the implementation of nation-wide lockdown since late March. For an analyses on these models, see Pinaki Chaudhuri and Gautam Menon, "How many deaths prevented?' *Indian Express*, June 4, 2020.
4. For some reports on this aspect, see Dylan Scott, 'Coronavirus is Exposing all of the Weaknesses in the US Health System,' *Vox*, 16 March 2020, available at https://www.vox.com/policy-and-politics/2020/3/16/21173766/coronavirus-Covid-19-us-cases-health-care-system; Prabhjot Singh, 'Why the US Health Care System Failed the Coronavirus Test?' *Foreign Policy*, 12 May 2020, available at https://foreignpolicy.com/2020/05/12/why-us-health-care-system-fail-coronavirus-test-cant-handle-covid19/; Melissa Godin, 'Why is Italy's Coronavirus Outbreak So Bad?' *Time*, 10 March 2020, available at https://time.com/5799586/italy-coronavirus-outbreak/; Denise Chow and Emmanuelle Saliba, 'Italy has a World-class Health System. The

Coronavirus has Pushed it to the Breaking Point,' *NBC News*, 19 March 2020, available at https://www.nbcnews.com/health/health-news/italy-has-world-class-health-system-coronavirus-has-pushed-it-n1162786; Selim Gonen, 'Europe's Healthcare System Fails in the Face of Coronavirus Emergency,' *Daily Sabah*, 26 March 2020, available at https://www.dailysabah.com/world/europe/europes-health-care-system-fails-in-the-face-of-coronavirus-emergency, accessed on 10 June 2020.

5. For an analysis, Dhwani Pandya, 'How Asia's densest slum Dharavi chased the Virus has Lessons for others,' *Economic Times*, 14 June 2020.
6. Community spread is in itself an ambiguous concept. As per the widely espoused meaning, community spread of the CoV-2 is supposed to have happened when such people who are mostly asymptomatic and have no history of contact with a COVID-19 patient or have travelled to an affected region, are infected with the virus. On the other hand, community spread can logically be seen as having happened when existing cluster(s) expands rapidly to swarm a neighbourhood or contiguous areas through secondary and tertiary transmission. At the initial stages of the virus spread in India, there were attempts made to understand extent of community spread by testing existing patients with benchmark conditions similar to COVID symptoms but without a history of contact or foreign travel.
7. Kairvy Grewal, 'How Kerala's Experience in tackling Nipah in 2018 will Help it Contain Coronavirus,' *The Print*, 3 February 2020, available at https://theprint.in/theprint-essential/how-keralas-experience-in-tackling-nipah-in-2018-will-help-it-contain-coronavirus/359037/, accessed on 10 June 2020.
8. Kerala had two subsequent waves of district-wide outbreaks in Kottayam (Italy-origin traveler as source) and Kasargod (Middle-East returnee as source) and numerous, but minor localized spreads including the latest instance of a major resurgence caused by infected in-bound travelers as daily cases in June traverse 80-110 on an average. For a recent analysis, see Julia Hollingsworth and Manveena Suri, 'The way these Indian states handled coronavirus shows where you live matters,' *CNN*, 13 May 2020, https://edition.cnn.com/2020/05/12/asia/india-coronavirus-kerala-flatten-curve-intl-hnk/index.html, accessed on 20 June 2020.
9. Among the seven versions, the SARS-CoV, MERS-CoV and SARS-CoV-2 are supposed to cause severe illnesses while the other versions, namely, HKU1, NL63, OC43 and 229E, display milder symptoms. See Kristian G. Andersen, et.al, 'The Proximal Origin of SARS-CoV-2,' *Nature Medicine*, no. 26, 17 March 2020, available at https://www.nature.com/articles/s41591-020-0820-9, accessed on 20 June 2020.
10. '"Solidarity" clinical trial for COVID-19 treatments,' WHO, available at https://www.who.int/emergencies/diseases/novel-coronavirus-2019/global-research-on-novel-coronavirus-2019-ncov/solidarity-clinical-trial-for-Covid-19-treatments, accessed on May 15, 2020. Also see Abantika Ghosh, "Solidarity Trial progress so far," *Indian Express*, 27 May 2020.
11. The claim about remdesivir is that it inhibits the enzyme (RdRp) and stops replication of the CoV-2 inside a human cell. The patient trials reportedly demonstrated ability of the drug to cure patients in 11 days compared to 15 days of placebo remedies. See Yeming Wang, et.al, 'Redmesivir in adults with severe COVID-19: a randomized, double-blind, placebo-controlled, multicentre trial,' *The Lancet*, 29 April 2020.
12. 'NIH Clinical Trial Shows Remdesivir Accelerates Recovery from Advanced COVID-19,' *National Institute of Allergy and Infectious Diseases*, 29 April 2020, available at https://www.niaid.nih.gov/news-events/nih-clinical-trial-shows-remdesivir-accelerates-recovery-advanced-Covid-19, accessed on 20 June 2020.

13. Jillian Mock, 'Short Course of Remdesivir May Benefit Moderately Ill COVID-19 Patients,' *Medscape*, 3 June 2020, available at https://www.medscape.com/viewarticle/931659, accessed on 20 June 2020.
14. Divya Rajagopal, 'India to Test Four Drugs for COVID-19 as part of the WHO Solidarity Trial,' *The Economic Times*, May 15, 2020, available at https://economictimes.indiatimes.com/industry/healthcare/biotech/healthcare/india-to-test-four-drugs-for-Covid-19-as-part-of-the-who-solidarity-trial/articleshow/75721525.cms?utm_source= contentofinterest&utm _medium =text&utm_campaign=cppst, accessed on 2 June 2020.
15. Joe C. Mathew, 'Coronavirus Cure: Cipla, Dr Reddy's in Race to Manufacture Gilead's Remdesivir in India,' *Business Today*, 7 May 2020, available at https://www.businesstoday.in/latest/trends/coronavirus-gilead-to-partner-with-local-firms-for-remdesivir-production-in-india/story/401387.html, accessed on 2 June 2020.
16. 'Four Indian Firms Ink Licensing Pact with Gilead for COVID-19 Drug Remdesivir,' *New Indian Express*, 14 May 2020; Teena Thacker & Divya Rajagopal, 'Indian Licensees Free to Price Remdesivir: Gilead,' *Economic Times*, 4 June 2020.
17. Viswanath Pilla, 'CDSCO Reviewing Remdesivir Applications on Priority Basis,' *Moneycontrol*, 15 June 2020, available at https://www.moneycontrol.com/news/business/companies/cdsco-reviewing-remdesivir-applications-on-priority-basis-5404141.html; Prabha Raghavan, 'Gilead's remdesivir now part of India's COVID Treatment Protocol, but licenses for 5 Firms are Stuck in Red Tape,' *Indian Express*, 14 June 2020.
18. See Joshua Geleris, et.al., 'Observational Study of Hydroxychloroquine in Hospitalized Patients with COVID-19,' *The New England Journal of Medicine*, 7 May 2020, available at https://www.nejm.org/doi/full/10.1056/NEJMoa2012410, accessed on 20 June 2020.
19. Mandeep R. Mehta, et.al., 'RETRACTED: Hydroxychloroquine or Chloroquine with or without a Macrolide for Treatment of COVID-19: A Multinational Registry Analysis,' *The Lancet*, 22 May 2020, available at https://www.thelancet.com/journals/lancet/article/PIIS0140-6736(20)31180-6/fulltext?utm_source=AusSMC+mailing+list&utm_campaign=a5c0a299a0-EMAIL_CAMPAIGN_2020_05_26_03_00&utm_medium=email&utm_term=0_90d9431cd5-a5c0a299a0-126967137, accessed on 20 June 2020.
20. Paul Ricard and Kelly MacNamara, 'The Lancet Casts Doubt over Hydroxychloroquine Study,' *The Medical Express*, 3 June 2020, available at https://medicalxpress.com/news/2020-06-lancet-hydroxychloroquine.html, accessed on 20 June 2020.
21. Anuradha Mascarenhas, 'After WHO move, 22 trial sites in India to stop HCQ research,' *India Express*, 19 June 2020.
22. For an analysis, see Jienchi Dorward and Kome Gbinigie, *Lopinavir/ritonavir: A rapid review of effectiveness in COVID-19*, The Centre for Evidence-Based Medicine, University of Oxford, 14 April 2020, available at https://www.cebm.net/Covid-19/lopinavir-ritonavir-a-rapid-review-of-the-evidence-for-effectiveness-in-treating-covid/, accessed on 20 June 2020.
23. While both attempts had shown encouraging results, the Italian citizen on whom it was tested in Rajasthan had later died, reportedly due to co-morbidities. See 'COVID-19: Anti-HIV drugs Administered on Italian couple at Jaipur hospital,' *Economic Times*, 11 March 2020, available at https://health.economictimes.indiatimes.com/news/industry/Covid-19-anti-hiv-drugs-administered-on-italian-couple-at-jaipur-hospital/74568247; 'For the first time in Kerala, doctors try anti-HIV drug on COVID-19 patient,' *Manorama Online*, 19 March 2020, available at https://english.manoramaonline.com/news/kerala/2020/03/19/first-time-in-kerala-doctors-try-anti-hiv-drug-on-Covid-19-patient.html, accessed on 20 June 2020.

24. Mohana Basu, 'HIV Drug Combo Approved by ICMR for Coronavirus Treatment Fails Clinical trials in China,' *The Print*, March 24, 2020, available at https://theprint.in/health/hiv-drug-combo-approved-by-icmr-for-coronavirus-treatment-fails-clinical-trials-in-china/386865/, accessed on 20 June 2020.
25. Favipiravir is a generic version of Fujifilm Toyama Chemical's Avigan and has been approved in Japan for the treatment of novel influenza virus infections. Glenmark Pharmaceuticals was permitted by Indian government to clinical trials on Favipiravir for COVID-19 patients in India, and on June 20, was permitted to undertake production by the Drug Controller of India. 'Glenmark initiates Phase 3 clinical trials on Favipiravir to check efficacy on COVID-19 patients,' *Economic Times*, 12 May 2020.
26. Nikhil Ghanekar, 'Govt Task Force Ranks Favipiravir, Tocilizumab as Most Promising Drugs Against COVID-19,' *News18*, 27 April 2020, available at https://www.news18.com/news/india/coronavirus-treatment-update-Covid-19-cure-medicines-favipiravir-tocilizumab-hydroxchloroquine-2595057.html, accessed on 20 June 2020.
27. Mohana Basu, 'Plasma therapy works only when donor has recently recovered from COVID-19, says study,' *The Print*, 16 June 2020, available at https://theprint.in/health/plasma-therapy-works-only-when-donor-has-recently-recovered-from-Covid-19-says-study/442614/, accessed on 18 June 2020.
28. In the initial assessment by ICMR covering the four months of the contagion from January to April, it was reported that around 69% of the COVID cases were asymptomatic as derived from 4 lakh tests and 18,601 positive sample. However, a subsequent survey by Indian Council for Medical Research (ICMR) covering 10.2 lakh tests and 40,184 positive samples massively revised this number to 28%. At the same time, other reports pegged the numbers at between 50-80% approximate. The status for May and June are awaited. See Sushmi Dey, '28% of COVID cases asymptomatic: ICMR,' *Times of India*, 31 May 2020. Also see, Chetan Chauhan, 'Coronavirus outbreak: 50 to 82% COVID cases in India are asymptomatic,' *Hindustan Times*, 19 April 2020.
29. The anti-SARS-CoV-2 human IgG ELISA antibody test kit, also called the COVID Kavach Elisa, is approved for mass production. Sumi Sukanya Dutta, "Zydus to produce India's first antibody testing kit," *Morning Standard*, 11 May 2020. 'India increases testing capability to 1 lakh a day,' *The Hindu*, 14 May 2020.
30. Sushmi Dey, 'India ramps up testing to 3 lakh samples/day,' *Times of India*, June 17, 2020; 'Testing may go up to about 5 lakh per day by July: Centre,' *The Morning Standard*, 29 May 2020.
31. TrueNat is designed by Goa-based MolBio Diagonistics. See Tabassum Barnagarwala, 'How India tests for COVID-19,' *Indian Express*, 15 June 2020.
32. Similar to NIV's Kavach, these new kits detect whether a person's immune system has produced antibodies against infection through immunoglobulin G (IgG) and M (IgM) sampling. Seven companies are known to be producing ELISA kits in India, besides India-US R&D venture permitted to design new ELISA kits. Ibid.
33. While antigen test also seeks to detect the virus instead of antibodies, the key difference with RT-PCR is its ability to interpret a positive or negative result in about 30 minutes unlike the 2-5 hours used up by the RT-PCR kits. For an assessment, see Kaunain Sheriff M, 'How Rapid Antigen Test Detects Coronavirus, where it will be used,' *Indian Express*, 16 June 2020.
34. Sushmi Dey, 'ICMR: Only 0.7% of population in 83 districts exposed to COVID,' *Times of India*, 12 June 2020.

35. While the news about the 83 districts appeared on June 20, the reports of a week earlier had a different data set of 69 districts thus creating confusion on whether there were different sero-surveys. See Jacob Koshy, 'India may have undercounted cases,' *The Hindu*, 14 June 2020; and 'Community Transmission of COVID-19 on in many parts of India, ICMR survey not reflective of current reality: Experts,' *Hindustan Times*, 13 June 2020.
36. Among the top vaccine quests are the ones by Moderna, an initiative supported by the US National Institute of Health; the joint project of the Oxford Vaccine Group and Jenner Institute, which is developing a recombinant adenovirus, christened as ChAdOx1 nCoV-19; the project funded by Bill and Melinda Gates foundation called the COVID-19 Therapeutics Accelerator; and venture of Hong Kong based firm CanSino Biologics, all of which have started initial trials, and the Oxford Group galloping towards human trials as it had base experience of the vaccine samples on earlier SARS variant.
37. While Italian firm Takis announced successful test of a COVID vaccine on mice, the Israeli Institute of Biological Research claimed to have isolated a "monoclonal neutralizing antibody" that attacks the novel coronavirus and neutralizes it in the body of the carrier. Claiming success in its initial two phases of human trials, Chinese company Sinovac Biotech Ltd had announced a swift progress to third phase of trials of its COVID-19 vaccine in the next few months. 'Italian firm claims to have developed vaccine that neutralizes coronavirus in human cells,' *Indian Express*, 6 May 2020; Shubham Sharma, 'Has Israel Developed a COVID-19 Vaccine? Here's what we know,' *Newsbytes*, 7 May 2020, available at https://www.newsbytesapp.com/timeline/Science/60745/284137/israel-develops-antibody-capable-of-neutralizing-novel-coronavirus; Victor Ordonez (et.al.), 'China company says its vaccine could be complete by 'autumn',' *ABC News*, 19 June 2020, available at https://abcnews.go.com/Health/china-company-vaccine-complete-autumn/story?id=71328018, accessed on 20 June 2020.
38. Chethan Kumar, 'Coronavirus: 14 projects in 8 cities lead India's vaccine hunt,' *Times of India*, 16 May 2020.
39. The Oxford Group's vaccine has directly moved to human trails as the safety of ChAdOx1 nCoV-19 was already proven in animal trials when it was earlier tested for MERS. Sudhir Suryawanshi, 'COVID-19 vaccine will be kept affordable: Serum Institute of India CEO,' *New Indian Express*, 1 May 2020.
40. Ian Sample, 'Why we Might not Get a Coronavirus Vaccine,' *The Guardian*, 22 May 2020, available at https://www.theguardian.com/world/2020/may/22/why-we-might-not-get-a-coronavirus-vaccine, accessed on 20 June 2020.
41. Gypsyamber D'Souza and David Dowdy, 'What is Herd Immunity and How Can We Achieve It With COVID-19?' *Bloomberg School of Public Health (John Hopkins University)*, 10 April 2020, available at https://www.jhsph.edu/Covid-19/articles/achieving-herd-immunity-with-covid19.html, accessed on 20 June 2020.
42. T J John and R Samuel, 'Herd Immunity and Herd Effect: New Insights and Definitions,' *European Journal of Epidemiology*, vol.16, no. 7, 2000.
43. R. Prasad, 'Aiming to Achieve Herd Immunity Naturally is 'Dangerous'," warns WHO,' *The Hindu*, 16 May 2020.

4

China and US Response Plans Against COVID-19

Xie Chao

Human history is full of stories about how deadly viruses spread and kills humans indiscriminately and until today the emergence of a new virus tends to wake up a common ancestral fear toward infectious diseases. The outbreak of COVID-19 is just one more example to remind the world of real threat and heavy lethality of an infectious disease. Proved and unproved arguments that the pharmaceutical industry sells the threat of infectious disease and benefits from the thus expanded public expenditures only further damage public trust in the government to do a proper response job.[1] Collateral damage from human greed and government corruption only leads to more infection and higher death tolls.[2] Hence human fears toward infectious disease persist and it doesn't necessarily disappear with the development of medical science.

This chapter tries to understand the logic and thus compare the response strategies of China and the US (United States of America) from the perspective of fear and trust. Regardless of government types, concrete measures should be taken to address and mitigate the stress thus caused to individuals by the pandemic. The first thing a spreading virus destroys is people's trust on the environment. Any working public health strategy should aim at maximizing the trust and minimizing the stress thus caused.[3] Government care is not necessarily in the place and in the case of Zika, studies find that individuals who suppress their fears would have higher levels of fear later.[4] For people with governmental care, it should be made based on their own culture and tradition. A failure in addressing public fear would only deepen people's suffering.

There are different logics on how to mitigate public fear and regain trust among the people and with the government. The discursive approach stresses that the government should carefully design narratives to calm down the public, and a functional approach that only concrete measures serving the control of disease matter. Be that as it may, the biggest challenge is how to strike a delicate balance between caring public sentiment and initiating exclusionary protective measures. For centuries, measures such as quarantine, lockdowns and contact tracing have been central to responding infectious disease outbreaks.[5] The same still applies today, albeit with much larger cities involved. In the case of COVID-19, the uncertainty lies in the fact that it is invisible, and it runs all the risks of infection if a human being is exposed to the environment. Public fear also comes from the certainty of a pandemic. Denial towards such a situation would not help the response measures. The failure to control the situation only increases and deepens the sense of fear.

China's Response Against COVID-19

China's response against COVID-19 witnessed setbacks with a heavy human loss at the initial stage and recognition when it finally controlled the situation. Discussions in summarizing useful experiences and lessons become extremely relevant when a second or even third wave of contagion might occur even before a working vaccine can be found.

1. Mask-Wearing and its Comforting Effect

There were debates in China whether people should wear masks in confronting COVID-19 and the Chinese government's positive suggestion generated a discussion on whether and how to wear face masks could help to control a highly contagious disease like COVID-19.[6] Similar discussions arise when other governments entertaining similar suggestions to their citizens.[7] The discussion does not have a solid conclusion yet from a medical science perspective. With all the valid questions on the measure, it is difficult to construct its positive logical links with the eventual control of pandemic, still, its psychological effects in addressing public fear and rebuilding the trust among people and with the government should be properly recognized.

Wearing masks does not change the particular fact that the invisible virus is making the environment dangerous. But wearing masks gives a psychological suggestion that others in the environment care about your sense of insecurity and none in the environment would intentionally or unintentionally spread the disease. It is not about its effectiveness. If there are no other effects, it means at least a comforting effect, which still is an effect. Subconscious measures like this would distract individual stress and thus mitigate the fear caused by environmental uncertainty. It works as an indicator to others that their chance of infection is reduced when people in the environment wear masks.

When the Chinese government suggested and the public was willing to wearing masks, the next question that arose was about meeting the demand. In China, the National Medical Products Administration (NMPA) is responsible for ensuring medical supplies and in 2009 it has established standard procedures for emergent medical supplies for public health needs.[8] On 7 February 2020, NMPA issued a further administration notice to expedite registration and approval procedures on PPE (Personal Protective Equipment) production.[9] Then provincial and further local levels take over to make detailed plans and local NMPA agencies establish guidelines and temporary measures on emergency and temporary approvals.[10] But facing a dramatic outbreak of COVID-19, it was chaotic as the fear drove people to store masks, the supply chain was further severed when most manufacturers were on holiday leaves for Chinese lunar new year. Only when big players like SINOPEC, an example of state-owned enterprises and BYD of private companies, launched mask manufacturing lines of massive capacities that the supply-demand gap was filled.

Transportation of PPEs to affected areas was equally challenging as major highways were closed due to holidays and forthcoming lockdowns. The lack of intra-provincial coordination only made the situation worse when local governments had started storing and competing for ready PPE products. Public opinion backfired when it was reported that some local governments were taking expropriation of pandemic prevention materials crossing their districts.[11] These obstacles could only be dealt with when the State Council stepped in by pressing provincial governments, and the latter pressing further local governments to ensure smooth transportation of anti-epidemic materials.

2. Lockdowns and Physical Separation

On 23 January Wuhan announced the lockdown. Later on, several other cities announced the same, and the subsequent nation-wide social distancing measures were implemented to prevent epidemic spreading. Eventually, a quasi-national lockdown remained in place for about two months. And the necessity of drastic measures was obvious. However, in the week-long holiday and month-long vacation meant numerous human flow and gatherings, and an immediate lockdown would slow down, if not cut the community transmissions, in a tangible way.

On every count, nation-wide lockdown and physical separation is a risky political decision. First, it might work to flatten the curve, but public stress would become more and more intense with the duration of lockdown and the rising confirmed cases. The sooner the curve goes to the other (declining) side, which nobody knows when, the lower would be political costs. Second, the Chinese new year means a lot of domestic and international travel and traditional processions and extensive visits of relatives and friends.[12] The power of tradition should be properly understood here, and one can understand it as asking people to stay at home during the festivals like Christmas. It is a huge task to get a public understanding of this and no one can guarantee public cooperation.

The lens of fear and trust can help to understand the logic of the Chinese government's choice of measures of high political costs such as massive quarantine and lockdowns.[13] A counter argument is that drastic measures themselves would create panic. However, its marginal effect would decrease to a minimum when there is a high level of fear in existence due to the contagion. With a spreading panic in sight, the counter-measure should be far harsher and a physical isolation strategy can serve as a stabilizer of public sentiment.[14] Such drastic measures carry a message that as long as people stay at home, they will be safe. With initial resentment, the public was quick to accept that it would be in their best interest to suspend social activities and thus cut short the transmission chains. Again, it helps to comfort the public in a time of high uncertainty.

Quarantine and lockdowns are indeed ancient tools to conquer epidemic disease, modern technology only transforms these into more powerful public health weapons. In China, people got used to online shopping during the SARS quarantines, and COVID-19 would only further drive the public ascribing an online living in a largely cash-less society developed since then.[15] Despite so, it is no easy task to ensure the basic supply of daily commodities and the sheer size of the population being affected is enough to demonstrate the scale of the challenge. After the initial mess, the big data technology and intelligent supply chain took the charge and the feature of door-to-door and zero-contact delivery help gain public trust in the environment.

3. *Epidemiological Source-tracking and Slow-down of Community Transmission*

Besides wearing masks and lockdowns, tracking close contacts are "probably the most important thing" as noted by Dr. Zhong Nanshan on 21 January 2020.[16] Dr. Zhong is the leading medical scientist to contain COVID-19 in China and a public health veteran who had led China's campaign against SARS. Modern technology again intervenes to make these ancestor toolkits more effective. In China, popular apps such as WeChat and Alipay are used to monitor and track the travel route, and possible contacts if needed. Colored health codes of green, yellow and red are generated after people filled out information about their temperature, whereabouts in the last 14 days in a quick health survey and these tools allow them to go to other cities or enter residential areas or official buildings.[17] Some apps develop functions for people to check nearby infection and transmission status so that depending on the status they could feel relieved or keep high alert. Despite all the controversies over privacy invasion, the massive surveillance measures proved to be a useful measure in tracking close contacts and places visited by confirmed patients.

Combined with source-tracking, testing all close contacts and admitting all suspected and confirmed cases for treatment are the ultimate tools to control the disease. Without proper testing, affected persons might have to delay seeking medical help and remain undetected in the community.[18] In the case of a pandemic, the number of tests in discussion could have easily discouraged most governments from entertaining such massive tests.[19] Demand spurt of testing caused a huge shortage of testing kits and a huge influx of confirmed patients that overwhelmed hospitals. Public health workers were overworked in pandemic epicenters such as Wuhan and Huangshi. In ordinary times, a city in China would only have dozens of beds, hundreds in the case of a megacity for infectious disease, but during the COVID-19 time, it was tens of thousands of confirmed patients we were talking, and the number would be multiplied if the suspect cases were added.

The situation was only partially addressed when differentiated and phase treatment plan was adopted that the situation stabilized. Suspected cases were quarantined in independent houses and hotel rooms; confirmed cases with light and modest syndromes went to temporary hospitals that were specially established to monitor and provide them basic medical care; and those with severe syndromes to designated hospitals with epidemiological experts and intensive care units.[20] At a later stage, health workers from cities and regions that had largely controlled the situation came to help, with each province assisting one city or region of Wuhan, the city hit first and most by the disease.

US's Response Against COVID-19

While China's response plan cares to strike a balance between discursive approaches of soothing sensitive public feelings and functional approach of enforcing exclusionary precautions, the US's response so far lacks a clear and coordinated plan to control the spreading virus and thus respond public sentiment of fear. With confirmed cases and the death toll in the country hiking to the highest among major countries, Trump administration against COVID-19 is thus under domestic and international criticism for its passive response strategy.

1. Social Taboo and Culture War on Mask-Wearing

Since March, community-related cases spiral up and it becomes certain that an inevitable outbreak in the US is on the way. To most people in the US, a passive pandemic prevention and control strategy by the government means they have to suppress and digest that sense of fear individually. President Donald Trump's remarks only drove up public fear when he expressed his wish that "One day – it's like a miracle – it will disappear."[21] President Trump might have expected his remarks to enhance public perceptions that the situation would become really worse and eventually mitigate public fear when they accept the status as it is, but it surely does not work that way. A parallel message that was perceived is that the American public has to rely more on themselves instead of government since their president and his administration are expecting a miracle like any individuals would do in a desperate situation.

Most Asian governments encourage wearing masks as a precaution, but Western culture tends to see the measure counterproductive and believes it actually generates fear among the public. This is a shared conviction in the US because wearing masks means you have covered your identity and thus cause damage to the public sense of safety and security. A social taboo is thus formed that only sick people wear masks.[22] Trump administration also questions the measure's efficacy and thinks it as a cowardly act.[23] To wear or not wear a mask thus becomes a highly politicized issue in the US and the contrasting ideas of different groups are so sharp that violence ensues. In Michigan, a supermarket security guard was shot dead when he asked a customer to wear a mask,[24] indicating a culture war over mask-wearing as a precautious measure. Trump administration's negative attitude and passive promotion of the measure only wastes a chance to educate and unite the American public for a common battle against the virus.

Regardless of government types, cultural and historical factors make big differences on public acceptance of wearing masks. It is understood that a higher public acceptance of wearing masks in China is due to its tradition and culture. Chinese culture is full of stories about how ancient kings like King Shennong tastes a hundred herbs and Dayu tames the flood to conquer diseases and natural disasters. Such cultural background makes the public more cooperative in tolerating the cost and observing government measures. In the case of the US's response against COVID-19, the Trump administration displays open reluctance and chooses to wage a cultural war against the recommendation of wearing-masks, making the social taboo stronger among the American public.[25] Without a proper plan to cater for public sentiment, it can be predicted that public resentment and refusal to cooperate would only make the situation worse.

2. *Partisan Differences on Social Distancing and Lockdowns*

Other countries' experience before the US has proved that social distancing is important to slow down the spread of COVID-19 and after initial reluctance, Trump administration announces a series of lockdown measures, including the use of cellphone location data to track the movements of people.[26] A Pew survey suggests high public awareness on protecting privacy and data safety: about half of Americans (52 percent) tend to accept the measure to track the location of those who have tested positive while 48 percent finding it somewhat unacceptable, and in a later survey on using cellphones to monitor people's compliance with social distancing recommendations, it finds lower percentage (38 percent) of respondents see the measure acceptable and greater percentage (62 percent) somewhat unacceptable.[27] The survey indicates a divided public opinion on accepting massive lockdowns as a core measure to contain the spreading virus.

Compared to public resentment on wearing masks in the US, public acceptance on tracking measures is more encouraging when it does help to track the locations of infected cases and thus mitigate public fear and distrust on the environment. Despite so, geolocation data finds a divided public opinion based on partisan lines. It finds that residents in Republican counties are less likely to strictly observe the stay-at-home order than those in Democratic counties.[28] Partisan differences are impacting the effectiveness of social distancing orders. Trump publicly expressed his objection that stay-at-home orders enforced in some states are "too tough" and gave his support to demonstrators in states such as Minnesota, Michigan and Virginia.[29] The resentment is also visible among Trump's hardline supporters on Dr. Anthony Fauci, who was promoting strict social distancing guidelines.[30]

In a comparative view, mass surveillance tools for source-tracking purposes are accepted as a temporary measure in China. While in the US, people are more critical of such measures and debate more on potential data abuse.[31] The argument can be understood in two ways: first, it does not mean Chinese people do not have second thoughts on the issue. However, with the real threat of a second wave of the pandemic, the social tracking measures including health codes are still in place in China to help restart the economy while the concerns for privacy abuses thus remain.[32] With the pandemic situation largely under control in China, public concerns regarding exit mechanisms for these tracking measures have emerged. Second, the US experience proves that public trust is vital for social tracking measures to really work to contain the virus.[33] Tracking the virus is only as effective as the public's willingness to hand over personal details of daily living.

3. Blame Game on Finding Scapegoats for Response Failure

Amid domestic and international criticism on its failing response against the pandemic, Trump administration develops another plan of blame game to divert the public attention, and China is an easy target. President Trump openly pushes for a mention of the "China virus," and only promises to stop using it when being pushed back by domestic and international opinions.[34] But the blame game goes on as a coordinated messaging campaign. In an incident, CNN found that US State Department pushed to insert the phrase of "Wuhan Virus" instead of its official name COVID-19 in the joint statement after foreign ministers from the Group of Seven met in March and US gesture is resented by European countries in the group.[35] The report also discloses that the talk points circulated by the National Security Council to coordinate government officials to put pressure on China and thus divert domestic public opinion on the US's passive response plan against COVID-19.

Labelling the virus is not the only content in the plan and there are frequent allegations by US officials that the virus is not only intentionally made but also released as a bioweapon from China. Australian researchers found evidence that rumor posts of such allegations have been shared and re-tweeted within conservative US right-wing groups to reach a wider audience online.[36] Blaming a foreign country cannot change the fact that the government is not testing enough and the pandemic situation in the US is only getting worse.[37] Considering all the time President Trump and his administration is spending on blaming China and the consistency and diligence with which this plan is devised and implemented, showcases their carelessness to public sentiment and lack of a consistent response strategy against COVID-19.

Since the current US administration prioritize other factors above the response campaign against COVID, it shows that they are fighting a totally different battle. James Mattis perhaps makes one of the best sum-up of his former boss's strategy by stating that "Donald Trump is the first president in my lifetime who does not try to unite the American people - does not even pretend to try. Instead, he tries to divide us."[38] Public sentiment and the mood of health workers are thus not situated at a better level to fight the pandemic. Despite the worsening pandemic situation, President Trump has switched into the re-election mode. He believes that he does not poll well because of the economic slowdown caused by massive lockdowns and decides to push for an early reopening amid the worsening pandemic situation.[39] As warmed by Dr Fauci, the decision to reopen is definitely pre-mature when the US is still on the left side of curve.[40] At the time of writing the chapter, the pandemic is far from over in the US.

Conclusion

Psychological perspective is just one of the lenses to understand government responses against COVID-19, and other factors should get fair credits too. For instance, a higher public saving rate in China allows the public to more likely get through the living hardship thus caused by the response measures. China did an effective fight against SARS in 2003 when rural areas were cordoned off and kept untouched even though they were most vulnerable to the epidemic disease.[41] Such a unique public memory assures a quick manner of public acceptance of similar measures. Chinese people tend to prioritize the rights of development and survival before they can enjoy freedom and liberty rights in social life, and most of them tend to accept that there will be limits for latter rights. In the West, individual freedom and liberty come on top of other rights. Thus, the public would defend and protest any attempt to sabotage their rights, and a pandemic will not simply change that belief.

It is understood that both unlimited and limited governments have records in succeeding and failing epidemic prevention and control. Whatever approaches the government adopts, they should aim at fostering public acceptance and unity in an overwhelming public health crisis like COVID-19. With a high cost, China has largely controlled the situation, but this does not mean its public health strategy can be simply copied by others. Besides domestic debates on the controversial decisions, China's response against COVID-19 is still under international criticism that it was using medieval tool kits in the 21st century.[42] Even now a haunting question for China is whether measures other than massive lockdowns could have the same effect. With the US's increasing attention to China as a strategic competitor, it is natural for US officials and strategists to impose their world views on the issue of COVID-19 response and at the same time increase the alert level against China. Politics matters in the discussion, but it does not mean questioning

China will help its domestic handling of an imminent public health crisis due to its passive response.

Human history evolves forward by conquering numerous disasters and diseases. COVID-19 would not be the last pandemic for human beings. Until a vaccine comes out, the danger of second or even third wave of the pandemic is real and for populous countries such as China and the US, there is no time to relax. Discussions on proper public health strategies that suit countries of different national characteristics and their tradition and culture are extremely relevant. With a comparative study on response plans of China and the US, this chapter suggests that governments should pay due attention in mitigating public fear and hence restoring the trust among the public and the public trust in the government. For the general public, one thing should be made clear that the enemy in this battle is not the government but the virus. There is no point to defend your rights from a virus that infects human beings indiscriminately. The same reminder goes to the government that the enemy is not the people and the people in a foreign land but the virus. A considerate and all-out response will be rewarded with high public support.

Postscript

After finishing the manuscript, there were 19 new coronavirus cases reported on 30 June in Beijing and more cases came out in the forthcoming days. As a Beijing resident, the author has the privilege to observe how real a COVID-19 comeback can be and what lessons and experience from the past months help the city. The new cases required special attention because for 56 consecutive days the capital city of China reported no new case. The first of such cases came from Xinfadi's wholesale market, which provides about 80 percent of agricultural goods for Beijing. This city has a population of more than 20 million. The report comes at night and in a press conference the next morning it is announced what actions are being taken like the undergoing reopening process is suspended; residents are suggested to stay at home and get back to social distancing mode; the market is closed immediately and social media is full of posts reminding people around who have visited the market after 30 May to have the test at the nearest testing station. Now, the daily testing capacity of Beijing has reached 230,000, effectively covering all residence areas wherever new cases and close contact are reported.

There is no official shutdown announced yet and people who have got tested and received a COVID-negative certificate can leave the city for their business. So far, no panic is registered, daily life goes on (of course mostly at home). Some choose to work from home while some have to commute to work. The price fluctuations of daily goods are acceptable and online deliveries are preferred. From the beginning of the June and until the 18th, there is one of the largest online shopping festivals in China and this year the contracted value of online shopping for Tmall reaching RMB 700 million yuan and JD.com 270 billion yuan, showing that people are spending and Beijing residents are part of the festival. While it is still early to confirm that the city has reached the left side of the curve, the reported cases are declining steadily into single digit per day. Unconfirmed sources show that the testing range will expand by following the trait of confirmed cases and their close contacts. The municipal government has no issue if a population test is thus needed. Again, concrete and swift measures are the ultimate tool to calm down the public and effective testing and treatment is gaining public cooperation. The implication from what happened in Beijing since June reminds the world that there is a real threat from the second-wave outbreak and any reopening plan should have procedures to guard against it.

* * *

A shorter version of this essay was published in the CBW Magazine, Vol. 13, No. 1, Jan-June 2020.

NOTES

1. M. A. Vance, 'Disease Mongering and the Fear of Pandemic Influenza,' *International Journal of Health Services*, vol. 41, no. 1, 2011, pp. 95-115.
2. M.A. Riva, M. Benedetti and G. Cesana, 'Pandemic Fear and Literature: Observations from Jack London's The Scarlet Plague,' *Emerging Infectious Diseases*, vol. 20, no. 10, 2014, p. 1753.
3. P. D. Harms, M. Credé, M. Tynan, M Leon and W. Jeung, 'Leadership and Stress: A Meta-analytic Review,' *The Leadership Quarterly*, vol. 28, no. 1, 2017, pp. 178-194.
4. Einav Keet, 'New Study Examines Public Fears During Disease Outbreaks,' *Contagion Live*, 11 July 2018, available at https://www.contagionlive.com/news/new-study-examines-public-fears-during-disease-outbreaks, accessed on 1 June 2020.
5. E. Tognotti, 'Lessons from the History of Quarantine, from Plague to Influenza A,' *Emerging Infectious Diseases*, vol. 19, no. 2, 2013, pp. 254-259.
6. 'Under Coronavirus, Do We Need to Wear Masks?' *Xinhua News*, 10 February, 2020, available at http://www.xinhuanet.com/politics/2020-02/10/c_1125554775.htm, accessed on 2 June 2020.
7. 'The Face Mask Debate Reveals a Scientific Double Standard,' *The Wired*, 8 April, 2020, available at https://www.wired.com/story/the-face-mask-debate-reveals-a-scientific-double-standard/, accessed on 2 June 2020.
8. 'Notice on Emergency Approval Procedures on Medical Apparatus and Instruments,' *NMPA*, 28 August 2009, available at http://www.nmpa.gov.cn/WS04/CL2197/324626.html, accessed on 1 June 2020.

9. 'Notice on Accelerating Registration and Approval of Manufacturing Medical Protective Gears,' *NMPA*, 7 February 2020, available at http://www.nmpa.gov.cn/WS04/CL2078/374630.html, accessed on 5 June 2020.
10. 'Collection of Emergency Approval Polices on Medical Masks and Protective Gears,' *China Regulatory Consulting for Medical Device*, 2 March 2020, available at http://www.cirs-group.com/md/news/news/12721.html, accessed on 5 June 2020.
11. 'Dali Apologizes for Requisition of Chongqing Masks,' *China Daily*, 6 February 2020, available at https://www.chinadaily.com.cn/a/202002/07/WS5e3c9eb2a3101282172759a6.html, accessed on 5 June 2020.
12. 'Chinese New Year Spring Movement Ends with 3.0 Billion Trips in 40 days in 2019,' *Xinhua News*, 1 March 2019, available at http://www.xinhuanet.com/politics/2019-03/01/c_1124181637.htm, accessed on 5 June 2020.
13. 'Wuhan Lockdowns Aims at Calming Down Public,' *The Beijing News*, 23 January 2020, available at http://www.bjnews.com.cn/opinion/2020/01/23/678263.html, accessed on 8 June 2020.
14. Belinda Luscombe, 'Why Overreacting to the Threat of the Coronavirus May Be Rational,' *Time*, 11 March 2020, available at https://time.com/5801010/coronavirus-overreaction/, accessed on 1 June 2020.
15. C. Shuyang, S. Meng and L. Haotong, 'The Comparative Study Between China and South Korea on Online Shopping,' in *2014 International Conference on Management of e-Commerce and e-Government*, IEEE, October 2014, pp. 16-19.
16. 'Timeline of China Releasing Information on COVID-19 and Advancing International Cooperation on Epidemic Response,' *National Health Commission*, 6 April 6, 2020, available at http://en.nhc.gov.cn/2020-04/06/c_78840.htm, accessed on 1 June 2020.
17. 'Beijing Rolls Out Colour-coded QR System for Coronavirus Tracking Despite Concerns over Privacy, Inaccurate Ratings,' *South China Morning Post*, 2 March 2020, available at https://www.scmp.com/tech/apps-social/article/3064574/beijing-rolls-out-colour-coded-qr-system-coronavirus-tracking, accessed on 10 June 2020.
18. B. Person, F. Sy, K. Holton, B. Govert and A. Liang, 'Fear and Stigma: The Epidemic within the SARS Outbreak,' *Emerging Infectious Diseases*, vol. 10, no. 2, 2014, p. 358.
19. There is no available data of how many tests China has done, but as a reference, as of 25 April Guangdong province alone accomplished 4.54 million tests. See 'As of 25 April, Guangdong Province Completed 4.54 million tests,' *Sina.com*, 28 April 2020, available at http://news.sina.com.cn/c/2020-04-28/doc-iirczymi8877014.shtml, accessed on 10 June 2020.
20. F. Peng, L. Tu, Y. Yang, P. Hu, R. Wang, Q Hu and C. Chang, 'Management and Treatment of COVID-19: The Chinese Experience,' *Canadian Journal of Cardiology*, vol. 36, no.6, 2020, pp. 915–930.
21. 'Remarks by President Trump in Meeting with African American Leaders,' *White House*, 28 March 2020, available at https://www.whitehouse.gov/briefings-statements/remarks-president-trump-meeting-african-american-leaders, accessed on 11 June 2020.
22. Hillary Leung, 'Why Wearing a Face Mask Is Encouraged in Asia, but Shunned in the US,' *Time*, 12 March 2020, available at https://time.com/5799964/coronavirus-face-mask-asia-us/, accessed on 11 June 2020.
23. Paul Waldman, 'Trump's Accidental Culture War Over Wearing Masks,' *Washington Post*, 27 May 2020, available at https://www.washingtonpost.com/opinions/2020/05/27/trumps-accidental-culture-war-over-wearing-masks/, accessed on 12 June 2020.
24. Meredith Spelbring, 'Security Guard, Father of 9, Shot and Killed in Michigan after Telling

Customer to Put on Face Mask,' *USA Today*, 4 May 2020, available at https://www.usatoday.com/story/news/nation/2020/05/04/family-dollar-security-guard-killed-after-telling-shopper-wear-mask/3081674001/, accessed on 12 June 2020.

25. Paul Krugman, 'On the Economics of Not Dying; *The New York Times*, 28 May 2020, available at https://www.nytimes.com/2020/05/28/opinion/coronavirus-economy-death.html, accessed on 12 June 2020.
26. Byron Tau, 'Government tracking how people move around in Coronavirus pandemic,' *The Wall Street Journal*, 28 March 2020, available at https://www.wsj.com/articles/government-tracking-how-people-move-around-in-coronavirus-pandemic-11585393202, accessed on 13 June 2020.
27. Brooke Auxier, 'How Americans see Digital Privacy Issues Amid the COVID-19 Outbreak,' *Pew Research Center*, 4 May 2020, available at https://www.pewresearch.org/fact-tank/2020/05/04/how-americans-see-digital-privacy-issues-amid-the-covid-19-outbreak/, accessed on 14 June 2020.
28. Marcus Painter and Tian Qiu, 'Political Beliefs affect Compliance with COVID-19 Social Distancing Orders,' *SSRN*, 6 April 2020, available at https://papers.ssrn.com/sol3/papers.cfm?abstract_id=3569098, accessed on 14 June 2020.
29. Morgan Chalfant and Brett Samuels, 'Trump defends demonstrators protesting social distancing restrictions,' *The Hill*, 17 April 2020, available at https://thehill.com/homenews/administration/493445-trump-defends-demonstrators-protesting-social-distancing-restrictions, accessed on 15 June 2020.
30. Tina Nguyen, 'MAGA world finds its coronavirus scapegoats,' *Politico*, 18 April 2020, available at https://www.politico.com/news/2020/04/18/trump-coronavirus-who-bill-gates-fauci-193379, accessed on 15 June 2020.
31. Bruno Macaes, 'Coronavirus and the Clash of Civilizations,' *National Review*, 10 March 2020, available at https://www.nationalreview.com/2020/03/coronavirus-and-the-clash-of-civilizations/, accessed on 16 June 2020.
32. Raymond Zhong, 'China's coronavirus tracking Apps stir privacy fears,' *The New York Times*, 26 May 2020, available at https://www.nytimes.com/2020/05/26/technology/china-coronavirus-surveillance.html, accessed on 14 June 2020.
33. Albert Fox Cahn, 'Surveillance and the City: Public Trust Needed for a Public Tracing System,' *Gotham Gazette*, 14 May 2020, available at https://www.gothamgazette.com/opinion/9381-surveillance-and-the-city-public-trust-needed-coronavirus-tracking-system, accessed on 15 June 2020.
34. Karen Leign, 'Trump says he'll stop using the term 'China Virus',' *Bloomberg*, 25 March 2020, available at https://www.bloomberg.com/news/articles/2020-03-25/trump-says-he-ll-stop-using-chinese-virus-easing-blame-game, accessed on 14 June 2020.
35. Alex Marquardt and Jennifer Hansler, 'US push to include 'Wuhan virus' language in G7 joint statement fractures alliance,' *CNN*, 25 March 2020, available at https://www.cnn.com/2020/03/25/politics/g7-coronavirus-statement/index.html, accessed on 14 June 2020.
36. Mark Scott, 'Trump supporters on Twitter spread Covid-19 rumors about China,"' *Politico*, 2 June 2020, available at https://www.politico.com/news/2020/06/02/trump-supporters-on-twitter-spread-covid-19-rumors-about-china-296808, accessed on 14 June 2020.
37. Maggie Fox, 'Coronavirus Testing is 'a mess' in the US, report says,' *CNN*, 21 May 2020, available at https://edition.cnn.com/2020/05/20/health/testing-coronavirus-cidrap-report/index.html, accessed on 18 June 2020.

38. Jeffrey Glodberg, 'James Mattis Denounces President Trump, Describes Him as a Threat to the Constitution,' *The Atlantic*, 3 June 2020, available at https://www.theatlantic.com/politics/archive/2020/06/james-mattis-denounces-trump-protests-militarization/612640/, accessed on 16 June 2020.
39. Dan Balz, 'America was Unprepared for a Major Crisis, Again,' *The Washington Post*, 5 April 2020, available at https://www.washingtonpost.com/politics/america-was-unprepared-for-a-major-crisis-again/2020/04/04/df85c0da-75d9-11ea-87da-77a8136c1a6d_story.html, accessed on 15 June 2020.
40. Lucy Sherriff, 'Dr Fauci warns Coronavirus 'isn't over yet' and that we 'are only at the Beginning of it',' *The Sun*, 9 June 2020, available at https://www.thesun.co.uk/news/11824775/dr-fauci-coronavirus-not-over-just-beginning/, accessed on 14 June 2020.
41. A. Ahmad, R. Krumkamp and R. Reintjes, "Controlling SARS: A Review on China's Response Compared with other SARS-Affected Countries," *Tropical Medicine & International Health*, vol. 14, no. 1, 2009, pp. 36-45.
42. Fabian Kretschmer, 'Wuhan Lockdown: China takes Extreme Measures to Stop Virus Spread,' *Deutsche Welle*, 23 January 2020, available at https://www.dw.com/en/wuhan-lockdown-china-takes-extreme-measures-to-stop-virus-spread/a-52120126, accessed on 18 June 2020.

5

Japan's Pandemic Politics: The COVID-19 Challenge to the *Reiwa* Era

Titli Basu

Japan's approach to the pandemic features amidst one of the success stories in East Asia along with Taiwan and South Korea. COVID-19, a transnational bio-security threat, posed one of the toughest challenges to Prime Minister Abe Shinzo's political legacy. The United Nations has called this global pandemic as a "human crisis" attacking societies at their core. Japan has opted for a declaration of emergency instead of lockdown. But the politics of pandemic that unfolded in Tokyo since the *Diamond Princess* episode that started in February 2020 underscored severe stress on the governance structures and institutions. The pandemic demanded decisive leadership as the resilience of the Japanese economy and good governance is put to litmus test.

This year is supposed to be the hallmark year in Prime Minister Abe Shinzo's historic political graph. The administration arranged the 2020 diplomatic calendar with two mega-events to seal Abe's legacy before his present tenure as Liberal Democratic Party president finishes in September 2021. First in the calendar was the maiden state visit by Chinese President Xi Jinping to Tokyo and the signing of a possible fifth political document and second, the Olympic Games. While the first was critically important not just for Sino-Japan bilateral relations but also for strategic stability in East Asia. This would have been the first state visit by Chinese President since 2008 (President Xi Jinping visited Japan for G20 Osaka Summit). The second was more aspirational. The Olympic Games is an opportunity to showcase the nation's recovery from the 2011 Triple Disaster and thus was pitched as the "Recovery and Reconstruction Games". Abe's deft manoeuvring has saved the Games from outright cancellation[1] but postponing the Games by a year is representative of the enormous economic and political challenges that wait for Japan.

Thus, Abe administration invested political energy on methodically preparing for the success of these events, possibly with an eye on an extraordinary fourth term in the LDP with the support of his factions. [2] However, the diplomatic calendar got hijacked by the unforeseen yet overwhelming challenge of the pandemic. Going ahead, Prime Minister Abe's critical policy choices will define the future course of the newly dawned *Reiwa* era.

Pandemic's Economic Dent

The scale and nature of the pandemic have inflicted an unprecedented dent on the global economy and pushed several countries into recession. International Monetary Fund (IMF) estimates have indicated that the adverse impact on economies may be similar or worse than in 2009.[3] Japan's economy is also officially in recession. The pandemic has wrecked the globalised markets, regional supply chains and production networks. It has further sparked a discussion on the merits of globalisation and the economic governance structure.

COVID-19 imposed a colossal challenge for the Japanese economy. Organisation for Economic Cooperation and Development (OECD) has lowered the global growth outlook from 2.9 to 2.4 percent and Japan is likely to grow at 0.2 percent in 2020.[4] Already reeling under the Sino-US trade tensions, waning demand from Beijing, and disorder in the vital supply chain, especially in manufacturing, following the pandemic is sternly testing the resilience of the Japanese economy. Even before the pandemic, the Japanese economy was already besieged under the pressure exerted by the northward movement of consumption tax in October 2019. Japan's Cabinet Office has confirmed that GDP for October-December 2019 indicates annualised contraction of 7.1 percent in real terms.[5] Furthermore, the economy contracted 0.9 percent in January-March 2020 or at an annualised contraction of 3.4 percent. Thus, Japan slipped into a recession prior to the imposition of a national emergency.

Japan has been pushed to shore up some of the boldest measures to manage the adverse impact of the pandemic. Tokyo initially injected about a trillion dollars or 20 percent of GDP in April 2020 as an economic stimulus package.[6] Subsequently, it padded it up with an additional trillion dollars plus package in May 2020. Thus, the total stimulus spending amounts to 2.2 trillion USD or 40 percent of the annual output of Japan's economy.[7] Additionally, Japan has allocated an economic stimulus package of 2.2 billion USD to help its manufacturing firms shift production out of China, where supply chains have been disrupted due to coronavirus outbreak. Out of 2.2 billion USD, the Japanese government proposes to allot 220 billion Yen (2 billion USD) to firms for shifting production back to Japan and 23.5 billion Yen to companies seeking to move manufacturing base to other countries. This decision was taken at a time when Chinese President Xi Jinping was expected to visit to Japan. It remains to be seen how this change in policy stance will affect Japan's relationship with China, which is one of its biggest trading partners.[8]

Earlier this year, Nomura Research Institute pointed out that inbound-related losses for COVID-19 will be about 776 billion Yen. Such evaluations are based on the assumption that the pandemic will be under control within a few months. Nonetheless, if it continues for a year, Japan will record a GDP loss of 2.47 trillion Yen.[9] Some evaluation proposes that delaying the Olympics may force the nominal GDP in 2020 to fall 0.36 percent.[10]

Tokyo was eyeing an economic turnaround with the Olympic Games. The Audit report points out that the nation has possibly spent 12.6 billion USD for the Olympics.[11] In the meantime, a few Japanese media prognoses suggest that the Olympics would cost Japan approximately 28 billion USD in total,[12] a significant upsurge from the original 7.3 billion USD estimates when Japan won the bid in 2013. Furthermore, Nikkei assessments reflect that rescheduling the Games will cost around 6 billion USD in economic losses.[13] Despite these assessments, Japanese government had agreed to reschedule the competitions for 23 July–8 August 2021, exactly one year after what was planned. The costs of a postponement come from maintaining venues, storing gear and materials, rehiring staff, and duplicating marketing efforts, all of which will need to be spent amid the broader economic fallout and recovery efforts from the pandemic.[14] Katsuhiro Miyamoto, an emeritus professor of economics at Kansai University, estimates that a one-year postponement will likely cost 6 billion USD on top of the money already spent by Japan. The IOC (International Olympic Committee) may cover a portion of these costs, but the vast burden will fall onto Japanese taxpayers.[15]

Japan depended on the Games to steer international tourism on the one hand and push construction investments on the other. Japanese businesses have paid out billions of dollars in sponsorship and broadcasting rights. But the economy now has to endure the severe adverse impact of the pandemic on the tourism industry. The pandemic severely affected the projections of Japan attaining the previously outlined target of hosting 40 million tourists in 2020. According to Japan Tourism Agency (JTA) records,[16] in 2019 foreign tourists augmented by 2.2 percent to 31.882 million and they spent approximately 44 billion USD. Amongst this, China sent 9.594 million tourists, who spent 36.8 percent of overall tourism expenditures.

Pandemic and Politics

Given the fact that the pandemic assumed unparalleled scale in terms of the spread of the infection, it demanded decisive leadership to initiate bold decisions. Yet, initial political inertia adversely affected coordination amongst bureaucratic silos. There are some who suggested that Prime Minister Abe's policy response to battle the virus was rather "too little too late"[17] and generated more confusion than giving clarity. Absence of initial leadership caused some discontent[18] and led some to suggest that Abe's policy choices are mostly intended at mending the dent to his political reputation, rescue the prospects of the Olympic Games and the strained economy.[19] With 18,476 positive cases on 30 June,[20] COVID-19 proved to be a formidable challenge for Japan. The US Forces Japan also issued a Public Health Emergency for the Kanto region, which was later extended to entire Japan on 15 April.

While the number of positive cases remained comparatively low when matched with the hotspots in Europe and also the US, Prime Minister Abe's mettle was tested as global attention shifted to Yokohama when the narrative on faulty quarantine practice implemented in the Diamond Princess Cruise ship gained momentum with the account of Kentaro Iwata.[21] US Centers for Disease Control and Prevention (CDC) in its evaluation indicated that quarantine procedures practiced in the Diamond Princess may not have been adequate to avert transmission of the virus.

As the virus made inroads into the major cities and business centre of the country, Japan recognised that the National Security Secretariat (NSS) structure is primarily focussed on traditional security threats and has struggled in dealing with non-traditional threats, for example, the current pandemic.[22] Subsequently, when Japan revisited its policy to regulate the movement of pathogenic agents and put in place strict immigration rules, it directed the newly instituted economic division at the NSS to oversee the implementation of constraints on the movement of people who qualify as potential risks to national security.[23] Meanwhile, the defence administration sent Japan Self-Defense Forces (JSDF) to Narita and Haneda International Airports in order to strengthen border control measures *against* the pandemic. As the virus started infecting more and more citizens, Japan incrementally extended its net of border control beyond Hubei and Zhejiang provinces in China, and Daegu and Cheongdo in North Gyeongsang province in South Korea.

Some suggested that as there was no "control tower", similar to American CDC which predominantly concentrates on gathering and analysing information, proposing expert advice vis-à-vis travel limitations, quarantines, and public communication, it affected effective response. At the House of Councillors Budget Committee meeting, suggestions emerged from the Japanese Communist Party to strengthen the National Institute of Infectious Diseases (NIID) to design a structure similar to CDC.[24] The Cabinet Secretariat's crisis management operation has steered government measures against the pandemic, but it does not have considerable experience in handling infectious virus countermeasures. Tokyo formed the COVID-19 task force two weeks after the maiden case detection and instituted an expert advisory group just about a month later. The Headquarters of Novel Coronavirus Disease Control issued Basic Policies in late February which was almost instantaneously followed by the Prime Minister's hasty statement on the subject of nationwide school closure.

In an attempt to demonstrate pragmatic leadership, Prime Minister Abe requested closure of elementary, junior and senior high schools to prevent dissemination of group infection. However, the decision generated considerable confusion as institutions, corporations and working parents struggled to adapt in a rather short notice. Moreover, some local authorities also expressed reservations. For instance, Hokkaido, Osaka, Ichikawa shut schools even before Abe's declaration, but Kyoto, Kanazawa wanted to keep the schools operational.[25] In addition, there were concerns about the impact of the pandemic on the micro, small and medium businesses given the scarcity of workers given parents had to take leave. To ease the effects, the government provided support through the Employment Adjustment Subsidies.

As discontent over this decision grew, it emerged that Prime Minister's decision to shut schools was rather a hasty one. It reflected not just lack of consultation but also internal political cracks in the Abe administration.[26] Despite the fact that Prime Minister Abe's tenure is characterised by centralisation of political power and administration around *Kantei* and the Cabinet, but recently differences between the Prime Minister and his Chief Cabinet Secretary Suga Yoshihide, the winning duo behind the political stability in the last seven years, became obvious over the pandemic response. Severe criticism on the decision to shut schools forced Abe to admit in the parliament that the pronouncement to close schools was his personal political decision which he took without discussing with Suga and also the Education Minister Haguida Koichi.[27]

Subsequently, in March, Prime Minister diverted all his political energy in generating consensus across party lines on revising special measures law to tackle a new type of influenza with the aim of including COVID-19, and thus creating the possibility to prepare for the worst case scenario and announce a state of emergency if required.[28] It permits the prefectural governors to give directives on the subject of preventive measures, for instance staying at home and so on. The special measures law empowers the prime minister to issue a state of emergency, with a detailed timeline and geographic scope, in case the virus poses a huge impact on people's lives and the economy. After the revision to the special measures law on 13 March, national debate strengthened on the topic of the declaration of emergency. This is conditional on fatality rates and the number of available hospital beds for COVID-19 patients.

The discussion intensified as influential voices from the medical community expressed concerns. These along with others in the political class urged Prime Minister Abe to issue an emergency. Kamayachi Satoshi, an executive board member of Japan Medical Association (JMA) who also sits on the government panel on coronavirus, suggested that because of the limitations on hospital beds, there was an urgency to issue an emergency. Yokokura Yoshitake, JMA President also indicated that given the fact that the number of beds available for corona infected patients nears capacity, the administration should weigh in the possibility of announcing a state of emergency.[29] In the meantime, Osaka Governor Yoshimura Hirofumi and Tokyo Governor Koike Yuriko insisted that Prime Minister should make a decision as Osaka and Tokyo are suffering escalation of corona cases.

Furthermore, opposition political parties, including Edano Yukio, leader of the Constitutional Democratic Party, acknowledged that as Japan entered a new phase, the decision on declaring an emergency is looming large. There were criticisms on the limited number of COVID-19 tests conducted and the shortage of masks in the country. Subsequently, the most powerful business lobby in the country, Keidanren extended support for the state of emergency on condition that it would not interfere with essential services like utilities, food supplies and medical care.

Afterward, as COVID cases saw an increase in early April, Prime Minister Abe declared a state of emergency including seven prefectures from 7 April. Subsequently, he extended the emergency encompassing the entire country. Tokyo urged people to focus on side-stepping the "three Cs" – closed spaces, closely gathering, and close conversation.[30] As Japan started showing considerable improvement with regards to the number of infections in a short span of time, Prime Minister Abe lifted the state of emergency on May 25, before the set deadline on May 31.

Moving Ahead

Abe has emerged as one of Japan's most consequential and longest serving Prime Minister since the inception of parliamentary politics during the Meiji Restoration. In December 2012, Abe arrived in Nagatacho following disarray in crisis management by then Democratic Party of Japan (DPJ) government on the heels of the 2011 Triple Disaster. At that point in time, Abe stepped up and provided political stability and turned Japanese politics away from its legacy of revolving-door prime ministers and leadership deficit. Today Abe stares at the colossal task of crisis-management with this global pandemic. Additionally, Abe administration is already reeling under a series of high-profile political corruption scandals, some involving Prime Minister and his wife. So much so, Abe's political mentor and former Prime Minister Koizumi Junichiro urged his resignation over rampant corruption. As Prime Minister Abe's present tenure nears its end, he banked on the Olympics glitz and glam to frame his achievement and distract public attention from his administration's challenges with reference to his political priorities including the Constitutional amendment, resolving the abduction issue with Chairman Kim Jung-un or settling the territorial dispute with President Putin. As regards Abe's political future, the biggest advantage is the weak political opposition. Nonetheless, factional politics within his own LDP may pose some tough questions. Political rival within LDP, Ishiba has leveraged the crisis by critiquing Prime Minister's policy approach towards the pandemic. Masuzoe Yoichi, who headed Japan's battle against the 2009 swine flu, criticised and pinned structural problems of the Abe administration for the "disastrous" crisis-management.[31] Abe has also been criticised for being removed from the troubles of ordinary Japanese.[32] The approval ratings of Prime Minister Abe in opinion polls also reflected a downward spiral. However, given that political survival is at stake, Prime Minister Abe shed his initial political inertia with bold policy projections. Even though the opposition parties barely exhibit encouraging policy alternatives, but for LDP contenders who wish to succeed Abe, treading into power in the middle of this unprecedented pandemic may be a deterrent.

Every crisis presents an opportunity. A leader's legacy is often defined by their ability to manage watersheds. Abe has adeptly utilised COVID-19 to mend Sino-Japanese relations with "mask diplomacy" even as the domestic discourse on

"Abenomask"[33] created some problems for him. In addition, Japan demonstrated regional leadership by assisting developing economies in dealing with the pandemic, such as Tokyo extended 1.86 million USD to Hanoi through an international organisation.[34] Also, Japan remains at the forefront in steering clinical research on developing a vaccine that may lead the world out of this pandemic. WHO indicated that some 110 coronavirus vaccine development projects are ongoing globally. Meanwhile, six such projects are ongoing in Japan. National Institute of Infectious Diseases has also engaged in such endeavours. Clinical trials will reportedly start in July. Meanwhile, the government has indicated to enable large-scale manufacturing of vaccines with support of subsidy programmes for the producers.[35] As the pandemic altered much of Japan's political power dynamics and the diplomatic slate, Prime Minister Abe's political fortune will be depending on how sharply he delivers on the economic and governance challenges posed by the COVID-19.

NOTES

1. Olympic Games suffered cancellation thrice in history during the World War I (1916) and twice during World War II (1940, 1944).
2. Currently, LDP allows only three consecutive terms for party presidents. There are speculations that LDP may amend rules yet again to extend Abe's tenure to four consecutive terms from the present three, to empower Abe to continue as party president and prime minister.
3. Kristalina Georgieva, 'Opening Remarks at a Press Briefing by Kristalina Georgieva following a Conference Call of the International Monetary and Financial Committee (IMFC)', *International Monetary Fund*, 27 March 2020, available at https://www.imf.org/en/News/Articles/2020/03/27/sp032720-opening-remarks-at-press-briefing-following-imfc-conference-call, accessed on 6 April 2020.
4. 'OECD Interim Economic Assessment Coronavirus: The World Economy at Risk', *OECD*, 2 March 2020, available at https://www.oecd-ilibrary.org/economics/oecd-economic-outlook/volume-2019/issue-2_7969896b-en;jsessionid=2Np6Hyin_bp4EjjlzT83EcBs.ip-10-240-5-50, accessed on 6 April 2020.
5. 'Japan's Q4 GDP Revised Downward', *NHK World*, 9 March 2020, accessed on 6 April 2020.
6. 'Japan Set to Roll out $1 Trillion Package,' *NHK World*, 6 April 2020, available at http://www.newsonjapan.com/html/newsdesk/article/126755.php, accessed on 6 April 2020.
7. 'Japan Probes the Limits of Economic Policy,' *The Economist*, 4 June 2020, available at https://www.economist.com/finance-and-economics/2020/06/04/japan-probes-the-limits-of-economic-policy accessed on 4 June 2020.
8. Isabel Reynolds and Emi Urabe, 'Japan to Fund Firms to Shift Production Out of China,' *Bloomberg*, 8 April 2020, available at https://www.bloomberg.com/news/articles/2020-04-08/japan-to-fund-firms-to-shift-production-out-of-china, accessed on 12 April 2020.
9. 'Coronavirus to Deal a Blow to Japan's GDP Due to Fewer Chinese Visitors', *Nippon.com*, 6 February 2020, available at https://www.nippon.com/en/japan-data/h00654/coronavirus-to-deal-a-blow-to-japan's-gdp-due-to-fewer-chinese-visitors.html, accessed on 6 April 6, 2020.

10. Takahide Kiuchi, 'Postponing the Tokyo Olympics could Lead Japan's 2020 GDP to Fall 2 trillion yen, or 0.36%,' *NRI*, 26 March 2020, available at https://www.nri.com/en/knowledge/blog/lst/2020/fis/finsights/Market_0326, accessed on 6 April 2020.
11. 'OLYMPICS/ Audit Report says Costs Higher than $12.6 billion,' *The Associated Press*, 20 December 2019, available at http://www.asahi.com/ajw/articles/AJ201912200052.html, accessed on 6 April 2020.
12. Ibid.
13. Rurika Imahashi and Francesca Regalado, 'Olympics Delay to Cost Japan $6bn in Economic Losses,' *Nikkei Asian Review*, 24 March 2020, available at https://asia.nikkei.com/Spotlight/Tokyo-2020-Olympics/Olympics-delay-to-cost-Japan-6bn-in-economic-losses, accessed on 6 April 2020.
14. Eric Margolis, 'The Logistical Hell of Postponing the Olympics for One Year,' *Slate*, 14 April 2020, available at https://slate.com/culture/2020/04/tokyo-olympics-postponed-logistics-plans-costs.html, accessed on 26 April 2020.
15. Ibid.
16. 'Records Set for Foreign Tourists, Spending for 7th Straight Year,' *The Asahi Shimbun*, 18 January 2020, available at http://www.asahi.com/ajw/articles/AJ202001180030.html, accessed on 6 April 2020.
17. Hiromi Murakami, 'A Japan Divided over COVID-19 Control,' *East Asia Forum*, 8 March 2020, available at https://www.eastasiaforum.org/2020/03/08/a-japan-divided-over-covid-19-control/, accessed on 24 April 2020.
18. Koichi Nakano, 'Japan Can't Handle the Coronavirus. Can It Host the Olympics? How Leaders' Sense of Entitlement Breeds Indifference and Incompetence,' *The New York Times*, 26 February 2020, available at https://www.nytimes.com/2020/02/26/opinion/coronavirus-japan-abe.html, accessed on 28 April 2020.
19. Satoshi Sugiyama, 'Abe's Bold School Closure move Appears Spurred by Criticism of Virus Response,' *The Japan Times*, 28 February 2020, available at https://www.japantimes.co.jp/news/2020/02/28/national/abe-closes-school-coronavirus#.Xut_GG5uKse accessed on 28 April 2020.
20. About Coronavirus Disease 2019 (COVID-19), Ministry of Health, Labour and Welfare, 16 June 2020, available at https://www.mhlw.go.jp/stf/seisakunitsuite/bunya/newpage_00032.html, accessed on 19 June 2020.
21. Reiji Yoshida, 'COVID-19 spread on Diamond Princess before Quarantine, Report Suggests,' *The Japan Times*, 20 February 2020, available at https://www.japantimes.co.jp/news/2020/02/20/national/coronavirus-diamond-princess-before-quarantine/#.XuuAY25uKse, accessed on 28 April 2020.
22. Toshiya Takahashi, 'Japan's COVID-19 National Security Problem,' *East Asia Forum*, 18 March 2020, available at https://www.eastasiaforum.org/2020/03/18/japans-covid-19-national-security-problem/, accessed on 28 March 2020.
23. 'Japan Puts National Security Office In the Forefront of Fight Against Infectious Diseases,' *The Sankei Shimbun*, 14 March 2020, available at https://japan-forward.com/japan-puts-national-security-office-in-the-forefront-of-fight-against-infectious-diseases/, accessed on 14 March 2020.
24. 'Lack of 'Control Tower' in Japan's Coronavirus Response Deals Blow to Abe Administration,' *Mainichi Shimbun*, March 9, 2020, available at https://mainichi.jp/english/articles/20200309/p2a/00m/0na/006000c, accessed on 14 March 2020.
25. 'Abe's Abrupt call to Close Schools Amid Virus Triggers Confusion,' *Kyodo*, 28 February 2020, available at https://english.kyodonews.net/news/2020/02/ce71c062614b-abes-abrupt-call-to-

close-schools-amid-virus-triggers-confusion.html, accessed on 14 March 2020.

26. Corey Wallace, 'Abe Departs from His Own Winning Formula in Battling COVID-19,' *Australian Institute of International Affairs*, March 5, 2020, available at http://www.internationalaffairs.org.au/australianoutlook/abe-departs-from-his-own-winning-formula-in-battling-covid-19/, accessed on 28 March 2020.
27. Francesca Regalado, 'Japan's Bid to Save the Olympics has an Air of Desperation', *Nikkei Asian Review*, 6 March, 2020, available at https://asia.nikkei.com/Spotlight/Tokyo-2020-Olympics/Japan-s-bid-to-save-Olympics-has-an-air-of-desperation2, accessed on 28 March 2020.
28. Emergency empowers prefectural governors to take away buildings to accommodate medical facilities and make producers and retailers supply food and medicine.
29. 'Calls Grow for Japan PM Abe to Declare State of Emergency Over Virus,' *Kyodo*, 31 March 2020, available at https://english.kyodonews.net/news/2020/03/ce4960a6b1cc-calls-grow-for-japan-pm-to-declare-state-of-emergency-over-virus.html, accessed on 1 June 2020.
30. 'Message from Governor Koike on the Novel Coronavirus,' *The Governor's Corner*, 13 May 2020, available at https://www.metro.tokyo.lg.jp/english/governor/act/2020/0206_00.html, accessed on 1 June 2020.
31. Ben Dooley, 'Shinzo Abe, Japan's Political Houdini, Can't Escape Coronavirus Backlash', *The New York Times*, 5 March 2020, available at https://www.nytimes.com/2020/03/05/world/asia/japan-abe-coronavirus.html, accessed on 28 March 2020.
32. Koichi Nakano, See note no. 24.
33. Yuki Fujita, 'Abe faces calls for decisive action after 'Abenomask' blunder', *Nikkei Asian Review*, 3 April 2020, available at https://asia.nikkei.com/Spotlight/Coronavirus/Abe-faces-calls-for-decisive-action-after-Abenomask-blunder, accessed on 28 May 2020.
34. 'The Coronavirus in Asia and ASEAN', *ASEAN Briefing*, 4 April 2020, available at https://www.aseanbriefing.com/news/coronavirus-asia-asean-live-updates-by-country/, accessed on 28 May 2020.
35. 'Japan to Subsidize Mass Production of Eventual Coronavirus Vaccine', *Kyodo*, 22 May 2020, available at https://www.japantimes.co.jp/news/2020/05/22/national/science-health/japan-subsidies-coronavirus-vaccine/#.XuuFsm5uKsd, accessed on 28 May 2020.

6

Effective Management of COVID-19 in Iran

Ali Karami

On 30 December 2019, a cluster of viral pneumonia cases of unknown origin emerged in Wuhan, Hubei Province of China which soon spread across the world.[1] From the first COVID-19 case in Iran, the Iranian President ordered health minister to set up a national committee for managing coronavirus epidemic. In his decree, President urged the Iranian Health Minister to use all his power to prevent the spread of coronavirus as well as uproot it from the country.

In response to the COVID-19 situation, Iran established a National Corona Virus Management Committee (NCVMC). The NCVMC consists of ministers of road and urban development, interior, education, science, tourism, and culture, as well as chief of staff of Iran's Armed Forces, head of budget and planning organization, IRIB chief, Iran's Attorney-General, head of pilgrimage and hajj organization, government spokesman and police chief. The committee is responsible to hold meetings, make policies in presenting services on health, treatment and pharmaceutical field, and inform people.

Understanding Biological Composition of COVID-19

On 30 December 2019, a cluster of viral pneumonia cases of unknown origin emerged in Wuhan, Hubei Province of China. Coronaviruses are 65–125 nm in diameter and its genome pool contained a single-stranded RNA from 26 to 32kbs length.[2]

Most coronaviruses contain three major proteins: the phosphorylated nucleocapsid protein (N); a small membrane-embedded glycoprotein (M); and a large club-shaped glycoprotein (S) which is projected spikes with 20 nm length.

The M protein is synthesised on ribosomes bound to the endoplasmic reticulum and accumulates in the Golgi apparatus. Researchers believed that the site of virus budding in the infected cell is affected by subcellular localisation of M protein to the Golgi. The S-protein involved in many of the biological processes of the virus, such as attachment to cell receptors, penetration, cell-fusion, and it is the major target for virus-neutralizing antibodies.[3]

Four subgroups are reported for coronaviruses family including alpha (α), beta (β), gamma (γ) and delta (δ) coronavirus.[4] The International Committee on Taxonomy of Viruses (ICTV) named the virus as SARS-CoV-2 and the disease as COVID-19.[5]

Middle East respiratory syndrome coronavirus (MERS-CoV),[6] SARS-CoV[7] like COVID-19 cause acute lung injury (ALI) and acute respiratory distress syndrome (ARDS) which leads to pulmonary failure and subsequently to a fatality.[8]

Two prominent genomic characteristics have been reported for COVID-19. First, structural studies revealed that SARS-CoV-2 seems to have a great affinity for binding to Angiotensin-converting enzyme 2 (ACE2) human receptors.[9] ACE2 is highly expressed on the luminal surface of intestinal epithelial cells, it acts as a co-receptor for nutrient uptake, in particular for amino acid resorption from food.[10] The receptor binding domain (RBD) in the spike protein is the most variable part of the coronavirus genome. Six RBD amino acids are known to be critical for binding to ACE2 receptors and for determining the host range of SARS-CoV-like viruses.[11] In summary, the SARS-CoV-2 spike protein directly binds with the host cell surface ACE2 receptor facilitating virus entry and replication.

Second, the spike protein of SARS-CoV-2 has a functional polybasic cleavage site at the junction of two spike subunit (the S1–S2 boundary) through the insertion of 12 nucleotides, which additionally led to the predicted acquisition of three O-linked glycans around the site. This allows effective cleavage by Furin and other proteases and has a role in determining viral infectivity and host range. These sites have not been reported in although other human beta-coronaviruses.[12]

Due importance of genome sequence currently there are more than 11,346 full genome sequence of viruses from clinical samples around the World in https: //www.epicov.org and GeneBank with one full genome from Iran Accession ID: EPI_ISL_424349.

Coronavirus Cases in the World and Iran (Last updated 30 June 2020)

The number of people diagnosed with coronavirus in Iran reached 227,662, of whom 10,817 have died and 188,758 recovered.

Figure 1: Global Statistics

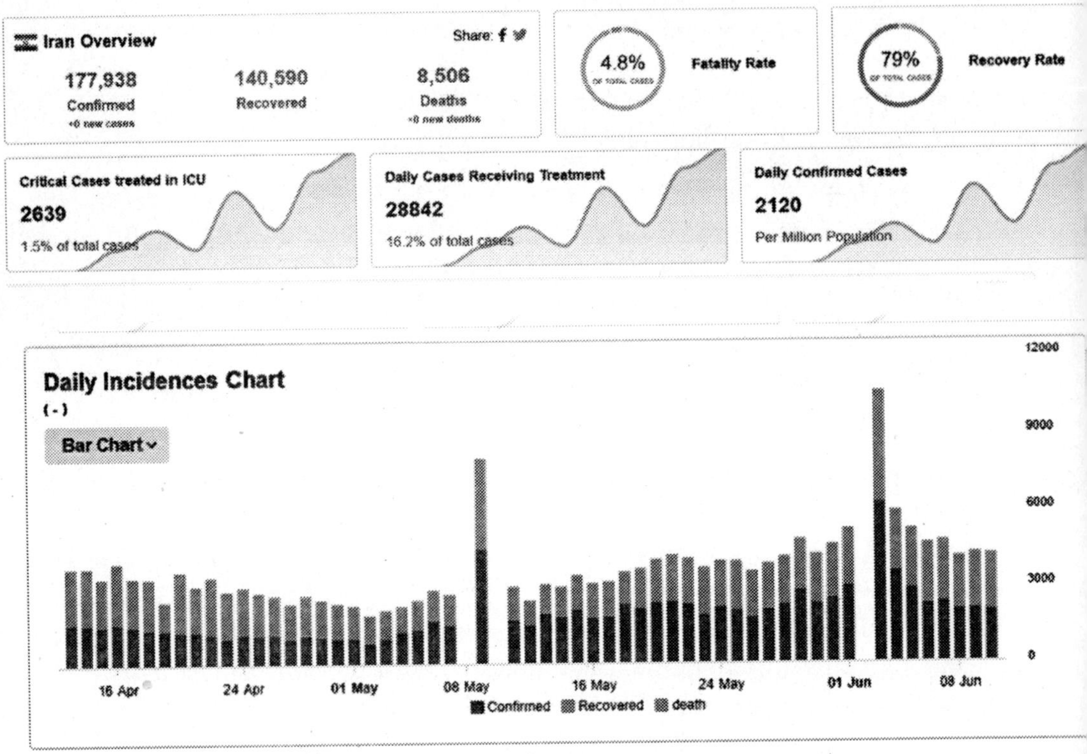

Country	Total Confirmed	Total Recovered	Total Deaths
USA	2,066,401	808,551	115,130
Brazil	775,184	396,692	39,797
Russia	493,657	252,783	6,358
UK	290,143	135	41,128
Spain	289,360	7,015	27,136
India	287,155	140,979	8,107
Italy	235,763	169,939	34,114
Peru	208,823	98,031	5,903
Germany	186,866	170,700	8,844
Iran	177,938	140,590	8,506
Turkey	173,036	146,839	4,746

Iran ranks 10 in the above data

Diagnostic

There are various methods to diagnose a COVID-19 infection. Diagnosis through CT imaging of chest and counting white blood cell and or, preparation of a laboratory sample for definitive diagnosis by molecular methods.

Low-dose CT-scan, that is a widely available and almost inexpensive imaging test in Iran, is beneficial for the diagnosis of COVID-19 suspicious cases.[13]

Sharif University of Technology engineers has provide a new diagnostic system by utilizing artificial intelligence algorithms via CT scans, this COVID-19 diagnostic system can be used when there are large number of patients in hospitals or there is no access to a radiologist. Such a system can double up as a doctor too.[14]

Figure 2: Mobile Biological Lab of the Iranian Army

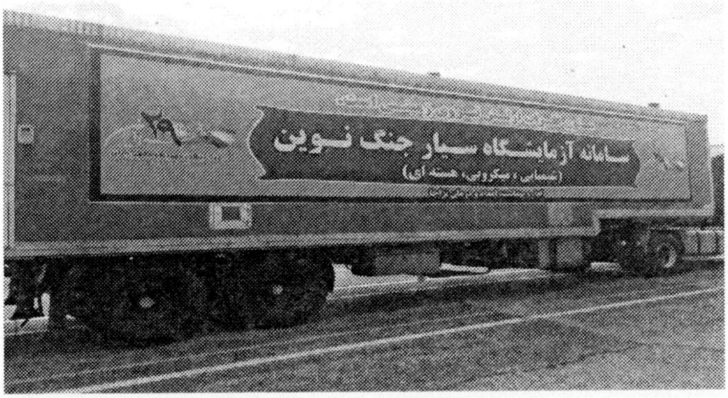

Islamic Revolutionary Guards Corps (IRGC) also unveiled a Bio-detection kits and Mobile Labs which is designed and manufacture in Iran and is capable of detecting the coronavirus named "MOSTA'AN" that is currently under evaluation process.[15]

Figure 3: Mobile Lab Made by Basij

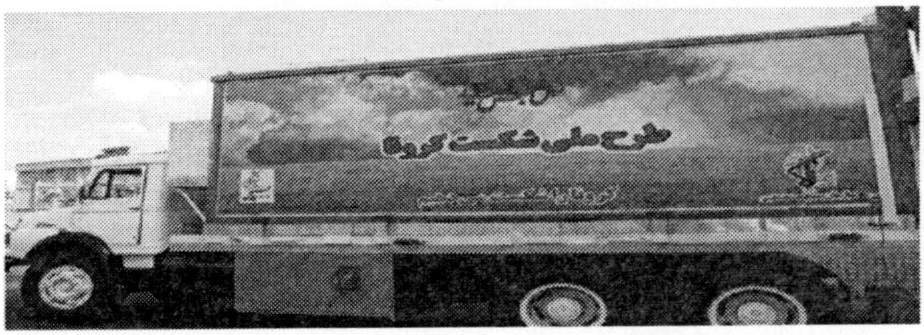

The diagnosis of COVID-19 should be confirmed by molecular examinations the most usual one, reverse-transcription polymerase chain reaction (RT-PCR), or by gene sequencing of respiratory or blood specimens., Although these methods are crucial standard tools for COVID-19 detecting, they are time-consuming as well as may not be accessible widely.[16] This delay in diagnosis and treatment subsequently results in a higher risk of infecting a larger population.

Several knowledge-based companies like Pishtaz Teb Company successfully designed and manufactured COVID-19 diagnostic kits.[17]

Iran's Defense Ministry has begun the mass production of rapid coronavirus test kits (RT-PCR and serologic test). In late February, the Pasteur Institute of Iran approved the ministry's testing kit after examining them and comprising the result to foreign ones.[18]

Anti COVID-19 Treatment Assessment

(a) Vaccine

The development of a safe and effective vaccine for this highly transmittable respiratory virus is an important epidemic control. To date, no efficient vaccine has been developed against COVID-19.[19] Recombinant protein, mRNA, DNA and inactivated whole virus vaccines are being developed and some are now entering the clinical trial stage. The first COVID-19 vaccine in China is expected to be ready for the clinical trials by the end of July 2020, according to Xu Nanping, China's vice-minister of science and technology. Invio Pharmaceuticals plans to begin clinical trials on a coronavirus vaccine in April 2020.[20] The most advanced candidates have recently moved into clinical development, including mRNA-1273 from Moderna, Ad5-nCoV from CanSino Biologicals, INO-4800 from Inovio, LV-SMENP-DC and pathogen-specific aAPC from Shenzhen Geno-Immune Medical Institute.[21]

Three independent groups are researching to produce a vaccine for COVID-19 in Iran and the country's health ministry concluded six contracts with knowledge-based companies for this approach.[22,23]

The Head of IRGC's Baqiyatallah University of Medical Sciences, Brigadier General Alireza Jalali said that Baqiyatallah University focused the research on virus behaviour that was the latest scientific material to be observed. Baqiyatallah University also focused on developing the Coronavirus vaccine, Diagnostic kits and drugs which is a complex and complicated process.

(b) Antibody

The first treatment for COVID-19 that anyone receives, is from their own immune system. Monoclonal antibodies are the major class of bio-therapeutics for passive immunotherapy to come up against viral infection. Monoclonal antibodies are a versatile class of pharmaceuticals that have been successfully used by the pharmaceutical industry. Monoclonal antibodies can perform efficient therapeutic intermediation with a highly specific treatment against a particular disease or agent.[24]

Cytokine storm occurs by COVID-19 infection a result of the release of proinflammatory cytokine including interleukins (IL)-6.[25] In the biopsy samples at dissection from a patient who died from the severe infection of COVID-19, histological examination showed bilateral diffuse alveolar damage with cellular fibromyxoid exudates. Mononuclear inflammatory lymphocytes were seen in both lungs.[26] These studies suggested that a cytokine or inflammatory storm has occurred. Further investigation on the immune characteristics of patients with COVID-19 showed that pathogenic T-cells and inflammatory monocytes quick activation leads to a large number of cytokines production and ultimately inflammatory storms occur. Among them, IL-6 is the key cytokines, that cause inflammatory storm which may lead to increased alveolar-capillary blood-gas exchange dysfunction, notably impaired oxygen diffusion, and finally, result in pulmonary fibrosis and organ failure.[27] Therefore IL-6 might play a crucial role in the inflammatory storm and interfering with IL-6 by Immunomodulating drugs such as IL-6 inhibitors might be a potential therapeutic agent for severe and critical COVID-19.

One of the effective IL-6 inhibitors is Tocilizumab. It was effectively tested for the patients diagnosed as severe or critical COVID-19 in the First Affiliated Hospital of the University of Science and Technology of China (Anhui Provincial Hospital) and Anhui Fuyang Second People's Hospital. As a recombinant humanized anti-human IL-6 receptor monoclonal antibody, Tocilizumab can specifically bind IL-6 receptors and inhibit signal transduction.[28] Tocilizumab rapidly resolved some of the clinical symptoms of COVID-19, such as fever and oxygen saturation while may decline the severity of the pulmonary complications of COVID-19, including respiratory failure, but there is no evidence that it has anti-viral potential.[29] By 11 March, the Iranian version of the Swiss-made "Actemra" has been used at one of Isfahan's hospitals (and then by 500 patients in different centers) and a relative improvement after 48 hours in the patient's symptoms has been observed. The mass production of this medicine was marketed in about three weeks.[30,31]

(c) Antivirals

Antiviral treatments are crucially needed to diminish the burden on healthcare systems worldwide. Effective therapeutics are expected to decrease fatality and hospitalizations. In the absence of a vaccine, antiviral agents could also be applied to protect vulnerable populations. The latest version is at exposed to the virus.

Remdesivir (RDV, formerly GS-5734) is an investigational broad-spectrum small-molecule antiviral drug that its activity against RNA viruses in several families, including *Coronaviridae* has been determined.[32] RDV is a phosphoramidate pro-drug of a 1'-cyano-substituted nucleotide analogue. Its triphosphate form (RDV-TP) resembles adenosine triphosphate (ATP) and is substrate for viral RNA-dependent RNA polymerase (RdRp) enzymes.[33] RDV showed a positive effect on 14 Americans who severer acute COVID-19. The first two of the five clinical trials testing, RDV have completion dates in early April. Both of phase trials are being run by Chinese groups.[34]

One of the four drugs that Iran has joined to WHO to complete of clinical phase is RDV. Iran has one of the biggest medical research capacities in the Middle East region and also among the Islamic countries has joined WHO clinical trials with 12 research teams in 100 patients.[35,36]

(d) Convalescent Plasma

Apart from supportive care such as oxygen supply, no specific effective drug or vaccines for COVID-19 are available. Several agents, like RDV are under research moreover, the antiviral efficacy of these drugs is not known yet.[37]

Immunotherapy by transferring the convalescent plasma (CP) from recovered patients to patients suffering from COVID-19 may be effective in humans to overcome the virus infection.[38] The use of CP was recommended as an experimental strategy during the outbreak of the Ebola virus in 2014.[39] In another study, 80 patients with SARS, performing CP was associated with a higher rate of hospital discharge at day 22 from symptom onset compared with patients who did not receive the same.[40] The early administration of CP from recovered patients that contains significant antibody titers may cause a reduction in viral load and disease fertility. Based on current findings a hypothesis raised that, utilizing a transfusion of recovered patients could be profitable in cases infected with SARS-CoV-2. However, some crucial challenges need to be considered before using CP as a therapeutic option such as the availability of sufficient donors, clinical condition, viral kinetics, and host interactions of SARS-CoV-2.[41]

Two independent studies in china (245 patients in Xinhua and 10 patients in Wuhan) showed CP as a therapeutic option that could potentially enhance the clinical issue through overcoming severe COVID-19 cases.[42,43] Some countries like Iran, Italy and the US also are using CP in the clinical phase.[44]

Masih Daneshvari Hospital in Tehran is the first medical center in Iran to collect plasma from recovered coronavirus patients to use as a possible treatment for the disease. 300 persons have donated their blood plasma, and the result was a 40 percent decline in the number of deaths due to COVID-19.[45] Now the trial phase continues in Baqiyatallah, Jondyshpoor, Mazandaran, Shiraz and Mashhad medical universities.[46]

(e) Cell-based Treatment

Severe respiratory consequences of the COVID-19 pandemic have inspired a potential need for novel therapies.[47] The most critical phase of COVID-19 is severe acute respiratory, thereby preventing this phase can be advantageous for the treatment and reduction of mortality rate.[48]

Cell-based approaches, primarily using Mesenchymal stem (stromal) cells (MSCs), have been determined as secure and efficient option in cases with the acute respiratory distress syndrome (ARDS).[49]

There are many advantages for preforming MSC therapy in comparison with other treatments, such as (i) They are accessible and can be isolated from various tissues such as bone marrow and adipose tissues, including in umbilical cord, dental pulp, menstrual-blood, fetal liver, etc.; (ii) MSC are multipotent stem cells; (iii) They can easily develop to clinical volume in an appropriate period of time; (iv) MSCs can be saved for repeated therapeutic utilization; (v) Clinical trials of MSCs so far have not shown harmful reactions to allogeneic MSC; (vi) several clinical trials have reported that MSCs therapy is safe and effective. However, the cost-effective and speed of therapeutic preparation are the capable discussed topic for MSC-based therapy for COVID-19.

Recently, published reports show that some countries like the USA, China, Jordon, and Iran have started cell therapy in the clinical trial phase. A case study reported in China on a female case with an acute COVID-19 syndrome. 21 days after the treatment with umbilical cord MSCs, results of laboratory tests and CT images indicate a significant improvement in her health condition.[50] By clearing phase one of the clinical study, phase II started in China on 6 February 2020 with 10 cases between the ages of 18-75 years old. This phase is expected to be completed by September 30, 2020.[51] In Iran, the clinical trial phase of MSC therapy on COVID-19 infected patients is being tested.[52]

(f) Other Drugs

Research thus far has revealed more than 30 agents including natural products may have potential efficacy against COVID-19. Some of these agents have been rapidly tested in the clinical phase and determined primary efficacy against COVID-19. Antivirals including interferon á (IFN-á), lopinavir/ritonavir, chloroquine phosphate, ribavirin, and arbidol have been suggested by the National Health Commission (NHC) of China for experimental treatment of COVID-19.[53]

The sulfate and phosphate salts of chloroquine have both been commercialized as antimalarial drugs. Hydroxychloroquine has also been used as an antimalaria but is now widely utilized to overcome autoimmune diseases such as rheumatoid arthritis. Notably, chloroquine and hydroxychloroquine are known to have side-effects. Lots of care must be taken while considering the effective dosage of this drug because chloroquine poisoning has been reported with cardiovascular disorders that can be life-threatening. Chloroquine and hydroxychloroquine use should be controlled with strict rules, and self-treatment must be forbidden.[54] On February 17 2020, the State Council of China revealed that chloroquine phosphate, an old drug for the treatment of malaria, had remarkable efficacy and suitable safety in treating COVID-19 associated pneumonia.[55] This drug now is in phase IV of clinical trial and is being tested on 50 patients with confirmed severe COVID-19. The final result is expected by April-June 2020.[56]

As per the reports of Health ministry, Iran joined WHO for clinical trials of this drug on 24 March.[57] On the other hand, Shahid Beheshti researchers showed that rheumatologic patients who take 200 mg per day hydroxychloroquine, as well as the medical workers who received the same dose for prophylaxis against COVID-19, revealed that hydroxychloroquine with a 200 mg/day dose can have a relative prophylactic effect on COVID-19.[58]

Volunteers Play a Significant Role

Even in Iran, the fear of COVID-19 led to mass hoarding of anti-corona products and masks. However, the country was quick to make up for those shortages. Almost all of the people reached out to volunteer in doing whatever could help to fail the disease. Volunteers offered services to the patients and medical staff, as well as aided in producing face masks, scrubs, and disinfectants. Many of these volunteers were housewives who sewed face masks and distributed them among the public and health workers. Furthermore, Iranian youth started producing disinfectants in universities, knowledge-based companies and religious places like a mosque. Many anti-corona products have been distributed among the financially weaker sections of the societies.

Many students and volunteers have also been working in hospitals and helping the medical staff. They help in feeding patients and sometimes encourage the patients and medical staff by reciting poems and songs. The medical staff has become so popular in Iran that they are being called "heroes of health".[59,60,61,62,63,64]

Under the 'Equality and Sincere Assistance Maneuver' command of Supreme Leader of Iran Ayatollah Seyed Ali Khamenei, seeks to receive cash aid from Iranian charities and philanthropists and deliver them to those low-income earners of the society. The maneuver is scheduled to be performed from Ramadan month till the end of the lethal virus outbreak in Iran in different phases. Jihadi and other volunteer forces aimed to attend to this maneuver and Basij would do the maneuver in its 54,000 bases all across Iran.[65] Along with the people, the officials also participated in this maneuver.[66] Parliamentarians, senior judiciary officials and the commanders of the IRGC, including those in the headquarters as well as the provincial chiefs have decided to allocate 20% of their next month's salary to those families affected by the economic consequences of the COVID-19 outbreak in the country.[67,68]

Further, the government announced that it will allocate 50,000 billion Rials (305 million USD) to the unemployment insurance fund to support those who have lost their jobs amid the outbreak of coronavirus.[69]

Meanwhile, Iran has tried to help other countries so that they can take steps to defeat Corona. A flight carrying Iran's humanitarian aid for the COVID-19 epidemic to Venezuela landed at Caracas airport.[70] Iran has already sent five petrol tankers to Venezuela despite US sanctions. This was considered by experts as a great success for Iran. Iran along with Russia urged sending humanitarian aid to Syria and Yemen amid the COVID-19 crisis.[71]

The Iranian health minister also expressed the country's readiness to share its experiences in the fight against the novel coronavirus, extensive research, and scientific projects with Qatar, the UAE, Kuwait, and Oman.[72]

Knowledge-based Companies, Researchers Come to the Scene

Since Iran has been imposed with sanctions, obtaining drugs and equipment from other countries is costly and time-consuming. Therefore, Iranian researchers and companies have come together to make an effort to overcome these conditions.

Iran soon achieved the technology to produce kits for COVID-19 diagnoses. Two types of diagnostic kits are now mass-produced by knowledge-based companies and defense ministry. First the RT-PCR kits of which around 8 million kits are being produced per month. The second is serology-based kits – a total of 400,000 are being manufactured monthly and may reach up to 2 million.[73] In addition, 40 advanced ventilators are manufactured daily in the medical equipment sector. This device is designed at a low-cost and easy-to-build technique by engineers in Tehran University Iran.[74]

Some companies like Pars Nano are capable of producing high-tech Nanofiber mask. There are some other companies which produce Nano filters that are altering their lines to produce Nano masks and increasing the capacity to manufacture from 100,000 masks each day to 300,000 in a few days. Iran also plans to export masks to some countries.[75,76] Iran is also producing ozone generator (produce Ozone to replace carcinogenic disinfectants) and disinfection gate.[77]

According to a professor of Sharif University of Technology, some African, American and European countries have used an Iranian smart software that is useful for diagnosing the COVID-19 with the help of artificial intelligence by analyzing computed tomography (CT) scans. Notably, the system is useful when a large number of patients are taken to a medical center, since the software does not require trained manpower to test the CT scans.[78]

Efforts of Iranian researchers in a knowledge-based company result in not only providing Iran medical centers but also exported a homegrown test kit that detected the coronavirus in saliva within 55 minutes.

Amirkabir University of technology have provided the advanced test kit using a real-time polymerase chain reaction (RT-PCR) system. They have received purchase orders from the Republic of Azerbaijan, Turkey, Romania, Spain and the UK, and has applied for permission for exports to Europe. The accuracy of this homegrown test kits is 2.5 to 10 times higher than that of the ones imported from abroad.[79]

Domestic production of various supplies by Iranian knowledge-based companies for the battle with COVID-19 has obviated the need for the import of the medical goods. He noted, "Our country does not currently need to import any equipment for the battle with the coronavirus, as all needs of the country are fulfilled domestically." Iranian knowledge-based companies have governed to manufacture a broad range of medical supplies and hospital equipment.[80]

Insisting on South-South collaboration to address the challenges of the COVID-19 pandemic, the Science and Technology Exchange Program (STEP), organized by Mustafa Science and Technology Foundation of Iran, together with the cooperation of other members, managed the 7 STEP summit virtually on 18 and 28 May 2020.

The first day of the summit was focused on "Sharing Experiences and

Observations of the Islamic Countries Medical Staff in Dealing with COVID-19."

The second day was focused on "Scientific discoveries, Technological innovations and Strategies Facing Coronavirus Challenges." It attempted to provide the best possible base by a virtual thematic meeting on the coronavirus and synergize the capacities and capabilities of scientists and experts in the Islamic world to help overcome this global disaster. Jorge Chediek, United Nations Office for South-South Cooperation Director, gave an inaugural message in the 7 STEP stating that "We are putting together some of the best minds in the Islamic world to confront the challenges brought about by coronavirus". STEP is an excellent example of the scientific community's efforts to overcome the pandemic and establish a long-lasting network among Muslim scientists.[81] Furthermore, MSTF laboratory network on 1 June 2020 managed a virtual workshop, the practical experiences and challenges of coronavirus PCR and serology-based testing were examined.[82]

The research center of corona management operations headquarters announced, the performance of more than 2,300 research projects to find an effective treatment for COVID-19, preceded by Iranian researchers. So far, 10,000 articles have been published on COVID-19 all around the world, out of which 280 articles are from Iranian researchers. Additionally, 215 corona clinical trials are currently underway to provide better services to patients.[83]

Health Work Forces

The Iranian health ministry has taken some steps to improve the quality of services provided to COVID-19 patients. Few of them are listed below:

1. On 01 March 2020 recruitment of front-line nurses to assist patients suffering from COVID-19 was done. Additionally, retired nurses and nursing students were invited to enhance the strength of specialized manpower in dealing with this epidemic and also help COVID-19 patients.
2. On 11 March 2020 nursing postgraduate students were invited to advise people on the 4030 portal. Call for volunteer doctors and paramedics to go to certain areas for control and treatment of COVID-19, providing quarantine and nursing accommodation in designated places, Sampling at a specific time of day by laboratory experts.
3. On 14 March 2020 payment was given to nurses for overtime. Nurses were admitted nationwide exams without passing departmental processes, the salary of front-line medical staff have been increased.[84]

65 percent of the 200,000 Iranian nursing community has been at the forefront of coronavirus pandemic in the country, as reported by the deputy health minister for nursing. Since the beginning of the epidemic, about 1,733 nurses, including faculty, graduate nursing students, retired and volunteer nurses, have offered to take care of COVID-19 patients as well as perform counseling and training services at hospitals and a total of 673 volunteer nurses are offering specialized counselling.[85]

Taghriri and colleagues manage an investigation about COVID-19 related knowledge, self-reported preventive behaviors and risk perception among Iranian medical students. The investigation was operated in the first week after the onset of the outbreak in Iran. A total of 240 medical students completed the questionnaire. The average age of participants was 23.67 years. The mean of true answers of knowledge was 86.96 percent; and 79.60 percent for women and men respectively, which had a high level of related knowledge. The average rate of practicing preventive behaviors was 94.47 percent; and 94.2 percent for women and men respectively that had high level of performance in preventive behaviors. The cumulative score of risk perception was in a moderate range. Generally, it was seen that there was a high level of COVID-19 related knowledge and self-reported preventive behaviors and moderate risk perception among Iranian medical students.[86]

The Islamic Revolution Guards Corps (IRGC) and Army

Soon after the spread of pneumonia secondary to COVID-19 in Iran, Armed forces mobile hospitals prepared for emergency admission of COVID-19 patients on 26 February. Iran's two defense arm (army and IRGC) managed it like a national biological defense exercise. The operation ran after the Iranian Supreme Leader Ayatollah Ali Khamenei, without evidence, which Iran had been subject to a "biological attack" following the outbreak of the virus.[87]

All medical centers of the IRGC Ground Force were used at full capacity during the exercise and the disinfectant operations took place in 3,000 locations across the country, including 100 in the capital of Tehran. The exercise also involved 100 units of the IRGC Ground Force across 10 bases to carry out the cleaning operations.[88]

On the other hand, Iran's Army established 300 medical centers in order to increase the capacity of COVID-19 infected cases identification and prevent the spread of the disease.[89] Army has transformed the Tehran exhibition center to a mobile hospital with 2000 beds in only two days.[90]

Besides, these operations, dedicated attention was put towards manufacturing a great mass of diagnostic kit as mentioned before. They also started mass production of face masks, disinfectants, and protective clothes from the early days that the coronavirus pneumonia in Iran. They also unveiled advanced thermal cameras used for screening infected cases in crowded places.[91]

By 29 May 2020 the deputy commander of IRGC ground force launched two new PCR centers in the country in order to fight against COVID-19. He noted, "Regarding the allocation of medical equipment to the hospitals of Armed Forces, Ministry of Health and Medical Education, Ministry of defense and also military hospitals cooperated and interacted with each other to provide necessary equipment in battling coronavirus in the country".[92]

Chief of staff of IRGC major general Mohammad Bagheri announced Iran's readiness to share its experiences of battling against coronavirus outbreak with regional countries. He also made the remarks in separate letters to defense ministers of Iraq, Azerbaijan, Afghanistan, Pakistan, Oman, Qatar, Kuwait, Syria, and Lebanon. He mentioned in his letter "Successful performance of the Islamic Republic of Iran in controlling the virus can offer solutions to other Islamic countries and friendly neighboring states".[93]

Some organisations like Khatam al-Anbia Construction (base in close cooperation with Imam Khomeini Relief Foundation), Astan-e Quds Razavi, the IRGC, etc; took action regarding the preparation and distribution of food packages and hot foods, in all regions of the country.[94] Only IRGC made efforts to provide aid to 3.5 million Iranian families most affected by the coronavirus outbreak.[95,96]

Social and Media Role for COVID-19 Prevention

To decrease the rate of infection, Social Distancing Plan including not holding gatherings and prohibiting unnecessary travels were implemented (as early as 27 March and continue until 3 April). According to the plan, inter-city trips will be prevented and only locals would be allowed to enter cities. Also, all parks, tour centers as well as any sites that might have large crowds, including pools, promenades, etc, was closed, even religious places like holy shires and mosques were closed.[97]

Informing media from the first day of COVID-19 pneumonia, put lots of its attention on training people about the Coronavirus confrontation approach. In fact, national TV and the Media are in charge of increasing public awareness for all people and teams involved in the campaign against COVID-19.[98]

Response to Iran's coronavirus outbreak in late February, one of the government's first actions was to close schools and universities on 5 March 2020.[99]

The prolonged closure was a major challenge for students, parents and teachers. To decrease the effect of the school closures on the education system, Iran's Education Ministry introduced an online app, the Social Network of Students (Shad in Persian), and presents daily lessons for different grades on state TV. Two state TV channels in Iran are broadcasting educational programs. These two channels supported distance learning for mathematics, history, and social sciences that are taught by teachers.[100]

Conclusion

The global spread of coronavirus has caused many casualties, financial and social losses. However, Iran has used all its capacity and experiences and knowledge of civilians and armed forces to combat the spread of the virus. Researchers, managers and the public have made a collective effort to combat the disease.

They have tried to turn the Corona crisis into a status for their scientific and social advancement. Due to long combat Experiences of defense forces consisting, the Army, Revolutionary Guards Corps (IRGC) and Basij or Mobilization Resistance and law enforcement police, Civil societies, volunteers, Red Crescent Movement against weapons of Mass Destruction especially Chemical and Biological warfare. All stages from surveillance to decontamination played an important part along with Medical and health staff to Control the epidemic.

By collaboration of all organisations and people's cooperation many people were able to recover from the infectious disease in Iran. Thus, the Leader of the Islamic Revolution sincerely expressed his gratitude to the Minister, all staff of the Ministry of Health and Medical Education in the country involved in the controlling virus and treatment of the patients with coronavirus and noted: "These highly valued efforts will elevate the status of the medical and nursing community in the society and will have divine merit and virtues."

After 41 years of various difficulties and crisis from, 8 years of war, sanctions and hardships, Iran emerged as one of the most resilient nation in the world to fight any natural or man-made disasters or crisis. Our knowledge and practical Experiences of Fighting WMD especially Chemical and Biological Weapons and Biological incidents due to more than 100,000 chemically injured military and Civilians' and continuous threats from enemies made nations defense forces to investigate and train to develop capabilities to fight against Biological incidents or crisis.

As the Iranian leader said at the beginning of the epidemic we will turn this threat into an opportunity and as commander of the chief ordered the armed forces to use this environment as an example of Biological attack maneuver and try to manage the crisis and evaluate your capabilities and weakness and work hard to develop and expand Biodefense capabilities for future threats. Fortunately, with effective collaboration between civilians and defense forces Iran has been able to control the coronavirus.

* * *

A shorter version of this essay was published in the CBW Magazine, Vol. 13, No. 1, Jan-June 2020.

NOTES

1. Jan-Wei Wang, Bin Cao, and Chen Wang, 'Science in the Fight Against the Novel Coronavirus Disease,' *PubMed*, vol. 133, no. 9, May 2020, pp. 1009-1011.
2. Muhammad A. Shereen, Suliman Khan, Abeer Kazmi, Nadia Bashir and Rabeea Siddique, 'COVID-19 Infection: Origin, Transmission, and Characteristics of Human Coronaviruses,' *Journal of Advanced Research*, vol. 24, July 2020, pp. 91-98.
3. Jody D. Berry, Steven Jones, Michael A Drebot, and et. al, 'Development and Characterisation of Neutralising Monoclonal Antibody to the SARS-coronavirus,' *Journal of virological methods*, vol. 120, no. 1, 2004, pp. 87-96.
4. See note 2.
5. See note 2.
6. N.S. Zhong, B. J Zheng, Y. M. Li, Poon, Z. H. Xie, K. H Chan, and et. al, 'Epidemiology and Cause of Severe Acute Respiratory Syndrome (SARS) in Guangdong, People's Republic of China, in February 2003,' *The Lancet*, vol. 362, no. 9393, pp. 1353-1358.
7. Nianshuang Wang, Xuanling Shi, Liwei Jiang and et. al, 'Structure of MERS-CoV Spike Receptor-Binding Domain Complexed with Human Receptor DPP4' *Cell research*, vol. 23, no. 8, July 2013, p. 986.
8. See note 2.
9. Kristian G. Andersen, Andrew Rambaut, Ian Lipkin, et al., 'The proximal Origin of SARS-CoV-2,' *Nature Medicine*, vol. 26, March 2020, pp. 450-452.
10. Haibo Zhang, Josef M. Penninger, Yimin Li, and et al 'Angiotensin-converting Enzyme 2 (ACE2) as a SARS-CoV-2 Receptor: Molecular Mechanisms and Potential Therapeutic Target' *Intensive care medicine*, vol. 46, March 2020, pp. 586-590.
11. See note 9.
12. See note 9.
13. Arash Mahdavi, Nastaran Khalili, Amir H. Davarpanah et al., 'Radiologic Management of COVID-19: Preliminary Experience of the Iranian Society of Radiology COVID-19 Consultant Group (ISRCC),' *Iranian Journal of Radiology*, (In Press), March 2020.
14. Iran Press, 'COVID-19 Detecting System Unveiled in Iran the Most Accurate in World,' *International News Agency, 04* April 2020, available at https://iranpress.com/en/iran-i145615-covid_19_detecting_system_unveiled_in_iran_most_accurate_in_world, accessed on 8 April 2020.
15. Callum Paton, 'Iran's 'Amazing' COVID-19 Detectors Identified as Repurposed Fake Bomb Scanners,' *The National*, 16 April 2020, available at https://www.thenational.ae/world/mena/

iran-s-amazing-covid-19-detectors-identified-as-re-purposed-fake-bomb-scanners-1.1006918, accessed on 20 April 2020.

16. Yang Yang, Minghui Yang, Chenguang Shen, and et al., 'Evaluating the Accuracy of Different Respiratory Specimens in the Laboratory Diagnosis and Monitoring the Viral shedding of 2019-nCoV Infections,' *MedRxiv*, February 2020.
17. 'Iran Starts Mass Producing PCR, Serologic COVID-19 Diagnostic Kits,' *ifpnews*, 11 April 2020, available at https://ifpnews.com/iran-starts-mass-producing-pcr-serologic-covid-19-diagnostic-kits,accessed on 20 April 2020.
18. 'Iran Mass-Produces Homegrown Rapid Test Kits for COVID-19,' *Tasnim News Agency*, 31 March 2020, available at https://www.tasnimnews.com/en/news/2020/03/31/2233785/iran-mass-produces-homegrown-rapid-test-kits-for-covid-19, accessed on 20 April 2020.
19. Alex Philippidis, 'COVID-19: Top 60 Drug Treatments in Development,' *Genetic Engineering & Biotechnology News*, vol. 40, no. 4, April 2020, pp. 10-13.
20. Sumita Agrawal, Akhil Danesh Goeland Nitesh Gupta, 'Emerging prophylaxis strategies against COVID-19,' *Monaldi Archives for Chest Disease*, vol. 90, no. 1, 2020.
21. Tung Thanh Le, Zacharias Andreadakis, Arun Kumar et al., 'The COVID-19 Vaccine Development Landscape,' *Nature Reviews Drug Discovery*, vol. 19, April 2020, pp. 305-306.
22. 'Six Contracts Inked for Producing COVID-19 Vaccine: VP,' *Mehrnews Agency*, 20 April 2020, available at https://en.mehrnews.com/news/157806/Six-contracts-inked-for-producing-COVID-19-vaccine-VP accessed on 25 April 2020.
23. 'Three Iranian Teams Working on COVID-19 Vaccine: VP,' *IFP News*, available at https://flipboard.com/topic/s:ifpnews.com/three-iranian-teams-working-on-covid-19-vaccine-vp/a-9LCx88gpT16NW1ExV4Ojng%3Aa%3A221756309-f3be3ac2be%2Fifpnews.com, accessed on 25 April 2020.
24. Balamurugan Shanmugaraj, Konlavat Siriwattananon, Kittikhun Wangkanont and Waranyoo Phoolcharoen, 'Perspectives on Monoclonal Antibody Therapy as Potential Therapeutic Intervention for Coronavirus Disease-19 (COVID-19),' *Asian Pacific Journal of Allergy and Immunology*, vol. 38, no. 1, 2020, pp. 10-18.
25. Yan Li, Ming Chen, Hongwei Cao, Yuanfeng Zhu and et. al, 'Extraordinary GU-rich Single-strand RNA Identified from SARS Coronavirus Contributes an Excessive Innate Immune Response,' *Microbes Infect*, vol. 15, no. 2, 2013, pp. 88-95.
26. Zhe Xu, Lei Shi, Yijin Wang and et al. 'Pathological Findings of COVID-19 Associated with Acute Respiratory Distress Syndrome,' *Lancet Respir Med*, February 2020, vol. 8, pp. 420-422.
27. Yonggang Zhou, Binqing Fu, Xiaohu Zheng and et al, 'Aberrant Pathogenic GM-CSF+T Cells and Inflammatory CD14+CD16+ Monocytes in Severe Pulmonary Syndrome Patients of a New Coronavirus, *BioRxiv*, February 2020.
28. Xiaoling Xu, Mingfeng Han, Tiantian Li, and et al, 'Effective Treatment of Severe COVID-19 Patients with Tocilizumab,' *Proceedings of the National Academy of Sciences*, vol. 117, no. 20, May 2020.
29. Daniela Marotto and Piercarlo Sarzi-Puttini, 'What is the Role of Rheumatologists in the Era of COVID-19?' *Autoimmunity Reviews*, vol. 19, no. 6, June 2020.
30. 'Iran Testing Own Version of 'Actemra' to Treat COVID-19,' *IFP News*, 11 March 2020, available at https://ifpnews.com/iran-testing-own-version-of-actemra-to-treat-covid-19 accessed on 20 April 2020.
31. Performance Report of the Deputy Minister of Research and Technology of the Ministry of Health and Medical Education, 11 April 2020, available at http://journals.research.ac.ir/files/med/site/covid-19_report_13990123.pdf accessed on 20 April 2020.

32. E. Susan Amirian and Julie K Levy, 'Current Knowledge about the Antivirals Remdesivir (GS-5734) and GS-441524 as Therapeutic Options for Coronaviruses,' *One Health*, vol. 9, June 2020.
33. Calvin J. Gordon, Egor P Tchesnokov, Emma Woolner, and et al, 'Remdesivir is a Direct-acting Antiviral that Inhibits RNA-dependent RNA polymerase from Severe Acute Respiratory Syndrome Coronavirus 2 with High Potency,' *Journal of Biological Chemistry*, vol. 295, no. 20, 2020.
34. See note 19.
35. See note 31.
36. 'Iran Joins WHO Clinical Trials on 4 anti-COVID-19 drugs,' *Islamic Republic News Agency*, 24 March 2020, available at https://en.irna.ir/news/83726343/Iran-joins-WHO-clinical-trials-on-4-anti-COVID-19-drugs, accessed on 30 March 2020.
37. Chenguang Shen, Zhaoqin Wang, Fang Zhao, and et al, 'Treatment of 5 Critically Ill Patients with COVID-19 with Convalescent Plasma,' *Jama*, March 2020.
38. See note 24.
39. Long Chen, Jing Xiong, Bao Lei, and et al, 'Convalescent Plasma as a Potential Therapy for COVID-19,' *The Lancet Infectious Diseases*, vol. 20, no. 4, February 2020, pp. 398-400.
40. Y. Cheng, R. Wong, Y.O.Y. Soo, and et al, 'Use of Convalescent Plasma Therapy in SARS Patients in Hong Kong,' *European Journal of Clinical Microbiology and Infectious Diseases*, vol. 24, no. 1, 2005, pp. 44-46.
41. See note 24.
42. Kai Duan, Bende Liu, Cesheng Li, Huajun Zhang, and et al, 'Effectiveness of Convalescent Plasma Therapy in Severe COVID-19 Patients,' *Proceedings of the National Academy of Sciences*, April 2020, vol 117, no. 17.
43. Arturo Casadevall and Liise-anne Pirofski, 'The Convalescent Sera Option for Containing COVID-19,' *The Journal of Clinical Investigation*, vol 130, no. 4, March 2020, pp.1545-1548.
44. Daniele Focosi, Julian Tang, Arthur Anderson, and Marco Tuccori, 'Convalescent Plasma Therapy for COVID-19: State of the Art,' *Preprints*, 2020.
45. 'Plasma Therapy Reduces Coronavirus Deaths in Iran by 40%,' *Tehran Times*, 14 April 2020, available at https://www.tehrantimes.com/news/446754/Plasma-therapy-reduces-coronavirus-deaths-in-Iran-by-40, accessed on 20 April 2020.
46. See note 31.
47. Bing Liang, Junhui Chen, Tao Li, Haiying Wu, and et al, 'Clinical Remission of a Critically Ill COVID-19 Patient Treated by Human Umbilical Cord Mesenchymal Stem Cells,' *ChinaXiv*, March 2020.
48. Ali Golchin, Ehsan Seyedjafari, and Abdolreza Ardeshirylajimi, 'Mesenchymal Stem Cell Therapy for COVID-19: Present or Future,' *Stem Cell Reviews and Reports*, April 2020.
49. See note 47.
50. Ali Golchin, Tahereh Z Farahany, Arash Khojasteh, Fatemeh Soleimanifar, et al., 'The Clinical Trials of Mesenchymal Stem Cell Therapy in Skin Diseases: An Update and Concise Review,' *Current stem cell research & therapy*, vol. 14, no. 1, 2019, pp. 22-33.
51. ZhiYong Peng, 'Umbilical Cord (UC)- Derived Mesenchymal Stem Cells (MSCs) Treatment for the 2019-novel Coronavirus (nCov) Pneumonia,' *ClinicalTrials.gov*, February 2020 available at https://clinicaltrials.gov/ct2/show/NCT04269525 accessed on 20 April 2020.
52. See note 31.
53. Liying Dong, Shasha Hu, and Jianjun Gao, 'Discovering Drugs to Treat Coronavirus Disease

2019 (COVID-19),' *Drug discoveries & Therapeutics*, vol. 14, no. 1, 2020, pp. 58-60.

54. Franck Touret and Xavier de Lamballerie, 'Of chloroquine and COVID-19,' *Antiviral Research*, vol. 177, 2020.
55. Jianjun Gao, Zhenxue Tian, and Xu Yang, 'Breakthrough: Chloroquine Phosphate has Shown Apparent Efficacy in Treatment of COVID-19 Associated Pneumonia in Clinical Studies,' *Bioscience Trends*, vol. 14, no. 1, 2020, pp. 72-73.
56. Shen Ning, 'Evaluation the Efficacy and Safety of Hydroxychloroquine Sulfate in Comparison with Phosphate Chloroquine in Severe Patients with Novel Coronavirus Pneumonia (COVID-19): A Randomized, Open-Label, Parallel, Controlled Trial,' *Chinese Clinical Trial Register*, 2020, available at http://www.chictr.org.cn/showprojen.aspx?proj=49482, accessed: 24 March 2020.
57. See Note 36.
58. Guitti Pourdowlat, Parnaz Panahi, Parichehr Pooransari, and Fariba Ghorbani, 'Prophylactic Recommendation for Healthcare Workers in COVID-19 Pandemic,' *Advanced Journal of Emergency Medicine*, vol. 4, no. 2, 2020.
59. Azam Raoofi, Amirhossein Takian, Ali Baba Akbari, Alireza Olyaeemanesh, and et al, 'COVID-19 Pandemic and Comparative Health Policy Learning in Iran,' *Archives of Iranian Medicine*, vol. 23, no. 4, pp. 220-234.
60. Huaxia, 'Iranian Volunteers Turn Theater Hall into Factory to Produce Face Masks Amid COVID-19 Pandemic,' *Xinhuanet*, 22 April 2020, available at http://www.xinhuanet.com/english/2020-04/22/c_138999148.htm, accessed on 28 April 2020.
61. 'Mosque Converted into Mask Factory in Virus-hit Iran,' *MSN News* 7 April 2020, available at https://www.msn.com/en-us/news/world/mosque-converted-into-mask-factory-in-virus-hit-iran/ar-BB12er3T, accessed on 28 April 2020.
62. 'Production Line for Disinfectant Gel in Isfahan,' *Fars News Agency*, 22 April 2020, available at https://en.farsnews.ir/imgrep.aspx?nn=13981212000468, accessed on 28 April 2020.
63. Forouzandeh Jannat, Ali Ardalan, Mokhtar Malekpour, and et al, 'Selection Criteria of Hospital Volunteers for the Provision of Health Services in Disasters,' فصلنامه سلامت در حوادث و بلایا, vol. 2, no. 3, 2017, pp. 139-144.
64. 'Basij Teams with 300 Members to Fight Coronavirus,' *International News Agency*, 21 March 2020, available at https://iranpress.com/en/iran-i145165-basij_teams_with_300_members_to_fight_coronavirus, accessed on 28 April 2020.
65. Haniyeh Sadat Jafariyeh, 'Iranians Start Performing 'Equality, Sincere Assistance Maneuver,' *Tehran Times*, 13 April 2020, available at https://www.tehrantimes.com/news/446715/Iranians-start-performing-Equality-Sincere-Assistance-Maneuver, accessed on 29 April 2020.
66. 'Lawmakers Offer 20% of their Wages to Corona-affected People,' *Tasnim News*, 20 April 2020, available at https://en.mehrnews.com/news/157649/Lawmakers-offer-20-of-their-wages-to-corona-affected-people, accessed on 30 April 2020.
67. 'Senior Judiciary Officials to Grant 20% of their Monthly Wages to Corona-hit Iranians,' *Tasnim News*, 13 April 2020, available at https://en.mehrnews.com/news/157562/Senior-judiciary-officials-to-grant-20-of-their-monthly-wages, accessed on 1 May 2020.
68. 'IRGC Chiefs Allocate 20% of Own Wages to Coronavirus Combat,' *Tasnim News*, 12 April 2020, available at https://en.mehrnews.com/news/157526/IRGC-chiefs-allocate-20-of-own-wages-to-coronavirus-combat, accessed on 30 April 2020.
69. 'IRGC forms Center to Aid 3.5m Families Affected by Coronavirus,' *Tehran times*, 14 April 2020, available at https://www.tehrantimes.com/news/446775/IRGC-forms-center-to-aid-3-

5m-families-affected-by-coronavirus, accessed on 28 April 2020.

70. 'Plane Carrying Iran's COVID-19 Aid Arrives in Venezuela,' *International News Agency*, 8 June 2020, available at https://iranpress.com/america-i148241-plane_carrying_iran's_covid_19_aid_arrives_in_venezuela, accessed on 10 June 2020.
71. 'Iran, Russia Urge sending Humanitarian Aid to Syria Amid COVID-19 Crisis,' *International News Agency*, 26 May 2020, available at https://iranpress.com/iran-i147697-iran_russia_urge_sending_humanitarian_aid_to_syria_amid_covid_19_crisis, accessed on 10 June 2020.
72. 'Iran Ready to Help Neighboring Countries in COVID-19 Management: Health Min,' *International News Agency*, 20 May 2020, available at https://iranpress.com/iran-i147484-iran_ready_to_help_neighboring_countries_in_covid_19_management_health_min., accessed on 10 June 2020.
73. Faranak Bakhtari, 'How Iran could Curb COVID-19 Despite Sanctions, Restrictions?' *Tehran Times*, 19 April 2020, available at https://www.tehrantimes.com/news/446956/How-Iran-could-curb-COVID-19-despite-sanctions-restrictions, accessed on 20 April 2020.
74. 'Iran Makes Ventilator to Fight COVID-19,' *Islamic Republic News Agency*, 22 April 2020, available at https://en.irna.ir/news/83732273/Iran-makes-ventilator-to-fight-COVID19, accessed on 31 April 2020.
75. 'Official: 70,000 Nano Masks Produced in Tehran Each Day,' Fars *News Agency*, 1 March 2020, available at https://www.msn.com/en-xl/middleeast/top-stories/official-70000-nano-masks-produced-in-tehran-each-day/ar-BB10Bfoa, accessed on 20 April 2020.
76. Ghanbar Naderi, 'Iran Boosts Production of Protective Face Masks,' *Press TV*, 14 April 2020, available at http://french.presstv.com/Detail/2020/04/14/623006/Iran-boosts-production-protective-face-masks, accessed on 20 April 2020.
77. 'Iran Unveils High-tech Products to Fight COVID-19,' *Tehran Times*, 18 April 2020, available at https://www.tehrantimes.com/news/446916/Iran-unveils-high-tech-products-to-fight-COVID-19, accessed on 20 April 2020.
78. 'Foreign Countries Using Iranian AI-Assisted Software for COVID-19 Diagnosis,' *Tasnim News Agency*, 30 May 2020, available at https://www.tasnimnews.com/en/news/2020/05/30/2275787/foreign-countries-using-iranian-ai-assisted-software-for-covid-19-diagnosis, accessed on 01 June 2020.
79. 'Iran to export COVID-19 Instant Salvia Test Kit,' *Tasnim News Agency*, 31 May 2020, available at https://www.tasnimnews.com/en/news/2020/05/31/2276714/iran-to-export-covid-19-instant-saliva-test-kits, accessed on 2 June 2020.
80. 'VP: Iran Self-sufficient in Coronavirus-related Supplies,' *Tasnim News Agency*, 29 May 2020, available at https://www.tasnimnews.com/en/news/2020/05/19/2269234/vp-iran-self-sufficient-in-coronavirus-related-supplies, accessed on 2 June 2020.
81. '7th STEP Meeting Addresses Ways to Combat COVID-19,' *Tasnim News Agency*, 28 May 2020, available at https://www.tasnimnews.com/en/news/2020/05/28/2274986/7th-step-meeting-addresses-ways-to-combat-covid-19, accessed on 2 June 2020.
82. 'Scientists from Pasteur, Royan institutes shared COVID-19 Testing Experiences in Virtual Workshop,' *Tasnim News Agency*, 4 June 2020, available at https://en.mehrnews.com/news/159415/Scientists-from-Pasteur-Royan-institutes-shared-COVID-19-testing, accessed on 2 June 2020.
83. 'Iranian Researchers Conduct above 2,000 COVID-19 Projects,' *International News Agency*, 27 May 2020, available at https://iranpress.com/iran-i147741-iranian_researchers_conduct_above_2_000_covid_19_projects, accessed on 2 June 2020.

84. See note 59.
85. Faranak Bakhtiari, '65% of Iranian Nurses at Forefront of Corona Fight,' *Tehran Times*, 12 May 2020, available at https://www.tehrantimes.com/news/447806/65-of-Iranian-nurses-at-forefront-of-corona-fight, accessed on 2 June 2020.
86. Mohammad Hossein Taghrir, Roham Borazjani and Ramin Shiraly, 'A Survey on Their Related-Knowledge, Preventive Behaviors and Risk Perception,' *Archives of Iranian medicine*, vol.23, no. 4, pp. 249-254.
87. See note 63.
88. Ben Kew, 'Iran's IRGC Terrorist Group to Stage 'Biological Defense Exercise.' Against Coronavirus,' *BREITBART*, 24 March 2020, available at https://www.breitbart.com/national-security/2020/03/24/irans-irgc-terrorist-group-stage-biological-defense-exercise-against-coronavirus/, accessed on 20 April 2020.
89. 'Iran Army Holding Biological Defense Exercise,' *Tasnim News Agency*, 15 March 2020, available at https://www.tasnimnews.com/en/news/2020/03/15/2223572/iran-army-holding-biological-defense-exercise, accessed on 20 April 2020.
90. See note 63.
91. 'Army Chief Lauds Defense Ministry for Coronavirus Fight,' *Tehran Times*, 22 April 2020, available at https://www.tehrantimes.com/news/446822/Army-chief-lauds-Defense-Ministry-for-coronavirus-fight, accessed on 30 April 2020.
92. 'IRGC Ground Force launches two new "PCR" Centers in Battling COVID-19: Cmdr,' *Mehrnews Agency*, 2 May 2020, available at https://en.mehrnews.com/news/159197/IRGC-Ground-Force-launches-two-new-PCR-centers-in-battling, accessed on 20 May 2020.
93. 'Iran Ready to Share Anti-corona Experiences with Friend Countries: cmdr' *Mehrnews Agency*, 2 May 2020, available at https://en.mehrnews.com/news/158247/Iran-ready-to-share-anti-corona-experiences-with-friend-countries, accessed on 20 May 2020.
94. See note 69.
95. '9000 Food Package Distribution by KAA, Imam Khomeini Relief Foundation,' *International News Agency*, 2 May 2020, available at https://iranpress.com/iran-i146716-9000_food_package_distribution_by_kaa_imam_khomeini_relief_foundation, accessed on 20 May 2020.
96. Amin Berenjkar, '8200 Food staffs Packages Distributed in Shiraz,' *Mehrnews Agency*, 17 June 2020, available at https://en.mehrnews.com/photo/158516/82-000-foodstuff-packages-distributed-in-Shiraz, accessed on 20 May 2020.
97. 'Iran Coronavirus Battle: Implementing Social Distancing Plan to Start Friday,' *Tasnim News Agency*, 26 March 2020, available at https://www.tasnimnews.com/en/news/2020/03/26/2230948/iran-coronavirus-battle-implementing-social-distancing-plan-to-start-friday, accessed on 20 April 2020.
98. See note 63.
99. Yusef Jalali, 'Iran Launches Online Learning Application Amid Virus,' *Press TV*, 21 April 2020, available at https://www.presstv.com/Detail/2020/04/21/623509/Iran-launches-online-learning-application-amid-virus, accessed on 30 April 2020.
100. 'Iranian Students Continue Education through TV Channels Amid Corona Threat,' *Tehran Times*, 9 March 2020, available at https://www.tehrantimes.com/news/445935/Iranian-students-continue-education-through-TV-channels-amid, accessed on 20 April 2020.

North and South America

7

US Response to COVID-19

Cherian Samuel and Munish Sharma

Pandemic at the Gates

The conventional wisdom is to see the disastrous response to the Coronavirus in the United States largely through the prism of it being an election year in the United States. The previous year had ended with President Trump coming out unscathed from the attempts to impeach him for abuse of power and obstruction of Congress. As late as February, even as the Coronavirus was spreading its wings and many countries had begun to impose restrictions on international travel, he had made a trip to India at the invitation of the Prime Minister.[1]

By then, the first known case of coronavirus infection in the United States had already surfaced on 21 January when a 35-year-old man returned from a visit to his family in the Wuhan region. That one case is believed to be responsible for a quarter of all cases in the United States, showing not only how contagious the virus was, but also how the belated response lead to its dispersion across the length and breadth of the country. Even as he appointed a task force under the Vice-President in late February, the President downplayed it, going to the extent of calling it a hoax put out by the Democrats.[2]

The United States, at the time of writing, accounts for the most number of COVID-19 infections and the resultant deaths in a single country. Since the Centers for Disease Control and Prevention (CDC) confirmed the first case of infection reported on 20 January 2020 in Snohomish County, Washington[3], at the time of writing (30 June 2020) the number of cases had surpassed a total of 2 million (Figure 1) claiming more than 1,30,000 lives across all 50 states (Figure 2). The

Figure 1: Total COVID-19 Cases in the United States

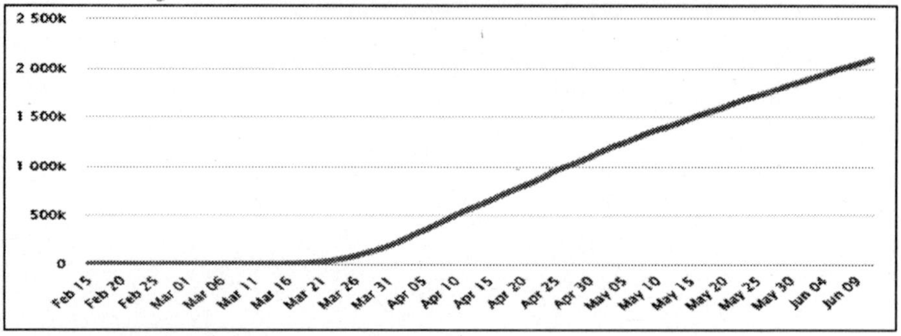

Source: www.worldometers.info

Figure 2: Total COVID-19 Related Deaths in the United States

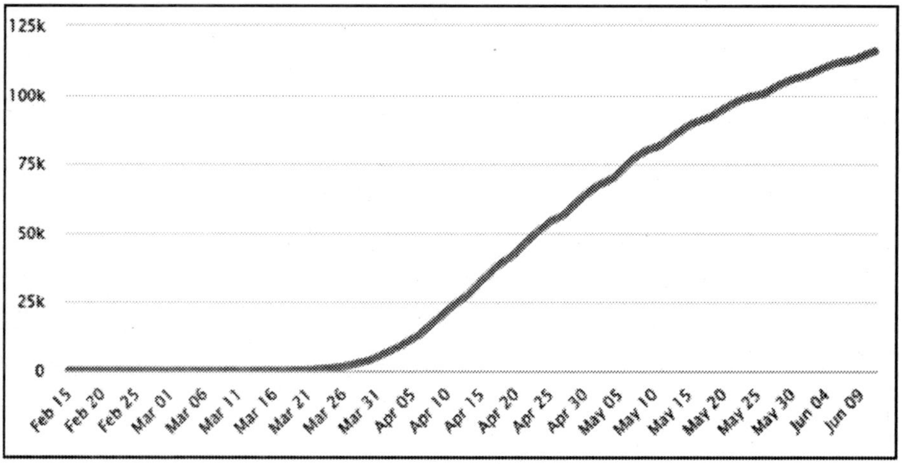

Source: www.worldometers.info

death rate from COVID-19 in the case of the United States at 340 per million residents is 100 times more than the rate in China (Figures 3 and 4). Since the March-end, the numbers of daily cases in the United States have incessantly remained between 20,000 and 30,000, though shooting above the 30,000 mark on around 18 occasions (Figure 5). The government has faced sharp criticism over its handling and management of the pandemic ever since it knocked at the door of the United States.

The early American public health response was the standard one for epidemics; designed to contain and slow down the outbreak, including isolation and quarantine measures, social distancing norms, closing of educational institutions and public places, ban on large-scale gatherings, and international as well domestic travel restrictions. The Secretary of Health and Human Services declared a public health

Figure 3: Total Confirmed COVID-19 Deaths per million People in the United States

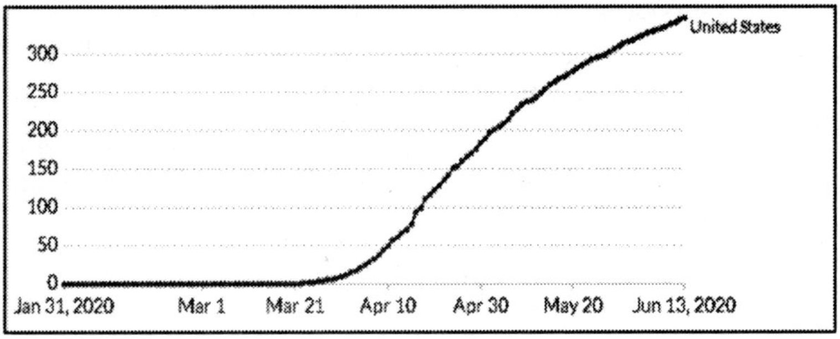

Source: www.ourworldindata.org

Figure 4: Total Confirmed COVID-19 Deaths per million People in China

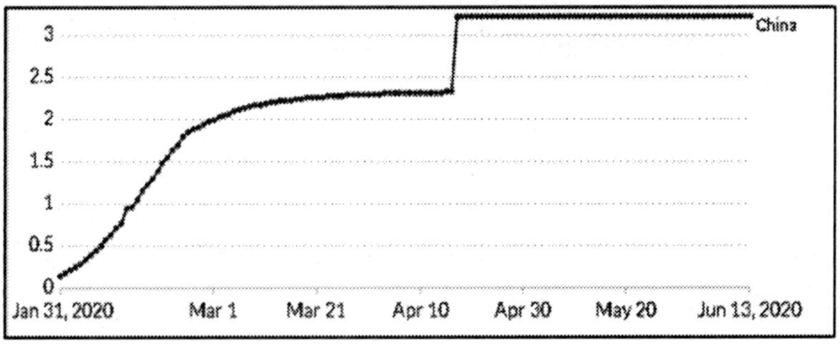

Source: www.ourworldindata.org

Figure 5: Daily New Cases in the United States

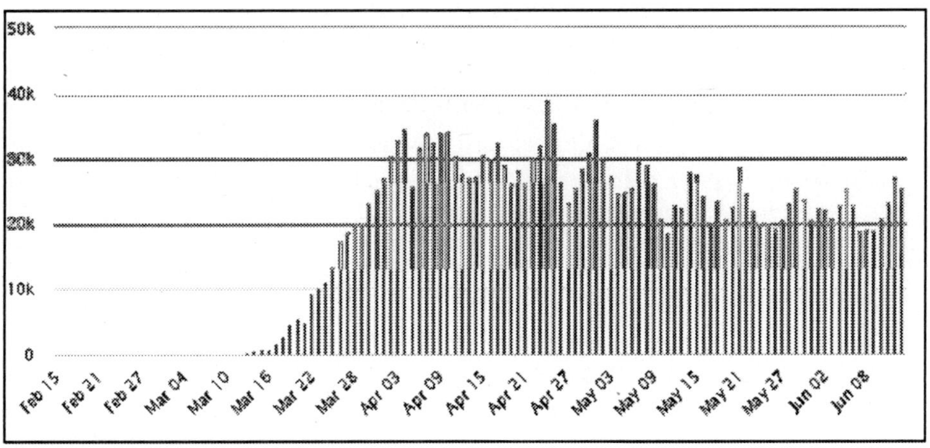

Source: www.worldometers.info

emergency on 31 January[4] and the government issued a series of travel restrictions for foreign nationals with a travel history to the impacted jurisdictions as early as 2 February, beginning with China, the first epicentre of the outbreak.[5] On 16 March, President Trump announced recommendations – called the "15 Days to Slow the Spread" – for physical distancing, self-isolation, personal hygiene, and protection for the elderly and individuals with underlying health conditions.[6] Given the limited know-how of the disease and no established management protocol, the government had no other option but to continuously correct its course of action. Just like the rest of the world, the United States too was caught off guard in the initial stages to contain a pandemic of such a scale and severity. However, while the developed world was able to largely reduce the impact of the pandemic through interventions such as lockdowns and other targeted measures, the US has found itself unable to flatten the all-important curve to show that the outbreak has been brought under control.

From the beginning of the outbreak in the United States, the CDC had restricted the eligibility criteria for COVID-19 testing to (a) people who had recently travelled to certain countries affected by the outbreak, or (b) people with respiratory illness serious enough to require hospitalization, or (c) people who have been in contact with a person confirmed to be positive. It was not until 4 March when the CDC expanded the evaluation criteria to include a wider group of symptomatic patients.[7]

The early hiccups in the response to contain COVID-19 spread such as manufacturing defects in the CDC test kits[8], narrow testing criteria, limited testing capacity[9] and sluggish scale-up of testing[10] indicate the government was slow to respond and implement stringent measures.[11] The government was cornered for downplaying the threat since the very onset as hospitals were reporting shortages of diagnostic test kits, test swabs, chemical reagents,[12] and personal protective equipment such as masks, gloves, face shields, eyewear, and gowns for health personnel.[13] There were delays in the procurement of medical equipment too, and to meet the demand, the government had to invoke the Defense Production Act to direct industries to produce medical equipment, especially ventilators and N95 respirator masks at war-footing.[14] This Korean War-era law gives powers to the President to mobilize the domestic industry to maintain supplies of essential materials and services necessary for the national defence, compelling companies to prioritize the government's order over those of other clients.[15] In the face of such an unprecedented healthcare emergency, the existing supply chains for medical equipment and protective gears failed to meet the rapid surge in demand, calling for unprecedented decisions to tackle the multiple issues that arose, from assuring medical supplies to containing the economic fallout of COVID-19.

Tackling the Virus

By late March, President Trump signed into law the Coronavirus Aid, Relief, and Economic Security (CARES) Act, providing massive 2 trillion USD economic relief package in a bid to safeguard the citizens from public health and economic impacts of the pandemic.[16] Dubbed as the largest rescue package in the history of United States, this federal government response aids various agencies such as Health and Human Services (HHS) in the development of diagnostics, therapeutics and vaccines; National Institutes of Health for prevention and preparation; Centers for Disease Control and Prevention for emergency health response; Food and Drug Administration for manufacturing for medical products; National Science Foundation for rapid response research; and also the Departments of Defense, Energy and Agriculture for a host of activities.[17] It also earmarked 3.5 billion USD to the Biomedical Advanced Research and Development Authority (part of the HHS) to facilitate the large-scale manufacturing, production, and purchase of vaccines, therapeutics, and diagnostics.[18]

In the absence of drugs or other therapeutics for COVID-19, the United States Food and Drug Administration (FDA) had recommended clinical management and supportive care, including supplemental oxygen and mechanical ventilator support for the patients.[19] By mid-May, the FDA created a special emergency program – the Coronavirus Treatment Acceleration Program (CTAP) – for possible therapies, while continuing to support clinical trials on the safety and efficacy of new treatments for COVID-19.[20] The National Institutes of Health sponsored one of the trials to evaluate the usage of anti-malarial drug hydroxychloroquine, together with the antibiotic azithromycin, to prevent hospitalization and death from COVID-19.[21] The US, in the meantime, imported around 50 million tablets of hydroxychloroquine from India followed by a request by President Trump to New Delhi.[22] As far as vaccine development is concerned, a vaccine candidate from the United States-based biotechnology company Moderna has shown some promising results in the first phase of clinical trials.[23] The Walter Reed Army Institute of Research of the Army Futures Command's Medical Research and Development Command is also playing a key role in the American pursuit of vaccines and therapeutic treatments. The vaccine candidate from the Institute is all set to enter the human clinical trials phase.[24]

Trumpian Follies

The response to the Coronavirus was played out in full public glare, almost like a soap opera, with daily news conferences by the President which he considered as a substitute bully pulpit to the mega rallies that he was accustomed to holding on a regular basis. Like with the rallies, these press conferences were designed to appeal to his support base, and simultaneously rile up the opposition. So, at a time when the country was supposed to come together to face the greatest threat to humanity, the President was seen to be sowing division and confusion, pitting Republicans against Democrats, and the federal government against state governments. He even asked his supporters in Democrat-led states like Michigan, Minnesota and Virginia which had implemented strict lockdown measures to "liberate" these states.[25] He peddled his own theories about the virus, pushing unscientifically proven solutions just to continue the illusion that he was in charge. The only substantial act, that of banning flights from China, was repeated *ad nauseum* as evidence that he had acted faster and more decisively than other world leaders, never mind the fact that much of the subsequent infections were spread by passengers arriving from European cities.[26] Though actions were promised against China and the WHO, the latter accused of being under China's thumb and actively engaged in suppressing facts about the virus under its tutelage, these ultimately never materialised.

Perhaps the most egregious was the failure of the federal system, exacerbated by what was seen as the President's attempts to set state against state, and the federal government against the state governments, as well as his propensity to blame the previous administration for any lacunae that became visible. The national stockpile of critical medical supplies such as ventilators was given out grudgingly, and as late as June, state governors were requesting the President to invoke the Defense Production Act to ensure a reliable supply of medical supplies like test kits.[27] The lack of support from the Federal government meant that states often had to make their purchases from private manufacturers, where they were competing against other states, thus driving prices up.[28]

The President was obsessed with re-opening the economy, starting first with an Easter deadline, even as states like New York were seeing an exponential rise in cases.[29] The President kept upping the ante, threatening to use the real (and some imaginary) powers of the Presidency, such as withholding funds (fiscal starvation) and other resources, to force states to open up their economies and reduce lockdown restrictions.[30] Even though the US Constitution gave the states the power to regulate health and welfare issues, the President could use his authority to administer funds to compel states to act in certain ways, sometimes detrimental to the health of residents, such as loosening lockdown measures before the virus had been brought under control.

Where also, it was part of the mystique of the Presidency that it was expected of the President to lead by example, he was often seen in public without a mask, and continuously brushed aside opinions of experts or contradicted them in public meetings, thus making their own jobs that much more difficult. It is no surprise then, that large swathes of the US population dismissed attempts to enforce restrictive measures such as lockdowns and social distancing, leading not only a continued rise in cases overall but a resurgence of cases in states where the spread had been successfully contained.[31] Part of the blame must also be apportioned to the individualistic nature of the US populace who have seen as these measures as an affront on their individual rights and freedom. Others have been taken in by conspiracy theories such as Coronavirus being a plot by Bill Gates to implant chips in all Americans, to 5G towers being used to spread the virus.[32]

Critics also pointed to many of the longer-term policy measures of the presidency, from defunding crucial institutions such as the state-run CDC, once seen as the "the gold standard for global disease detection and control" and disbanding the Global Health Security and Biodefense unit, the pandemic response unit that was set up in the National Security Council under the Obama Administration. This was seen to be of a piece with Trumps deliberate neglect of the healthcare system which had been one of the priorities of the Obama Administration. However, in-depth analysis of these criticisms showed that they were only partially true; the pandemic response unit, for instance, had only been folded into other existing units at the NSA (National Security Agency). Similarly, the budget of the CDC had not been reduced, but actually increased, though, in keeping with Trumps motto of America First, its global budget had been halved over the years.[33]

A 2014 article in the Lancet Medical journal titled *Global health and the US Centers for Disease Control and Prevention* began putting forth the rhetorical question "Why is an article about global health included in a special issue on health in the USA?" and answered it thus "The Centers for Disease Control and Prevention (CDC) has engaged in global health for more than 60 years. Although tackling infectious disease threats has been a constant, the agency has also provided humanitarian assistance in natural disasters, refugee crises, and famines; improved child survival; and strengthened scientific measurement of health metrics. CDC's workforce includes more than 300 internationally deployed public health professionals in addition to around 1330 locally employed staff working in about 60 countries (figure). CDC's global health strategy aims to: achieve optimum health effects; strengthen global health capacity; improve global health security....[34] The CDC had stepped up its global monitoring program after the Ebola outbreak in 2014 with a one-time budgetary provision of 600 million USD by the United States Congress.[35] The CDC's decision to cut down on the infectious disease monitoring programs in 39 out of 49 outposts it had worldwide including in China, in 2018 could well prove to be one of the reasons that the virus wasn't stopped in time. Other reports point out that it was not just the CDC but United States global health funding as a whole that had been halved in the 2020-2021 financial year even as the pandemic is raging around the world.

Figure 6: US Global Health Funding from FY 2006 to 2021 (Request)

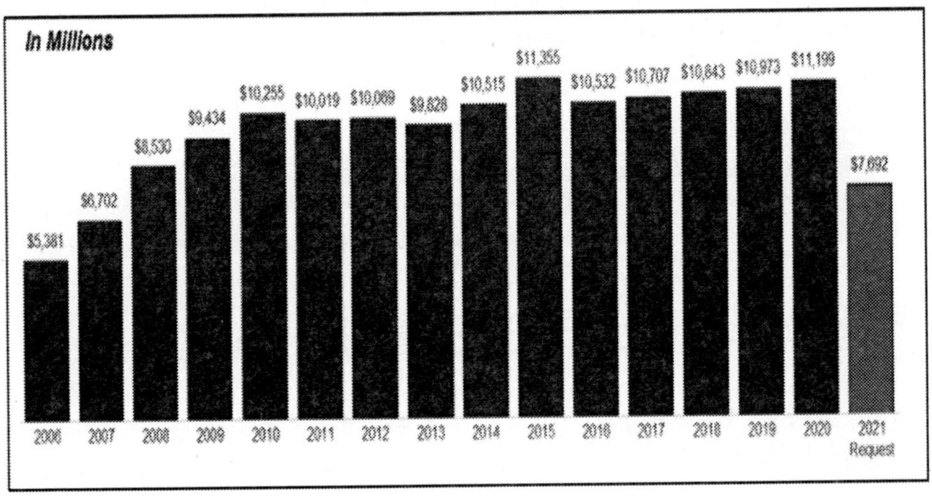

Source: Kaiser Family Foundation.

In a May 2020 editorial, the same Lancet magazine which had praised the role of the CDC in global health monitoring in 2014 lambasted the Trump Administration in an editorial for having "chipped away at the CDC's capacity to combat infectious diseases". It went to the extent of saying that "Americans must put a president in the White House come January 2021, who will understand that public health should not be guided by partisan politics."[36]

America First has impacted the fight against the coronavirus both in the short-term as well as the long term. In the short term, this has played out through multiple instances such as ham-handed efforts by the United States Administration to give a French drug maker millions of dollars for research in return for first preference when it came to obtaining the drug.[37] The same company, Sanofi, had been the subject of controversy just the previous month that President Trump's advocacy of Hydroxychloroquine (HCQ) was because he had a stake in Sanofi which was the distributor for the drug in the United States.[38]

Trump has also used the pandemic to push through on his favourite issue, immigration, signing an executive order on 23 April to block the issuance of green cards to most categories of prospective immigrants, and a subsequent order on 22 June suspending entry into the United States of H1B visa holders.[39] The latest proclamation has resulted in a humanitarian crisis of sorts for family members who were out of the country when international travel was stopped and now face the prospect of being apart indefinitely.[40] This was on top of the existing hardships faced by H1B holders in the United States who were now facing the risk of going out-of-status and being deported if they went over the limit of being unemployed for more than 60 days.[41]

In short, the Trump Administration and the Coronavirus have been playing a biological version of Mutually Assured Destruction (MAD) with the coronavirus presently ahead with the loss of over 116,000 American lives, more than the United States death toll during the entire course of the 2nd World War, and no vaccine in sight.[42] As a writer in the Atlantic magazine aptly put it:

> In the fullness of time, many books will be written about why a country as rich, powerful, and scientifically advanced as the United States failed quite so badly at coping with a public-health emergency that experts had predicted for many years. As is always the case, competing explanations will quickly emerge. Some will focus on the incompetence of the Trump administration, while others will draw attention to the country's loss of state capacity; some will argue that the United States is an outlier, while others will put its failure in the context of other countries, such as Brazil and Russia that are also faring poorly.[43]

The reality, no doubt, is much more complex and nuanced than the foibles of one individual or the idiosyncrasies of the Administration in office, but, without a doubt, the United States, the focal point of scientific and technological prowess on the planet, could have performed much better in it fight against the virus, than it has done so far. In the long march of history, the US response to the Coronavirus will come to be seen as a monumental tragedy of errors, resulting in a huge and unnecessary loss of life due to the incompetence exhibited by the US leadership in a time of crisis.

NOTES

1. Politicians of rival parties in India even held the visit responsible for the large number of COVID-19 infections in the state subsequently. 'Namaste Trump' Event Behind COVID-19 Spread In Gujarat: Sena MP Sanjay Raut,' *Outlook India*, 31 May 2020, available at https://www.outlookindia.com/website/story/india-news-namaste-trump-event-behind-covid-19-spread-in-gujarat-sena-mp-sanjay-raut/353864, accessed on 29 June 2020
2. Lauren Egan, 'Trump Calls Coronavirus Democrats' 'New Hoax',' *NBCNews.com*, 29 February 2020, available at www.nbcnews.com/politics/donald-trump/trump-calls-coronavirus-democrats-new-hoax-n1145721, accessed 15 June 2020.
3. Centers for Disease Control and Prevention, 'First Travel-related Case of 2019 Novel Coronavirus Detected in United States,' available at www.cdc.gov/media/releases/2020/p0121-novel-coronavirus-travel-case.html, accessed 05 June 2020.
4. HHS Press Office, "Secretary Azar Declares Public Health Emergency for United States for 2019 Novel Coronavirus", January 31, 2020, at /www.hhs.gov/about/news/2020/01/31/secretary-azar-declares-public-health-emergency-us-2019-novel-coronavirus.html, accessed June 05, 2020.
5. Dakin Andone, "US travel restrictions go into effect to combat coronavirus spread", *CNN*, February 03, 2020, at www.edition.cnn.com/2020/02/02/us/coronavirus-us-travel-restrictions/index.html, accessed June 05, 2020.
6. The White House, "15 Days to Slow the Spread", March 16, 2020, at www.whitehouse.gov/articles/15-days-slow-spread/, accessed June 05, 2020.
7. Centers for Disease Control and Prevention, 'Overview of Testing for SARS-CoV-2,' available at /www.cdc.gov/coronavirus/2019-ncov/hcp/testing-overview.html?CDC_AA_refVal= https%3A%2F%2Fwww.cdc.gov%2Fcoronavirus%2F2019-ncov%2Fhcp%2Fclinical-criteria.html, accessed 05 June 2020.
8. David Shepardson, 'U.S. Agency Investigating Production of Faulty Coronavirus Test Kits,' *Reuters*, 2 March 2020, available at www.in.reuters.com/article/china-health-test-kits/u-s-agency-investigating-production-of-faulty-coronavirus-test-kits-idINKBN20P0C8, accessed 05 June 2020, see also Steve Eder, Megan Twohey and Apoorva Mandavilli, "Antibody Test, Seen as Key to Reopening Country, Does Not Yet Deliver", *The New York Times*, 19 April 2020, available at www.nytimes.com/2020/04/19/us/coronavirus-antibody-tests.html, accessed 05 June 2020.
9. Julia Belluz and Brian Resnick, 'The Coronavirus Diagnostic Testing Snafu, explained,' *Vox*, 29 February 2020, available at www.vox.com/science-and-health/2020/2/28/21155917/preparing-for-coronavirus-in-the-us-cdc-diagnostic-testing, accessed 05 June 2020, see also Joe Hasell, 'Testing early, Testing Late: Four countries' approaches to COVID-19 Testing Compared,' Our World in Data, 19 May 2020, available at www.ourworldindata.org/covid-testing-us-uk-korea-italy, accessed 05 June 2020.
10. Stefan Thomke, 'Why Is the U.S. Behind on Coronavirus Testing?,' *Harvard Business Review*, 30 March 2020, available at www.hbr.org/2020/03/why-is-the-u-s-behind-on-coronavirus-testing, accessed June 05, 2020, see also Brian Resnick and Dylan Scott, 'America's shamefully slow coronavirus testing threatens all of us,' *Vox*, 12 March 2020, available at www.vox.com/science-and-health/2020/3/12/21175034/coronavirus-covid-19-testing-usa, accessed 05 June 2020.
11. Rebecca L. Haffajee and Michelle M. Mello, 'Thinking Globally, Acting Locally – The U.S. Response to COVID-19,' *The New England Journal of Medicine*, 28 May 2020, available at

www.nejm.org/doi/full/10.1056/NEJMp2006740, see also Jacquelyn Corley, 'U.S. Government Response To COVID-19 Was Slow. But How Does It Compare To Other Countries?,' *Forbes*, 10 April 2020, available at www.forbes.com/sites/jacquelyncorley/2020/04/10/us-government-response-to-covid-19-was-slow-but-how-does-it-compare-to-other-countries/#66b3410a6dc2, accessed 05 June 2020.

12. Centers for Disease Control and Prevention, 'Strategies to Optimize the Supply of PPE and Equipment,' available at www.cdc.gov/coronavirus/2019-ncov/hcp/ppe-strategy/index.html, accessed 05 June 2020, see also Matthew Herper and Helen Branswell, 'Shortage of Crucial Chemicals creates New Obstacle to U.S. Coronavirus Testing,' *Stat News*, 10 March 2020, available at www.statnews.com/2020/03/10/shortage-crucial-chemicals-us-coronavirus-testing/ , accessed 05 June 2020, see also Chris Canipe and Travis Hartman, 'The COVID-19 Testing Challenge,' *Reuters*, 13 May 2020, available at www.graphics.reuters.com/HEALTH-CORONAVIRUS/TESTING/azgvomklmvd/, accessed 05 June 2020.
13. US Food and Drug Administration, 'FAQs on Shortages of Surgical Masks and Gowns during the COVID-19 Pandemic,' available at www.fda.gov/medical-devices/personal-protective-equipment-infection-control/faqs-shortages-surgical-masks-and-gowns-during-covid-19-pandemic, accessed 05 June 2020.
14. Anshu Siripurapu, 'What Is the Defense Production Act?,' *Council on Foreign Relations*, 29 April 2020, at www.cfr.org/in-brief/what-defense-production-act, accessed 05 June 2020, see also Yelena Dzhanova, 'Trump Compelled these Companies to make Critical Supplies, but most of them were Already doing it,' *CNBC*, 04 April 2020, available at www.cnbc.com/2020/04/03/coronavirus-trump-used-defense-production-act-on-these-companies-so-far.html, accessed 05 June 2020.
15. Zolan Kanno-Youngs and Ana Swanson, 'Wartime Production Law Has Been Used Routinely, but Not with Coronavirus,' *The New York Times*, available at www.nytimes.com/2020/03/31/us/politics/coronavirus-defense-production-act.html, accessed 5 June 2020.
16. US Department of the Treasury, 'The CARES Act Works for All Americans,' available at www.home.treasury.gov/policy-issues/cares, accessed 10 June 2020.
17. Tony Samp, Steven R. Phillips and Nathaniel J. Bell, 'US $2T stimulus COVID-19 Package Includes significant R&D Funding,' *DLA Piper*, 10 April 2020, available at www.dlapiper.com/en/us/insights/publications/2020/04/us-2t-stimulus-covid-19-package-includes-significant-randd-funding/, accessed on 10 June 2020.
18. Miranda A. Franco, Lisa Hawke, Robert H. Bradner and Ethan Jorgensen-Earp, 'Coronavirus Response - CARES Act Summary,' *Holland and Knight*, 30 March 2020, available at www.hklaw.com/en/insights/publications/2020/03/coronavirus-response-cares-act-summary, accessed on 10 June 2020.
19. Centers for Disease Control and Prevention, 'Information for Clinicians on Investigational Therapeutics for Patients with COVID-19,' 25 April 2020, available at www.cdc.gov/coronavirus/2019-ncov/hcp/therapeutic-options.html, accessed on 10 June 2020.
20. US Food and Drug Administration, 'Coronavirus Treatment Acceleration Program (CTAP),' 12 May 2020, available at www.fda.gov/drugs/coronavirus-covid-19-drugs/coronavirus-treatment-acceleration-program-ctap, accessed 10 June 2020.
21. US Department of Health and Human Services – National Institutes of Health, 'NIH begins clinical trial of hydroxychloroquine and azithromycin to treat COVID-19,' 14 May 2020, available at www.nih.gov/news-events/news-releases/nih-begins-clinical-trial-hydroxychlo roquine-azithromycin-treat-covid-19, accessed on 10 June 2020.

22. Neha Arora and Sumit Khanna, "India exports 50 million hydroxychloroquine tablets to U.S. for COVID-19 fight", *Reuters*, 30 April 2020, available at www.in.reuters.com/article/health-coronavirus-india-hydroxychloroqu/india-exports-50-million-hydroxychloroquine-tablets-to-u-s-for-covid-19-fight-source-idINKBN22C2M6, accessed on 10 June 2020.
23. Moderna, 'Moderna's Work on a COVID-19 Vaccine Candidate,' available at www.modernatx.com/modernas-work-potential-vaccine-against-covid-19, accessed on 10 June 2020.
24. Jon Harper, 'COVID-19 NEWS: Army Identifies Leading Vaccine Candidate,' *National Defense*, 11 June 2020, available at www.nationaldefensemagazine.org/articles/2020/6/11/covid-19-news-army-making-progress-in-race-for-vaccine, accessed on 10 June 2020, see also Karen Jowers, 'Army COVID-19 vaccine candidate to be tested on humans,' *Military Times*, 11 June 2020, available at www.militarytimes.com/pay-benefits/2020/06/11/army-covid-19-vaccine-candidate-to-be-tested-on-humans/, accessed on 10 June 2020.
25. Bill Hutchinson, ''Operation Gridlock': Convoy in Michigan's Capital Protests Stay-at-Home Orders,' *ABC News*, 16 April 2020, available at www.abcnews.go.com/US/convoy-protesting-stay-home-orders-targets-michigans-capital/story?id=70138816, accessed on 15 June 2020.
26. Carl Zimmer, 'Most New York Coronavirus Cases Came From Europe, Genomes Show,' *The New York Times*, 09 April 2020, available at www.nytimes.com/2020/04/08/science/new-york-coronavirus-cases-europe-genomes.html, accessed on 15 June 2020.
27. Adam Kelsey, 'Arkansas governor calls on Trump to invoke Defense Production Act to increase testing capacity,' *ABC News*. 28 June 2020, available at https://abcnews.go.com/Politics/arkansas-governor-calls-trump-invoke-defense-production-act/story?id=71491985, accessed on June 28, 2020.
28. Rachan Pradhan, 'Abandoned by Trump's White House: Inside states' mad scramble to buy their own ventilators,' *Salon*, 16 June 2020, available at https://www.salon.com/2020/06/16/abandoned-by-trumps-white-house-inside-states-mad-scramble-to-buy-their-own-ventilators-_partner/, accessed on 29 June 2020.
29. Liptak, Kevin, et al., 'Trump Says He Wants the Country 'Opened up and Just Raring to Go by Easter,' despite Health Experts' Warnings,' *CNN*, Cable News Network, 25 March 2020, available at edition.cnn.com/2020/03/24/politics/trump-easter-economy-coronavirus/index.html, accessed on 29 June 2020.
30. Jonathan Chait, 'Trump Wants to Starve the States Into Opening Before It's Safe,' *New York*, 20 April 2020, available at https://nymag.com/intelligencer/2020/04/trump-coronavirus-open-state-governors-protests.html accessed on 29 June 2020.
31. 'Why is the US experiencing a Coronavirus Resurgence?,' *Economic Times*, 25 June 2020, available at https://economictimes.indiatimes.com/news/international/world-news/why-is-the-us-experiencing-a-coronavirus-resurgence/articleshow/76632122.cms, accessed on 29 June 2020.
32. Deccan Chronicle, Conspiracy theories thriving online accuse Bill Gates of starting the virus outbreak, 18 May 2020, available at https://www.deccanchronicle.com/technology/in-other-news/180520/conspiracy-theories-thriving-online-accuse-bill-gates-of-starting-the.html accessed on 29 June 2020.
33. Liz Alesse, 'Did Trump Try to Cut the CDC's Budget as Democrats Claim?: ANALYSIS,' *ABC News*, 29 February 2020, available at www.abcnews.go.com/Politics/trump-cut-cdcs-budget-democrats-claim-analysis/story?id=69233170, accessed on 15 June 2020.
34. Anne Schuchat et al., 'Global Health and the US Centers for Disease Control and Prevention,' *The Lancet*, vol. 384, no. 9937, 2014, pp. 98–101.
35. 'CDC to Cut by 80 Percent Efforts to Prevent Global Disease Outbreak,' *The Washington Post*,

01 February 2018, available at www.washingtonpost.com/news/to-your-health/wp/2018/02/01/cdc-to-cut-by-80-percent-efforts-to-prevent-global-disease-outbreak/, accessed on 15 June 2020.

36. 'Reviving the US CDC,' *The Lancet*, Elsevier, 16 May 2020, available at www.thelancet.com/journals/lancet/article/PIIS0140-6736(20)31140-5/fulltext, accessed on 15 June 2020.
37. "French Fury after Sanofi Says US to Get COVID-19 Vaccine First", *The Economic Times*, 14 May 2020, available at www.economictimes.indiatimes.com/news/international/business/french-fury-after-sanofi-says-us-to-get-covid-19-vaccine-first/articleshow/75735107.cms, accessed on 15 June 2020.
38. Peter Baker et al., 'Trump's Aggressive Advocacy of Malaria Drug for Treating Coronavirus Divides Medical Community,' *The New York Times*, 07 April 2020, available at www.nytimes.com/2020/04/06/us/politics/coronavirus-trump-malaria-drug.html, accessed on 15 June 2020.
39. 'Proclamation Suspending Entry of Aliens Who Present a Risk to the U.S. Labor Market Following the Coronavirus Outbreak,' *White House*, 22 June 2020, available at https://www.whitehouse.gov/presidential-actions/proclamation-suspending-entry-aliens-present-risk-u-s-labor-market-following-coronavirus-outbreak/, accessed on 29 June 2020
40. Ishani Dattagupta, 'Trump's H1-B order makes it impossible for many Indians to return to their lives in the US,' *Economic Times*, 29 June 2020, available at https://economictimes.indiatimes.com/nri/visa-and-immigration/trumps-h1-b-order-makes-it-impossible-for-many-indians-to-return-to-their-lives-in-the-us/articleshow/76663260.cms, accessed on 29 June 2020
41. Olivia Carville and Shelly Banjo, 'Over 200,000 H-1B Workers Could Lose Legal Status by June,' *Bloomberg*, 28 April 2020, available at www.bloomberg.com/news/articles/2020-04-28/200-000-h-1b-workers-could-lose-right-to-work-live-in-the-u-s, accessed on 15 June 2020.
42. Lance Lambert, 'The Coronavirus Death Toll in the U.S. Has Officially Surpassed That of WWI,' *Fortune*, 16 June 2020, available at www.fortune.com/2020/06/16/coronavirus-deaths-us-covid-19-death-toll-higher-wwi-total-how-many-dead/, accessed on 15 June 2020.
43. Yascha Mounk, 'The Virus Will Win,' *The Atlantic*, 12 June 2020, available at www.theatlantic.com/ideas/archive/2020/06/virus-will-win/612946/, accessed on 15 June 2020.

8

Economic and Political Implications of COVID-19 in Latin America

Syed Ali

In the last 100 years, more than 400 million lives have been lost to ten pandemics worldwide. Major outbreaks included the Spanish flu (1918-1920), Asian flu (1957-1958), Hong Kong flu (1968-1970), Swine flu (2009-2010), and the contagious COVID-19 virus. The spread of the COVID-19 or the Coronavirus has been exponential, infecting millions and affecting businesses worldwide. The faster mobility of the diseases is attributed to the access of connectivity for people; spreading germs through contact. As a result of this, the COVID-19 virus in Wuhan, China, has changed several hotspots, beginning with the country of origin and then shifting to Western Europe, the United States of America, and now Latin America. Latin America has had a traumatic relationship with pandemics because of its colonial past. The Spanish invasion also transmitted the smallpox virus wiping out almost 90 percent of the indigenous population.

Latin America has taken over the United States as the new epicenter of the COVID-19 pandemic, with Brazil as the hotspot of the outbreak with over 1.3 million cases. Mexico has reported over 200,000 cases, Peru has over 280,000 cases, cases in Chile are near 270,000 and over 55,000 in Ecuador. In Colombia, the number of confirmed cases is over 91,000, while Argentina has over 59,000 confirmed cases.[1] The worrying trend in the shifting of the epicenter is its descent from high-income countries to medium and low-income countries. As a result, Latin America is profoundly affected by the Coronavirus due to its struggling healthcare infrastructure, and the economic apprehensions which may engulf the region soon and prove to be more fatal than the Corona Virus itself. As of now, over half of the active coronavirus cases are in the Americas, predominantly concentrated in three countries; the USA, Brazil, and Peru. Subsequently, the World Health Organization (WHO) has designated Latin America as the new epicenter of the COVID-19 virus.[2] Brazil has the most number of cases followed by Peru, Chile, and Mexico. Moreover, Argentina, Chile, Colombia, Ecuador, Guatemala and Peru are each forecasted to see more than 10,000 fatalities. Unfortunately, with the rapid increase in infection and fatalities, testing is becoming a challenge in Latin America.

Figure 1: Rate of Testing for COVID-19 (July 2020)

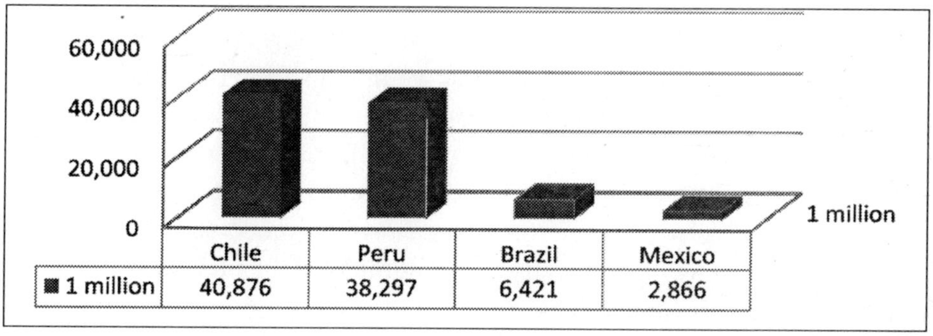

In Peru and Chile, political leaders who initially touted success in managing the pandemic now find their countries overrun by the virus with mounting discontent. The situation in Chile is peculiar, despite its advanced healthcare system, there is a surge in the number of infections as compared to its neighbors. The officials suggest they could soon distribute the world's first 'immunity passport', unfortunately, the health minister who proposed the initiative had to resign due to a further increase in infections. As of now, Chile's deaths per capita dramatically surpass those of Brazil and the United States, and its official number of cases eclipses those of Italy and Iran; erstwhile epicenters of the pandemic.[3] As Chile hunkers down due to the COVID-19 crisis, there is little to dissipate the popular discontent over inequality paralyzing the government last year, and resulting in the abandoning of the prominent UN COP summit. As is the case in much of the world, the spread of the virus has disproportionately affected the country's poor and only underscored societal and economic divisions.

In Brazil, a significant number of deaths have been of younger people, unlike in Europe and the United States, where the elderly were hardest-hit. Latin America faces the acute problem of inequality with sections of extreme poverty, where people live without health coverage and are often driven to work despite the threat of infection. Almost 130 million people in Latin America are part of the unorganized/ informal economy making them vulnerable to fall between gaps of the social security nets. In addition to this, fear of coronavirus and loss of jobs have started to create social unrest.

On 9 June 2020, Carissa Etienne, head of the Pan American Health Organization (PAHO), offered a clinical but dire assessment by moving through a chillingly long list that included countries from Mexico to Chile. She said, "In Mesoamerica, case counts are rising in Mexico, Panama and in Costa Rica, where we are seeing increased transmission around the Nicaraguan border," she said.[4] Costa Rica with one of the lowest COVID-19 infection rates is facing cross-border virus transmission from Nicaragua. In Nicaragua, the government under President Daniel Ortega and Vice President Rosario Murillo his wife, have neglected the pandemic. Despite the instructions from global health organizations to quarantine, wear masks, and adopt social distancing measures, Ortega and Murillo have done the complete opposite by simply ignoring the pandemic. On 13 March 2020, while neighboring countries like El Salvador, Costa Rica, and Honduras had called a state of emergency Vice President Murillo promoted a march titled "Love in times of COVID-19," declaring that in order to combat the virus one must do it "with love and faith" by keeping Businesses, schools, and government offices open.[5] Such disastrous decisions have led to the country having widespread community transmission. This is also having consequences for Costa Rica's Northern Zone sharing a 300 km unfortified border with Nicaragua.

The coronavirus outbreak in Guayaquil, Ecuador's largest city and economic engine, began in February, apparently with infected people returning from Spain. Despite the restrictions, the streets of Guayaquil were littered with corpses, warning how a full-blown outbreak may look like if restrictions are not imposed. Its rapid escalation prompted panicked officials to impose social isolation quickly as a containment strategy. Ecuador imposed strict restrictions on movement and urged its people not to leave their homes at all between the hours of 2 pm to 5 am. This is the second time in a year Quito residents have found themselves under lockdown. In October 2019, a nighttime curfew was established to quell massive protests against austerity measures that were imposed in exchange for a large loan from the International Monetary Fund.[6] Ecuador has been more proactive in responding to the epidemic than many neighboring countries. In Brazil President Jair Bolsonaro has largely downplayed the severity of the coronavirus, despite thousands of new COVID-19 infections reported every day. In Venezuela the power struggle between the government of Nicolás Maduro and the opposition government of Juan Guaidó is impeding a much-needed and coordinated pandemic response.

Most Latin American leaders who have taken decisive steps in combating coronavirus have imposed mobility restrictions to avoid the collapse of their fragile, underfunded health systems. Panama has limited outings based on gender, allowing men and women to leave their homes three days each and for Sundays this applicable to everyone. El Salvador's president sent soldiers to enforce a 48-hour full lockdown in the city of La Libertad and prohibited residents from leaving home including to get food or medicine. Argentina and Venezuela announced national lockdowns just a few days after the first cases were reported. Peru, Chile, and Colombia soon followed suit. By the end of March, eleven countries of the region were in firm lockdown, with others in strict isolation. Countries that took early action have slowed the progress of the virus. In comparison, Ecuador's botched response and Bolsonaro's catastrophic interventions have led to more severe outbreaks. Regardless, the virus continues to spread with alarming speed throughout the region, and in the absence of systematic testing catastrophic repercussions maybe underway. In Mexico, President Andres Manuel Lopez Obrador has also downplayed the need to shut down the economy in order to slow the spread of the virus and began pushing for a reopening weeks ago. He said he plans to resume his trips to smaller cities outside of the capital, where he frequently embraces fervent supporters of all ages flouting social distancing rules.[7]

Public healthcare infrastructure is the key to any country's capacity to deal with the pandemic. In some Latin America countries, the healthcare infrastructure is gutted due to the low expenditure, averaging at 3.7 percent of the GDP, well below the 6 percent mark as recommended by the WHO. This means less preparedness with fewer ICU beds, ventilators, and protection for healthcare workers. However, Cuba is an exception in the region, with its socialist disposition it has strengthened its healthcare system vastly, and it has also devised the policy of 'medical internationalism' and sent out medical assistance to more than a dozen countries. With its long experience of dealing with crisis, Cuba enacted a plan to shut down the tourist industry, shift production priorities to necessary supplies, and protect key workers before any cases had been announced.

In its April 2020 World Economic Outlook of the International Monetary Fund (IMF) predicted an economic contraction of 4.2 percent across the region. This forecast, which if anything was overly optimistic, already points to a far worse recession than the "lost decade" of the 1980s or the 2008–9 crash.[8] The biggest economies will be the worst hit: Mexico, with its reliance on US exports, oil, and remittances, faces a contraction of 6.6 percent; oil-dependent Brazil will contract by 5.3 percent, and Argentina by 5.7 percent, while facing the further challenge of having to renegotiate 98 billion USD in debts. As trade enters an unprecedented decline, corporations go into bankruptcy, currencies are devalued, households default on debts, and unemployment soars, Latin American economies are bracing for a deep and prolonged depression. Latin America has been the slowest-growing region in the Global South. To make things worse, the COVID-19 pandemic has struck at a time when Latin American economies were already facing some of the deepest slumps in recent history. Countries that a decade ago were striking a growth rate of 5 percent and above have fallen to 1 percent or less. Latin American economies are particularly vulnerable because their growth models are predesigned to trade and investment with mainly three countries; China, Europe, and the United States. Demand from these countries for primary commodities like oil, coal, copper, and zinc had been a blessing during the "commodities boom" of high prices, between 2002 and 2012. However, by mid-April 2020, 14 Latin American countries approached the IMF for emergency assistance.[9]

The exigency to rescue a floundering economy during the time of the Pandemic, gives rise to the discomforting conundrum, whether to resume the economy or not. As per Dr. Marcos Espinal, Director of Pan America Health Organization (PAHO), "It is not yet time to reopen, however, each country is sovereign". This debilitating dichotomy has enraged President Jair Bolsonaro, he downplayed the virus by referring it as the 'little flu' and lambasted his governors for imposing restrictions causing the economy to cripple further. Reopening the economy has its repercussion since major Latin American countries; Brazil, Chile, and Mexico, are experiencing daily infection increases of up to four or five percent. However, the economy is also on the ventilator along with its citizens. As described by the General Secretary of the UN Economic Commission for Latin America and the Caribbean (ECLAC) Alicia Barcena, "The crisis could provoke the region's 'worst recession in history", she further added, and "We're worried the region could come out of this crisis with more debt, poorer, hungrier and with more unemployment. And most of all, angry."[10] The Coronavirus has truly struck the very Demography of Latin America and has consequence that may transmit to other facets of its society.

NOTES

1. Robert Dillard, 'The COVID-19 Pandemic: Latin America the New Epicenter; Company Starts First Human Trial of Coronavirus Antibody Therapy; and More,' *Docwirenews*, 1 June 2020, available at https://www.docwirenews.com/home-page-editor-picks/the-covid-19-pandemic-latin-america-the-new-epicenter-company-starts-first-human-trial-of-coronavirus-antibody-therapy/, accessed on 26 June 2020.

2. Anthony Boadle, 'WHO says the Americas are new COVID-19 Epicenter as Deaths Surge in Latin America,' *Reuters*, 26 May 2020, available at https://www.reuters.com/article/us-health-coronavirus-latam/who-says-the-americas-are-new-covid-19-epicenter-as-deaths-surge-in-latin-america-idUSKBN2322G6, accessed on 26 June 2020.
3. Ishaan Tharoor, 'Latin America's Coronavirus Crisis is only Getting Worse,' *The Washington Post*, 26 June 2020, available at https://www.washingtonpost.com/world/2020/06/26/latin-america-coronavirus-crisis/?utm_campaign=wp_ world&utm_medium=referral&utm_source=rss, accessed on 27 June 2020.
4. Debbie Ponchner, 'Latin America Faces a Critical Moment in the Battle against COVID-19,' *Scientific American*, 17 June 2020, available at https://www.scientificamerican.com/article/latin-america-faces-a-critical-moment-in-the-battle-against-covid-19/, accessed on 27 June 30, 2020.
5. Nicaragua: Reckless COVID-19 Response, *Human Rights Watch*, 10 April 2020, available at https://www.hrw.org/news/2020/04/10/nicaragua-reckless-covid-19-response, accessed on 27 June 2020.
6. Dennis Altman and Juan Carlos Valarezo, 'Deaths and Desperation Mount in Ecuador, Epicenter of Coronavirus Pandemic in Latin America,' *The Conversation*, 24 April 2020, available at https://medicalxpress.com/news/2020-04-deaths-desperation-mount-ecuador-epicenter.html, accessed on 27 June 2020.
7. COVID-19 in Latin America and the Caribbean: An Overview of Government Responses to the Crisis, *OECD*, 4 May 2020, available at http://www.oecd.org/coronavirus/policy-responses/covid-19-in-latin-america-and-the-caribbean-an-overview-of-government-responses-to-the-crisis-0a2dee41/, accessed on 27 June 2020
8. World Economic outlook, IMF, April 2020, available at https://www.imf.org/en/Publications/WEO, accessed on 28 June2020.
9. Kyla Sankey, 'An Economic Storm Is Going to Devastate Latin America Very Soon,' *Jacobin*, 28 April 2020, available at https://jacobinmag.com/2020/05/latin-america-economy-coronavirus-pandemic/, accessed on 28 June 2020.
10. 'COVID-19 Roils Latin America as the Region Faces Recession,' *Hindustan Times*, 13 June 2020, available at https://www.hindustantimes.com/world-news/covid-19-roils-latin-america-as-the-region-faces-recession/story-5Zb4uaMlQkYZh1inHb8BbN.html, accessed on 28 June 2020.

Europe and Russia

9

France Response to COVID-19

Elisande Nexon and Frédéric Coste

France has a timely managed system for addressing public health crises, with capacities in terms of monitoring, alerting and care. Planning specifically takes into account the health system's preparedness and organization for exceptional health situations. However, the COVID-19 crisis has still proved to be a challenge, putting a strain on the healthcare system and society as a whole. It has highlighted vulnerabilities to be addressed but also assets to be strengthened as well as insufficiently explored capacities for resilience.

I. The French Public Health Crisis Management System

(i) Brief Outline of the Crisis Management System

Although France initially had a centralised administrative and political structure, it implemented a decentralization ("*déconcentration*") process. At the different territorial levels, a representative of the State, named prefect ("*préfet*"), acts as a guarantee for its effectiveness. This body of civil servants offers the advantage of being present on different scales of action, holding commensurate administrative and operational responsibilities. The decentralization policy involves delegating the minister's decision-making powers to the *départment*-level and regional prefects.[1] France also initiated a devolution policy ("*décentralisation*") by waves (1982-1983, 1986, 2003, 2005, 2010). Many State functions have directly been transferred to local government bodies ("Territorial authorities") in order to ensure a better balance of powers across the Nation and to produce policies more adapted to local particularities.

France has a four-tiered administrative structure: The State consists of 18 regions ("*régions*"),[2] each comprising between 2 and 13 departments (101 "*départments*"). These are in turn divided into municipalities (around 35, 500 "*communes*"). Regions, departments, and municipalities are self-governing communities – with regard to the specific fields devolved to them - administered by assemblies elected by the population concerned. They have their own body of administrative servants, separate from State administration, and responsibility for the interests of the population in their respective area of jurisdiction. The prefects are not involved in the work of these local policy makers, but they play an advisory and partnership role.[3]

Each commune has its own mayor who is chief of the various municipality services. The Mayor is responsible for the every-day public safety on the territory of its municipality (especially for the security and health of the constituents). In case of a crisis, in particular a disaster, the mayor is usually the first to step in. As "Emergency Operations Director", mayor engages the communal means, takes the decisions to safeguards lives, assesses the first damages, and – if necessary – finds shelter for the displaced people. As such, the mayor mobilizes public and private resources present on the territory of the municipality, coordinates communication between all the participants, and provides information to the population. The Mayor must also inform the defence and security zone prefects as well as the *département*-level prefects:

- When more than one municipalities are affected by a crisis,
- When municipality means are not sufficient for responding to the crisis,
- When the mayor officially asks for help,
- Or when the mayor did not take necessary decisions to safeguard the population,

In these cases, the *département*-level prefects take control of the rescue operations. Becoming "Emergency Operations Director", the prefects supports the mayor by mobilizing and coordinating departmental rescue and disaster response means (fire brigade, constabulary, road management and public transport, etc.) when necessary, and by assessing the disaster. However, the mayor is still responsible for the information, evacuation and shelter of the population within the territory of its commune.

Various past events have shown that the regions did not serve as an efficient level for the management of large-scale crises. Responses required more resources than those available at this scale. Thus, political authorities decided during the

2008-2010 period to reinforce an intermediary level: the Defence and Security Zone. The French metropolitan territory is divided into seven zones. When a major crisis involves several *départements*, the prefect of the Defence and Security Zone leading this special territorial jurisdiction may take control of the crisis management. This level is able to perform a more appropriate distribution of resources among the different *départements*, thus sparing the national level from having to respond too widely when a large geographical area is affected.

Each zone-level prefect is responsible for preparing and implementing national security measures, notably those regarding civil security and crisis management, and for supervising actions from *département*-level prefects. The zone-level prefects have been granted competencies to improve planning and crisis management capacities. Among other missions, they are tasked with the translation of governmental planning at the zone level, and with ensuring effective implementation at the level of the *département*. They organise operational surveillance and are responsible for the coordination with military authorities. They oversee civil security means and actions, including both public and private resources (they may requisition them if necessary).

At the national level, while the Prime Minister – as government head – coordinates the public action in case of a major crisis, each ministry is responsible for the preparation and implementation of measures in its competence field. Several have a specific centre dedicated to operational crisis management. However, the Ministry of Interior has a leading role at the Government level: it is responsible for preparing response measures and coordinating the repartition throughout the national territory of emergency resources coming from the State, territorial authorities, and public establishments.

(ii) Specifics of the Health Crisis Management System

During exceptional health emergencies, responsibility for the government's response falls largely under the Ministry of Interior and the Ministry in charge of Health. Among other things, representatives of these ministries play a major role within the inter-ministerial crisis unit ("*cellule interministérielle de crise*"), at the top of the chain of command. The main function of this governmental structure is to produce strategic orientations pertaining to crisis management. The different ministerial and prefect's operational centres must implement these general decisions.

Other public structures are involved in public health crisis management. Created in 2016, *Santé Publique France* ("Public Health France") is the French national health agency. Reporting to the Ministry of Health, this largely autonomous structure brings together functions previously divided among several agencies. Its missions are to:

- Coordinate and implement public health surveillance;
- Study the determinants of changes in trends of diseases;
- Alert national public health authorities on potential threats to health,
- Assist public health authorities in disease control, prevention and health promotion;
- Contribute to the response of health alerts and crises.

When it was founded, it integrated the activities of the *Health Emergency Preparedness and Response Agency* ("*Établissement de préparation et de réponse aux urgences sanitaires*", *EPRUS*) that was created in 2007 to respond to exceptional health situations in France or abroad. The EPRUS managed France's strategic health products stockpiles (pharmaceutical products and medical devices) and the health reserve, providing manpower, material, and logistical resources to reinforce the crisis response system if necessary.[4]

Public Health France is organised in departments, one of which is the infectious diseases department, which has about 60 staff members, including more than 40 epidemiologists. The department is responsible for: national surveillance of infectious diseases (mandatory notifications, laboratory networks, hospital-based networks, etc.); providing assistance to regional level actors in outbreak investigations, coordinating or conducting an investigation of outbreaks of national or interregional importance; conducting or coordinating planned studies (applied epidemiological research) on infectious disease risk factors to guide prevention and control strategies; and evaluating prevention activities or programmes.

Each region is responsible for the management of the regional health system, mainly through a Regional Health Agency ("*Agence Régionale de Santé*"; ARS). Since the mid-1990s, reforms have allowed the regional level a greater remit in governance and health policy decision-making, in particular in the field of planning. Several regional institutions were created, but in 2009-2010, most of these institutions merged into a single "one-stop shop" – ARS – with the aim of achieving better governance of the system, better responsiveness to needs, and higher efficiency. Cutting across the traditional boundaries of healthcare, public health and social care sectors for elderly and disabled people, ARSs which are not directly under the supervision of the ministry in charge of Health – have been created in order to improve the articulation between ambulatory, hospital and health and social care sectors, while respecting national health expenditure objectives.

France has a long tradition of emergency plans. Some of them pertain to specific risks and threats, including biological ones. For example, health authorities published a Pandemic Influenza Plan based upon the World Health Organisation's (WHO) Pandemic influenza risk management guidelines. Adapted to the national context, it contains mitigating measures against pandemic influenza with the aim of limiting casualties and preserving the functioning of society (especially economic activities).

Other plans focus on organisational requirements. Thus, at the national level, health crisis preparation is undertaken pursuant to the organisation plan for the health system response to public health emergencies (ORSAN). It defines care pathways for various emergency situations and determines coordination modalities among the actors, including assignment and management of response measures. Each region is required to have its own White Plan ("*Plan blanc*"), implementation of the national ORSAN plan that spells out exactly what should be done in the case of a mass influx of patients or victims or in the case of an exceptional health crisis situation. These White Plans are mandatory and bring together both public and private healthcare actors to ensure that sufficient resources are available. During a crisis, they are implemented and controlled by prefects. On the ground, each public and private healthcare facilities, especially hospitals, must adopt a declination of the regional White Plan. This emergency management plan contains gradual organisational measures intended to cope with an exceptional *health* situation or increased activity in *the structure*,[5] i.e. reorganisation of the activity and rescheduling of most programmed appointments and hospitalizations; cancellation of training activities in order to mobilize, when justified, the healthcare professionals in day-to-day care; the limitation of professional travel and cancellation of non-priority events.

II. The French Response to the COVID-19 Crisis

(i) Addressing an External Biological Threat

As the crisis worsened in China in January, medical freight was shipped to hospitals in Wuhan and Hubei province to express solidarity with China, with the support of a multinational luxury group and some contributions of civil society organisations. At this stage, the risk of importation of cases from Wuhan in France was still considered moderate and the risk of spread within the population low. From a national perspective, the main issue was the repatriation of French nationals present in the area of the outbreak. The French Ministry for Europe and Foreign Affairs' Crisis and Support Centre, in charge of responding to crisis situations abroad that affect French citizens, played a pivotal role in handling these actions that involved the ministries of Health, Foreign Affairs and Armed Forces.[6]

Several hundred French nationals were repatriated from Wuhan, in some cases along with other Europeans as efforts were coordinated. The first operation involved a French military aircraft from the squadron Esterel with a military medical team on board. Other rounds were operated via specially chartered civilian aircraft, in coordination with other countries to facilitate the repatriation of European citizens. All returnees were placed in quarantine fourteen days upon arrival on the national territory, under medical surveillance, and tested twice.

Then, as the outbreak expanded worldwide, French authorities first called on French nationals abroad to return to the national territory on commercial companies for as long as these were operating, then they had to manage the repatriation of tens of thousands of French nationals stranded abroad. In this context, French nationals living abroad were invited to stay put and to respect the lockdown rules of the host country. Coordinating with the other European States, authorities liaised with national and foreign airlines to organize repatriation by commercial or specially chartered flights. This operation obviously raised political and logistical challenges, for example, due to the closure of frontiers or of civil airports, or the need to bring together nationals scattered on the territory of foreign countries.[7] The Ministry of Foreign Affairs, in collaboration with the International Federation of French and French-Speaking Hosting Abroad (FIAFE), set up an assistance service called "SOS un toit" for nationals stranded on the spot without housing with the aim of putting them in touch with French people living abroad who may welcome them.[8]

The Ebola epidemic in West Africa had previously led to the strengthening of capacities for the repatriation of people likely to be contaminated and to a more in-depth reflection on the problem of evacuating a large number of nationals in the context of a large-scale public health crisis. Still, such an operation had so far remained unprecedented.

(ii) Responding to a Public Health Crisis with an Active Viral Circulation on the National Territory

(a) The Declaration of a State of Health Emergency

Article L3131-1 of the Public Health Code provides the legal framework. It states that "*in the event of a serious health threat requiring emergency measures, in particular in the event of the threat of an epidemic, the Minister responsible for health may, by reasoned order, prescribe, in the interests of public health, any measure proportionate to the risks involved and appropriate to the circumstances of time and place in order to prevent and limit the consequences of possible threats to the health of the population*". The adoption of an emergency law to deal with the COVID-19 strengthened the legal basis.[9] It established the state of health emergency which was subsequently extended by law. It allows the Prime minister to order by decree measures commensurate with the risks involved. They include measures restricting freedom of movement to and from work, freedom of enterprise and freedom of assembly, as well as possibilities to requisition all goods and services necessary to end the health disaster and temporary price control measures.[10]

To help inform public decision-making, the minister in charge of health, Olivier Véran, established on March 10 an *ad hoc* consultative COVID-19 Scientific Council, as required by law. The multidisciplinary group is tasked with providing the latest scientific information, as well as advice on the state of the health crisis and the measures envisaged to deal with it[11]. Jean-François Delfraissy, a clinical immunologist and past coordinator of the French Ebola Task Force, heads this Council. It has published COVID-19 oriented public opinions on matters such as the lockdown, the easing of lockdown, retirement and nursing homes, public health measures pertaining to the electoral process, or children and schools.[12]

If the European Union (EU) offers another framework for action to consider, it is worth recalling public health policies fall within the competence of the Member States, with action by the European Union complementing that of the Member States. Its field of action covers the improvement of public health and the prevention of human illness and disease, health information and education, the fight against major health scourges – by promoting research into their causes, transmission and prevention – as well as the monitoring, warning of and combating serious cross-border threats to health.[13] Still, France was the first country to urge the European Union to take the measure of the crisis, calling for an extraordinary European Council to be held on 10 March 2020 and for coordinated measures.[14]

(b) A Drastic Reorganisation of the Healthcare System to Withstand the Crisis

The organisation of the public health system's response to the emergence of COVID-19 is based on the ORSAN REB plan, which has been activated by the ministry of Health on February 23. Focusing on the epidemic and biological risks, developed, and implemented by each Regional Health Agency, this ORSAN component aims at limiting the SARS-Cov-2 progression and ensuring the care of suspected and confirmed patients. The containment strategy is based on the management of all patients classified as "possible cases" or "confirmed cases" in one of the authorized COVID-19 healthcare facilities. At the earlier stage, the containment strategy was based on the management of all patients classified as "possible" or "confirmed cases" in one of the authorized COVID-19 "frontline" healthcare facilities. When the virus began to circulate more widely, there was then a shift from a logic of individual care to one of collective action, relying on the protection of vulnerable people, ambulatory care of patients without any serious symptoms, and hospital care of severe cases.

In this context, health professionals have largely favoured teleconsultations, leading to a dramatic rise in their number and a trivialization of this practice. Hospitals have changed the organization of their services and adapted their practices, with barrier measures such a prohibition of visits barring derogation, actions aimed at trying to improve daily life for patients, and specific consideration of psychological issues. Non-emergency consultations and operations were postponed, and distance medical monitoring was organized. Local initiatives have been developed to help prevent hospital overcrowding, for example with the creation of COVID-19 care home for upstream triage.

While hospital treatments for patients with serious and chronic illnesses were globally not interrupted, the crisis still induced disturbances in some cases with a reorganisation of care having to balance treatment benefits and COVID-19 risks for patients. The number of medical consultations at hospitals or private doctors' practices also dramatically dropped during the lockdown and medical professionals raised the alert, urging patients to still consult when necessary. Many people cancelled or postponed medical appointments, with an estimated 65 per cent of senior citizens that did not consult their doctors during this period.[15] It has led to disturbances or even interruptions of medical monitoring and care, including for patients with chronic conditions. However, telemedicine is not a suitable alternative for some patients, including for many in the more vulnerable senior population, due to a lack of equipment, know-how, or even audition or cognitive problems. The post-lockdown challenge may thus include the necessity for the public health system to deal with patients requiring more complex medical care, with the risk of increased demands on specific capacities such as medical imaging.

As for other countries severely affected, the crisis has put a strain on the public health system, exacerbating already existing tensions at public hospitals. The health reserve has been solicited to reinforce the system. As of the end of May, crisis management and response have globally shown the resilience of the system, with the existence of real assets. The dedication of health professionals and carers must be commanded. But it has also dramatically highlighted some challenges pertaining to the overall public health system. It has notably put the spotlight on longstanding salary and organizational claims of professionals.

It also showed some vulnerabilities in terms of crisis response *per se* despite regularly updated plans. In addition to questions about the number of resuscitation beds that had to be increased under emergency conditions, the availability and distribution of masks to health professionals caused intense controversies when it became apparent that destroyed stocks had not been replaced leading to shortages. More broadly, supply constraints and shortages of protection equipment, tests or medical products of major therapeutic interest emphasised the need to reassess national requirements, supply chains and local industrial capacities. On another level, some administrative shortcomings may prompt considerations on the organisation of Regional Health Agencies and their adequacy to deal with such demanding circumstances.

(c) The Armed Forces in Support of the Civilian System

The Army Health Service (SSA) contributes to the public service healthcare offer and, because of its expertise, intervenes in the management of exceptional health crises. However, within the French political and administrative system, crisis management is first a civilian operation. Armed forces nevertheless contribute directly to civil security through three civil security military units placed under the authority of the Ministry of Interior. In addition, armed forces can be requested to aid, under the condition that public means are limited, inadequate, unavailable, or non-existent.

In the framework of the national COVID-19 response, the Ministry of Armed forces provides assistance to populations as well as support to public services. It launched the Operation Resilience on 25 March but had been involved since the beginning with the contribution to the repatriation of French citizens from Wuhan. Examples of significant actions include the deployment of the resuscitation military component to reinforce saturated hospital capacities in the East of France, the transportation of health professionals and evacuation of contaminated patients to hospitals in less affected areas, or the provision of health and logistical assistance in overseas French territories. In addition, the French Defence Procurement Agency is in charge of testing prototypes of reusable face masks for the general public sent by French textile manufacturers.

(d) A Broad Mobilisation of the Civil Society

Public health and social care professionals have been on the frontline, but it is also necessary to insist on the mobilisation of all those who allowed the continuity of essential activities (i.e. supply of food and other basic necessities, delivery services, security, refuse collection). Local elected officials also played a key role by launching community initiatives to support vulnerable people and health professionals. Many companies and their employees have also participated in the fight against COVID-19 by redirecting their activities to produce masks, protection equipment or hydroalcoholic gel, first for health professionals and then for the general population. In this respect, there are lessons to be learned from the organisation set up by the textile and clothing sector. The Fashion and Luxury Sector Strategic Committee have acted in cooperation with the General Directorate of Enterprises of the Ministry in charge of the economy, while the French standards association (AFNOR) has provided the barrier mask model and the French Defence procurement agency tests prototypes (DGA) sent by enterprises.

And more broadly, in the spirit of the 2004 law on the modernisation of civil security, if not knowingly, a majority citizens have in many ways become actors of their own security as well as of the collective effort by first accepting the constraints imposed by the lockdown, adapting their life and work practices, which was not a given beforehand.

(e) Imposing Lockdown

Authorities imposed a lockdown from 17 March followed by a gradual easing that was initiated on 11 May. The President of the French Republic, Emmanuel Macron, declared the introduction of lockdown in a televised speech on the evening of 16 March, repeatedly stating that France is at war (the lockdown was then extended twice, on 27 March and 13 April). At the same time, the external borders of the European area were closed, following approval of a European Commission proposal by the Heads of State and Government.

Restrictions took the form of a ban on leaving the place of residence. Motives of exceptions to this interdiction included work-related commuting and travels in case of necessity and in the absence of alternative arrangements, basic necessities purchases, compelling family reasons, assistance to vulnerable people, childcare, health reasons, short moves close to home related to individual physical activity and companion animal needs, and judicial or administrative summons or requests. It was mandatory to carry a handwritten or digital exemption movement certificate, and, for people commuting to go to work, a permanent certificate from the employer. A few days before the lockdown announcement, the government had already decreed the effective closure of all public places not essential to the life of the country, including nurseries, schools, and universities. The care of key workers' children had to be organised.

The imposition of lockdown triggered significant population movements. According to a statistical analysis of anonymized telephone geo-localisation data, nearly 1.2 million inhabitants left Paris and surrounding areas between 13 and 20 March, corresponding to approximatively 17 per cent of the population of this region.[16] Consequently, the population increased notably in some other regions. In addition to concerns related to viral propagation risks, it proved challenging in some tourist areas as public health services and store stocks were not dimensioned to welcome such an influx of people at this period of the year.

Regarding the respect of lockdown restrictions, Google Maps data indicate that, two weeks after the beginning of the lockdown, parks, grocery and pharmacy, and workplace visitation decreased by respectively 88 per cent, 72 per cent and 56 per cent among users that agreed to share their data[17]. Google and Apple data also show a slight relapse at the end of April after the President of the Republic announced on 13 April the end of containment as of 11 May, with a trend towards a gradual return to work and an increase in the frequentation of parks at weekends.[18]

As for the public health sector, the crisis combined with the constraints imposed by the lockdown logically led to the large-scale use of digitalised tools and solutions, but also any other possible means such as phone calls, to ensure as far as possible business and pedagogical continuity. Constraints resulting from restrictions of movements induced evolution of patterns of consumption, with an increase of e-commerce and the promotion of shorter local food supply chains. Despite a global decrease in consumption, some sectors continued to attract clients through the crisis, including do-it-yourself and hardware, household appliances and cycle stores, as well as garden centres.[19]

Despite a broad mobilisation of professionals and the availability of online resources, the virtual school has been especially fraught with challenges as many professionals – and pupils but also parents – had not been previously trained to work and interact in such a dematerialized way.[20] Specific digital workspaces and tools already existed but had not calibrated and tested to deal with such an influx of connections. Moreover, this approach implies that students should have access to the internet, and also adults should be available to help younger ones or those in difficulty. In addition, evaluation by continuous assessment has been preferred when possible while a number of examinations and competitive examinations have been postponed in order to avoid gatherings. For the academic community and in many enterprises, this change in usage was largely carried out under the strain from the crisis, in an extremely short period of time. This forced experience may have induced long-lasting significant modifications of practices. It will thus be necessary to assess their impact in terms of relevance and efficiency, and where appropriate to reflect how to integrate these evolutions in the most sustainable and adapted way possible.

On another level, the crisis disrupted the conduct of the municipal elections. Although the option of a postponement was considered, the government decided to hold the first round of elections on 15 May, after consultations with the political parties and the COVID-19 scientific council a few days before. This led to public health and politically driven controversies. A series of barrier measures was implemented but it did not include wearing masks. While some political leaders pressed for this first round to take place, a consensus emerged afterwards about the need to postpone the second round at least till June. Opinions differ, however, as to whether the results of the first phase should be annulled or kept and scores of actions for annulment have been filed. The epidemiological context undeniably discouraged many voters from going to polling booths. The Emergency Law to Confront the COVID-19 Epidemic stipulates that the election of municipal and community councillors elected in the first round is a foregone conclusion. However, these exceptional circumstances may raise among other issues the questions of representativeness of some future municipal teams.[21]

(f) Challenges Related to the Easing of Lockdown

The lockdown period ended on 11 May. Considering the incubation period, this easing process has been organised in several progressive phases till 22 June to verify that the easing of the restrictions would not result in an increase in contamination above a certain threshold. During the transition period between 11 May and 2 June, a regularly updated map helped to visualize the evolution of the situation with departments in red, orange, or green, with the aim of serving as a reference for the application of differentiated measures from 2 June onwards. It is based on four indicators - the epidemic activity, the rate of positivity of viral tests, the evolution of R0 and the occupancy rate in intensive care units – complemented by a risk analysis. At the end of May, the whole territory was in green except for the Ile-de-France, Guyana and Mayotte which remained in orange. Incidence and occupancy rates in intensive care units explain for example that an enhanced vigilance was still maintained in Paris and in the adjoining departments at the end of May.[22]

After 11 May, while authorities have not imposed the wearing of masks in public spaces, the obligation applies to public transport, schools and nurseries, and in professional environments where barriers cannot be respected. Gatherings in the public areas are limited to 10 people with respect to social distancing, the Constitutional Council refusing to authorise the extension of this prohibition to the private domain. Besides, outside of compelling health, family, or professional reason justified with a certificate, travelling further than 100 km outside the department of residence was also forbidden. The phase 2 on 2 June mostly entailed the reopening of bars and restaurants with the implementation of barrier measures such as wider distances between tables, preceded by the reopening of places of worship parks and gardens. However, 10-people limit remained for gathering in June. Travel is again allowed without limits throughout the country. However, prefects are allowed to restrict movements again, impose again a lockdown at the local level and order the closure of businesses, schools or places of worship, should the epidemiological situation warrant it.

Lockdown made it possible to significantly slow down the spread of the disease on the national territory, but the virus continues to circulate. In the context of the gradual resumption of activities, several challenges arise, the incidence of which is difficult to measure at this stage. On the one hand, there is a need to convince the population to continue to respect the rules of social distancing, since the switch to green areas should not be understood as an absence of risk. In such a context, official guidelines indeed recommend that teleworking remains the preferred option when feasible. On the other hand, there may also be a need to address the situation of people who now find it difficult to leave their homes. Childcare options linked to the reopening of nurseries and schools and the management of public transportation are amongst the key issues that have an impact on work resumption. They raise organizational issues. In many schools, the objective of re-establishing a direct contact at least once with each pupil before the end of the school year appears difficult to reconcile with the concrete implementation of barrier measures on their premises.

Considering the economic impact of the COVID-19 crisis, the massive support granted by the government has mitigated its effects in the short term compared with other countries. It encompassed a range of emergency measures including notably the partial unemployment scheme, state-guaranteed emergency bank loans for enterprises, exemptions from charges or a solidarity fund financed by the state and the regions to help the smallest businesses affected by the crisis.[23] To mitigate the middle and long-term consequences of the crisis, the government has launched a series of sectoral plans of investments to help recovery and transformation, focusing among others on the fields of tourism, automotive, aeronautics and catering.[24] The minister responsible for the budget summed it up by saying that the government has chosen debt over bankruptcy which will result in an increase in a public debt that is expected to exceed 100 per cent significantly contrary to pre-crisis forecasts.[25] This aid scheme has prevented an explosion in unemployment and should help economic recovery, as the purchasing power of French households has been globally less affected by the economic downturn than in other countries. However, the true extent of the impact on businesses can only be really assessed in the coming months. The minister in charge of the Economy indeed warned that a surge in bankruptcies and layoffs was to be expected in the months following the peak of the crisis.[26]

Like other countries where strict lockdown has been imposed, France faces the challenge of both economic recovery and the resumption of a collective life marked by new practices of social distancing, while preventing the occurrence of a new wave of contamination that could saturate hospital capacity once again. The COVID-19 crisis has highlighted the challenge of maintaining a prevention system in the long term as priorities evolve and the rationale behind decisions may no longer be relevant while gaining adaptability and flexibility capacities to address potential administrative, legal, and organizational hurdles in a constrained timeframe. But it has also shown society's ability to mobilise and adapt, from citizens to businesses, to deal collectively with a situation which, until recently, would have been difficult for many to envisage. All these strengths and weaknesses will have to be taken into account in order to adapt the system to cope with the next exceptional crisis.

NOTES

1. Local branches of central ministries are directly controlled by the prefect.
2. The 18 regions include 5 overseas territories.
3. Prefects are also responsible for the verification of the legality of the territorial authorities' decisions.
4. This corps of health reservists includes working and retired health professionals as well as students at the end of their studies, who are prepared to intervene on the ground if needed (with 6 000 voluntary reservists, mostly doctors and nurses).
5. White Plan covers general major emergencies, but every hospital adapts its contents to their local context. If the increase of activity involves several hospitals, an Extended White Plan is triggered to coordinate both impacted hospitals and the hospitals receiving the evacuees. The ARSs are one of main decision makers in the development and application of the Extended White Plan.
6. France Diplomatie, *Chine – Envoi de fret médical en solidarité avec la Chine à destination des structures hospitalières de Wuhan et de la province du Hubei*, 19 February 2020.
7. 'Coronavirus : le rapatriement des Français bloqués à l'étranger "est un travail politique et logistique"' *radioFrance*, 25 March 2020, available at https://www.francetvinfo.fr/sante/maladie/coronavirus/coronavirus-le-rapatriement-des-francais-bloques-a-letranger-est-un-travail-politique-et-logistique_3884461.html, accessed on 22 May 2020

8. Ministry of Europe and Foreign Affairs, available at http://www.sosuntoit.fr/, accessed on 23 May 2020.
9. Emergency law n°2020-290 of 23 March to respond to Covid-19, *JORF*, n°72, 24 March 2020.
10. Vie Publique, 'What is a state of health emergency?' available at https://www.vie-publique.fr/fiches/273947-quest-ce-que-letat-durgence-sanitaire accessed on 24 May 2020.
11. Règlement intérieur du Conseil Scientifique COVID-19, 30 April 2020, available at https://solidarites-sante.gouv.fr/IMG/pdf/reglement_interieur_cs.pdf accessed on 25 May 2020.
12. COVID-19: COVID-19 Scientific Council, available at https://solidarites-sante.gouv.fr/actualites/presse/dossiers-de-presse/article/covid-19-conseil-scientifique-covid-19 accessed on 28 May 2020.
13. Article 168 of the Treaty on the Functioning of the European Union.
14. European Solidarity with COVID-19, 17 April 2020, available at https://www.diplomatie.gouv.fr/fr/politique-etrangere-de-la-france/europe/evenements-et-actualites-lies-a-la-politique-europeenne-de-la-france/actualites-europeennes/article/la-solidarite-europeenne-face-au-covid-19, accessed on 31 May 2020.
15. ERGOCALL '65% of Seniors at Home have not Consulted a Doctor Since the Start of Confinement,' *Caducee. Net*, 29 May 2020, available at https://www.caducee.net/actualite-medicale/14951/65-des-seniors-a-domicile-n-ont-consulte-aucun-medecin-depuis-le-debut-du-confinement.html accessed on 31 May 2020.
16. Untersinger Martin, Confinement: plus d'un millions de Franciliens ont quitté la région parisienne en une semaine, *Le Monde*, 26 March 2020.
17. Dumoulin Sébastien, Confinement: Google publie des données de géolocalisation dans 131 pays, *Les Echos*, 03 April 2020.
18. Licata Caruso Damien and Alexandre Victor, Confinement: un léger relâchement observé fin avril, selon les données d'Apple et Google, *Le Parisien*, 05 May 2020.
19. Margaux Duguet, 'FRANCEINFO SURVEY. How the Rigidity and Slowness of the Administration Weighed Down French Management of the COVID-19 Crisis,' *FRANCEINFO*, 21 May 2020, available at https://www.francetvinfo.fr/sante/maladie/coronavirus/enquete-franceinfo-comment-la-rigidite-et-les-lenteurs-de-la-bureaucratie-ont-plombe-la-gestion-francaise-de-la-crise-du-covid-19_3962461.html accessed on 31 May 2020.
20. Cerisier Jean-François, Covid-19, ce que la continuité pédagogique nous apprend de l'école, The Conversation, 19 May 2020.
21. Emery Audrey, Pluie de recours contre le premier tour des municipales, *Le.Point.fr*, 28 May 2020.
22. France Government, 7 June 2020 available at https://www.gouvernement.fr/info-coronavirus/carte-et-donnees#activite-epidemique accessed on 8 June 2020.
23. The portal for the Economy, Finance, Action and Public Accounts, available at https://www.economie.gouv.fr/covid19-soutien-entreprises accessed on 31 May 2020.
24. AFP, Industrie aéronautique française: le dispositif de soutien se précise, *Le Journal de l'Aviation*, 28 May 2020.
25. Le coup de pouce supplémentaire de l'Etat aux secteurs les plus touchés par la crise, *Capital*, 25 May 2020.
26. 'Des faillites et des licenciements dans les mois qui viennent', prévient Le Maire, *Paris Match*, 25 May 2020.

10

Coronavirus in Spain

Maria J. Espona

The spread of COVID-19 surprised Spain in the worst way possible, shaking its healthcare system and its population in a way that reminded them of the 1918 Spanish Flu outbreak.

A National government recently formed, with some particularities, was able to cope with the situation, however, paying a price too high in human lives with the disease.

This chapter will analyze the situation in Spain, considering not only the specific aspects related to the pandemic but the social event so dear to the Spanish society that affected the evolution of the disease in the country.

Background

The Kingdom of Spain is located in southwestern Europe and bordering with Portugal and France and the Mediterranean Sea and the North Atlantic Ocean (Bay of Biscay).

In order to understand the response to the COVID-19 outbreak it is important to know how the country's administration is organized. Spain is a parliamentary monarchy, the Head of State is the King but the executive branch is constituted by a Council of Ministers led by the Prime Minister, nominated by the King after consultations with different parliamentary groups, then voted by the lower house and finally formally appointed by the Head of State.[1]

The Kingdom of Spain is a decentralized country: it has 17 different autonomous communities (Figure 1), each of them has its administrative structure including budget and resources and they manage their health and education system.

Figure 1: Autonomic Communities Map.[2]

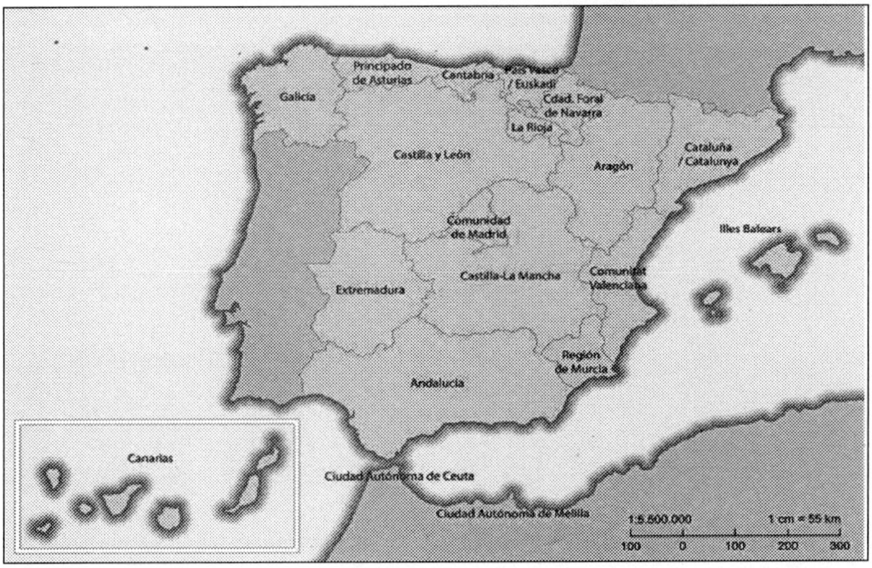

Not all the autonomic communities are organized equally and some of them are divided into provinces and others not. The variability in the country regarding the internal organization as well as infrastructure, economic activities and resources are extremely high. As we will see later, this consideration will have an impact on the response to the COVID-19 crisis.

COVID-19 in Spain

It is not really confirmed as to when COVID-19 arrived in Spain. However, there is a certain agreement about a case detected on 31 January.[3] The patient who tested positive, from German origin, was admitted to La Gomera with mild symptoms and he may have been in contact with a German infected businessman. Nine days after that, a new case was detected in Palma. And on 24 February, multiple cases were detected in other communities.[4]

After these couple of cases, the number of cases in Spain started to grow exponentially and reached a peak on 20 March 2020 (Many sources put the peak on the 31 March as well).[5]

Figure 2: Pandemic growth curve. TC: growth rate, TD: doubling rate, FP: peak date, TR: halving rate. Data obtained from individualized data reported to RENAVE (Red Nacional de Vigilancia Epidemiológica – Epidemiological Surveillance National Network).[6]

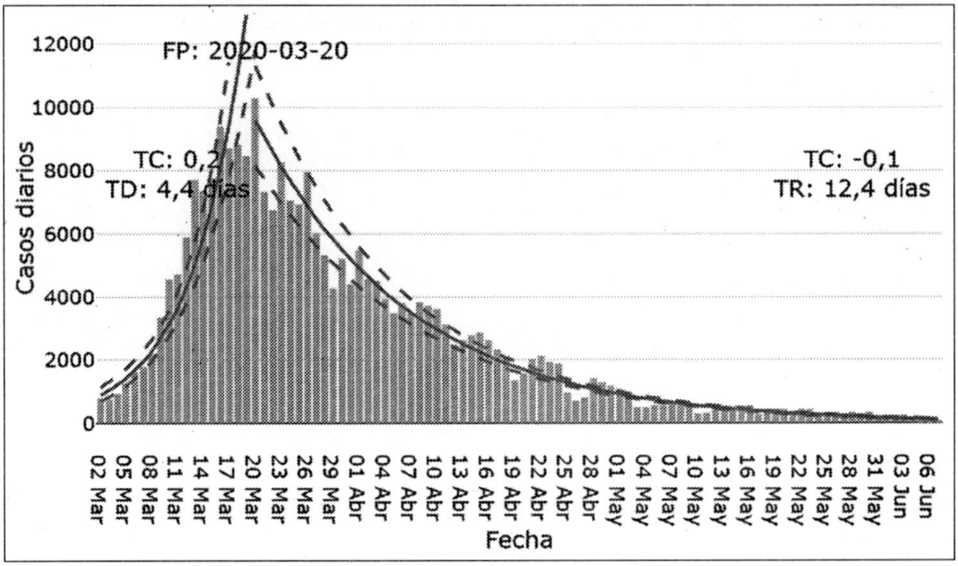

A scientific publication by Francisco Díez-Fuertes and other experts[7] mentions that a 'Phylogenetic analyses of the first 28 SARS-CoV-2 whole genome sequences obtained from patients in Spain revealed that most of them are distributed in G and S clades (13 sequences in each) with the remaining two sequences branching in the V clade. Eleven of the Spanish viruses of the S clade and six of the G clade grouped in two different monophyletic clusters (S-Spain and G-Spain, respectively), with the S-Spain cluster also comprising 8 sequences from 6 other countries from Europe and the Americas. The most recent common ancestor (MRCA) of the SARS-CoV-2 pandemic was estimated in the city of Wuhan, China, around 24 November 2019, with 95 percent highest posterior density (HPD) interval from 30 October to 17 December 2019. The origin of S-Spain and G-Spain clusters were estimated in Spain around 14 and 18 February 2020, respectively, with a possible ancestry of Spain in Shanghai'.

Because of this research, a conclusion was reached that 'multiple SARS-CoV-2 introductions have been detected in Spain and at least two resulted in the emergence of locally transmitted clusters, with further dissemination of one of them to at least 6 other countries. These results highlight the extraordinary potential of SARS-CoV-2 for rapid and widespread geographic dissemination.'[8]

Another analysis of the outbreak is by considering the number of new cases in the context of the announcements and public events that took place in Spain early in the pandemic.[9,10] But there is a huge problem when trying to do the above-mentioned analysis: different sources of information show different numbers for the health statistics under consideration, and it is very hard to find them.

Table 1: Main Events of the COVID-19 in Spain
(elaborated by the author with open sources)

Date	*Event*
31/1	First case is diagnosed in Spain
4/2	Council of Ministers approves creation of the Inter-ministerial Coordination Committee to face the threat to Public Health posed by the coronavirus
10/2	2nd case of coronavirus. A British citizen diagnosed in Mallorca
19/2	Valencia-Atlanta (Champions League, in Bergamo (Italy) with 2.500 fans from Valencia and 40.000 from Atlanta)
22/2	WHO recommends basic principles to reduce the risk of transmission and does not recommend specific sanitary measures for travelers
23/2	The Ministry of Health claims in Spain there was no local contagion
25/2	An Italian tourist test positive in a hotel in Tenerife. The first case of mass quarantine
26/2	From 26/2 to 01/03 takes place the Fair ARCO Madrid (93.000 participants)
	A patient from Seville is the first case of local contagion in Spain.
29/2	WHO updates its guide on travel restrictions
1/3	Football league: Real Madrid- FC Barcelona (Santiago Bernabéu)
	Ministry of Health affirms that it is a priority to locate and analyze cases of local contagion
2/3	The European Center for Disease Prevention and Control only recommends exceptionally canceling events with a high presence of attendees from risk areas
3/3	The Ministry of Health decides, with the Autonomous Communities, to hold professional sports competitions behind closed doors. Cancellation of congresses, seminars, workshops or courses in which healthcare professionals participate
	The first fatality due to coronavirus is known: a patient who died in Valencia on 13 February, the disease was detected at a necropsy
4/3	The authorities start talking about distance measures
6/3	The Civil Guard orders to quarantine a group of families from Haro (La Rioja) infected at a funeral. The lieutenant colonel in charge of this operation dies on 27 March due to coronavirus
7/3	WHO statement after over 100,000 cases of COVID-19: China and other countries are showing that the spread of the virus can be stopped through containment measures and control of activities.
	Football League: Atlético de Madrid-Sevilla vs Betis-Real Madrid 110.000 fans
8/3	Massive demonstrations are held because of Women's Day, public events of parties such as Vox and various sports are held normally
	Italy quarantines some 16 million people in Lombardy: confirmed cases exceed 5,800, with more than 230 deaths. The closed area includes Milan and Venice.
9/3	The WHO points out that in countries with community transmission, and depending on the context, the adoption of measures such as the closure of schools, cancellation of massive events and other measures can be considered.
	The Interterritorial Council of the National Health System agrees measures for areas that

Date	Event
	are in a phase of significant community transmission (Madrid/Vitoria/Labastida): Suspension of face-to-face teaching activity at all educational levels and complementary activities; labor flexibility (teleworking, time flexibility, shifts, videoconferences).
10/3	The Council of Ministers approves new measures: Ban direct flights from Italy to Spain from 11 to 25 March and suspension of IMSERSO (Institute for the Elderly and Social Services) travel. In Madrid, La Rioja, Vitoria and Labastida, suspension of activities in closed spaces that gather more than a thousand people.
	Champions League in Anfield (UK), Atlético de Madrid-Liverpool, with 3.000 Atlético de Madrid fans.
11/3	The WHO declares the global pandemic situation[11]
	Futurmoda, International Exhibition of Leather, Components and Machinery for footwear, at the Alicante Trade Fair Institution (about 3,100 professionals)
12/3	The Inter-territorial Council of the SNS[12] agrees to implement educational and social distancing measures throughout Spain, promote home care for the elderly and urge the population to avoid trips that are not necessary. First package of economic measures to cushion the impact on the activity of the coronavirus crisis (18,000 million euros).
13/3	The government announces that it is studying the state of Emergency statement. On this day were 7687 positive cases.
	The WHO states that: "Europe has become the epicenter of the pandemic."
14/3	Spain approves a declaration of a state of Emergency throughout the national territory for a period of fifteen days, starting tomorrow.[13]
15/3	The Ministry of Health establishes measures to reinforce health personnel and the supply of material. The Government launches the campaign #EsteVirusLoParamosUnidos (This Virus We Stop It United)
16/3	Spain decrees the reestablishment of land border controls.
17/3	The EU announces a 30-day ban on most inbound non-essential travel.
	The Second package of economic measures to cushion the impact on the activity of the coronavirus crisis (200,000 million euros).
19/3	The ECB announces a 750 billion Euro plan to help the economy in the eurozone.
20/3	The fatal victims exceed one thousand (1,002), and 10280 new cases. The country begins to organize field hospitals
22/3	The government announces that the state of Emergency will continue for another 15 days (it was approved by the Parliament later on 25 March)
28/3	The government decrees the hardening of the state of Emergency, with a ban on all non-essential activities.
29/3	New cases fall for the first time from a 10 percent daily increase.
	A recoverable paid leave is established for employed workers in sectors affected by the state of Emergency.
2/4	With 950 deaths recorded, this date is the hardest since the beginning of the crisis. The deceased reached 10,003, discharges 26,473 and registered cases, 110,238. However, these have three consecutive days slowing down the rate of increase.
7/4	The death toll rises after three days of relative decline and the total stands at 13,798
9/4	Prime Minister Pedro Sánchez gets parliamentary support for an extension of the State of Emergency until 26 April and declares that this will probably not be the last. The need for a pact between political and social actors is advanced. Sending patients from some Autonomous Communities to others to decongest ICUs. Registered cases slowed

Date	*Event*
	down again but stood at 152,446. The daily death toll falls to 64 victims the previous day but remains at 15,238
14/4	The provisional morgue of the La Nevera ice rink in Majadahonda is closed in Madrid.
17/4	The Government introduces changes in the accounting for the pandemic when inconsistencies are detected, in order to accurately plan the exit from the confinement. New cases remain below 3 percent mark.
18/4	Pedro Sánchez announces an extension of the confinement until 11 May, but with some relaxation measures from 26 April, such as the fact that children up to 12 years of age can leave their homes in a controlled manner from 27 April
23/4	Official announcement of activities for children like one-hour daily walks. The evolution figures of the disease remain stable.
28/4	Plan for Transition to a New Normality is announced [14]
1/5	The IFEMA campaign hospital in Madrid is closed. There is no shortage of controversy on the spot, due to the agglomeration of participants. It is announced that the Spanish GDP will fall this year by 9.2% due to the crisis
2/5	First day of easing lockdown which allowed outdoor activities, in a controlled manner and within stipulated times. The daily death toll stands at 276. For the seventh consecutive day, there are higher discharges than new cases confirmed by PCR
5/5	The Ministry of Health announces that 44,000 health workers have been infected with COVID-19 since the start of the crisis.
12/5	According to the first data from the serological study carried out, there would be no more than 15 percent of the population immune to the coronavirus in Spain. A 14-day quarantine is decreed for those who arrive in Spain.
23/5	Pedro Sánchez affirms that tourism would be allowed from July. The vital minimum income is approved. Car demonstrations against government management are taking place, called by the Vox party
24/5	Contagions reach a minimum of 246 in the last 24 hours. A British report notes that Liverpool-Atlético de Madrid caused 41 added deaths in the UK. Minister Illa announces that phase change dates may be made more flexible.
25/5	Accounting change that affects the statistics of deceased: only those who died in the last 24 hours will be included in it, although a figure is given for cases reported late in the last seven days.
29/5	The First Division League is announced to return on 11 June. More than 51,000 health workers are known to have been infected with coronavirus to date.
30/5	Prince Joaquín of Belgium attends a party in Seville, tests positive, and more than a dozen infections follow.
31/5	The government announces that it will request the sixth and last extension of the state of Emergency.

If we bear in mind the events that took place in Spain since the end of February 2020 until late May, and we study the Figure 3, it is possible to see graphically the positive impact of the measures taken by the government both when it comes to stop the academic activities and the starting of the State of Emergency.

Figure 3: Evolution of Coronavirus Curve (Blue: multiplication of cases; Black: multiplication of deaths).[15]

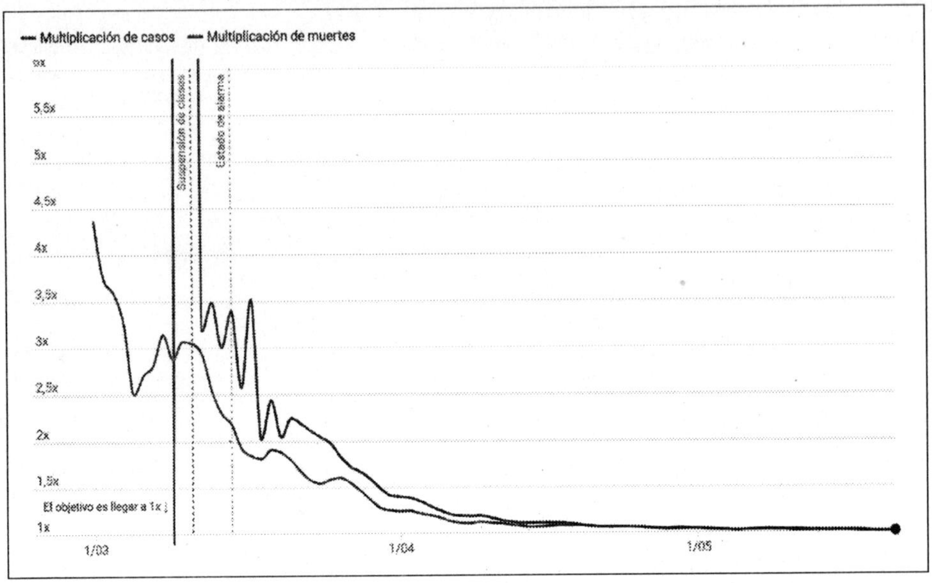

It is also interesting to note that the COVID-19 affected equally men and women, but when it comes to age distribution, the elderly population suffered the most (Figure 4).

Figure 4: Percentage of COVID-19 by Age Group[16]

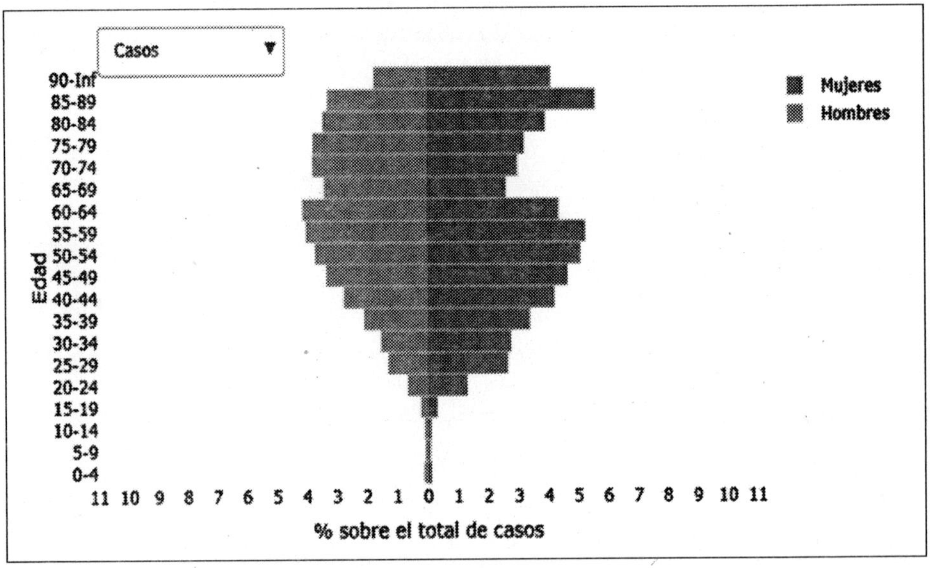

Another interesting analysis is the number of cases per 100,000 habitants and total cases and also the number of deaths per 100,00 and total deaths all by autonomous communities. In Figure 5 it is possible to see how the big cities and communities were the most affected (Madrid and Barcelona).

This figure also shows the importance of choosing the right metric: if we check the situation in La Rioja, considering the number of cases and deaths per 100,00 habitants looks much worse than Madrid, but if we go to the number of cases, we see that the impact is much lower. Something similar happens with Castilla la Mancha.

Figure 5: Statistics by Autonomous Communities[17]

CCAA	Casos por 100K hab.	Casos totales	Muertes por 100K hab.	Muertes totales
La Rioja	1.292	4.063	115	362
Madrid	1.048	70.051	130	8.691
C. La Mancha	868	17.702	144	2.045
Navarra	813	5.303	75	490
C. León	801	19.254	80	1.928
Cataluña	781	59.423	73	5.587
País Vasco	623	13.595	65	1.424
Aragón	439	5.812	62	826
Cantabria	400	2.327	35	202
Galicia	339	9.154	23	609
Extremadura	281	2.983	48	508
Asturias	238	2.431	31	314
C.Valenciana	228	11.381	27	1.332
Ceuta	193	163	5	4
Baleares	179	2.142	17	209
Andalucía	152	12.804	17	1.404
Melilla	145	122	2	2
Murcia	109	1.626	10	148
Canarias	107	2.371	7	151

Fuente: Ministerio de Sanidad · Creado con Datawrapper

Challenges to the Response and Next Steps

One of the challenges related to the Spanish response to the COVID-19 crises was posed by the degree of autonomy of each community:[18] some of them took decisions even beyond its competence, even when the Ministry of Health was in charge of the coordination of the overall response. The different perspective ranks from locating the sick people (if there were enough beds at the hospitals) to reorient factories for producing medical supplies, massive testing, contingency planning, etc., among other measures.[19] These measures did help to cope with the situation but also created chaos in the sense of not having complete coordination with the national authorities, thus, hindering the implementation of a national response.

The Spanish government elaborated on the Plan for transition to 'New normality'[20] or de-escalation plan as a way forward to move from the State of Emergency to the next stage. This plan has 4 phases that could be summarized as follows:

- *Phase 0 or Preparatory:* The economic activity will gradually begin, and also the professional training. The signalization of the public places will begin and other protective measures in preparation for the next phase.
- *Phase 1 or Initial:* Since 11 May, the provinces which meet the criteria, some activities will be allowed to start, especially commercial and with special timeframes for elderly people. Restaurants, hotels and other tourist places could open but with restrictions. Shopping malls will remain closed. Churches and worship centers can open but only could have one-third of its capacity.
- *Phase 2 or Intermediate:* Restaurants bigger than $70m^2$ in area would open with one-third of its capacity, with guaranties of social distancing. Schools will start in September. Other recreational activities, like cinema, theater, hunting and fishing, conferences and other activities would start but at one-third of its capacity. Churches and worship centers can open but only at half of its capacity.
- *Phase 3 or Advanced:* Until back to the new normality, once all the requirements are met, people can move freely in the public places but with protective masks. For commercial activities, the capacity of the paces is limited to a half, plus social distancing between people.

Each province should meet a series of criteria in order to change phases, and the criteria are linked to:

- The capacity of the healthcare system;
- The epidemiologic situation in the area;
- Collective protective measures are taken; and
- Economic and mobility data.

The latest update about the situation regarding the phases is included in Figure 6.

Figure 6: Status on 19 June[21]

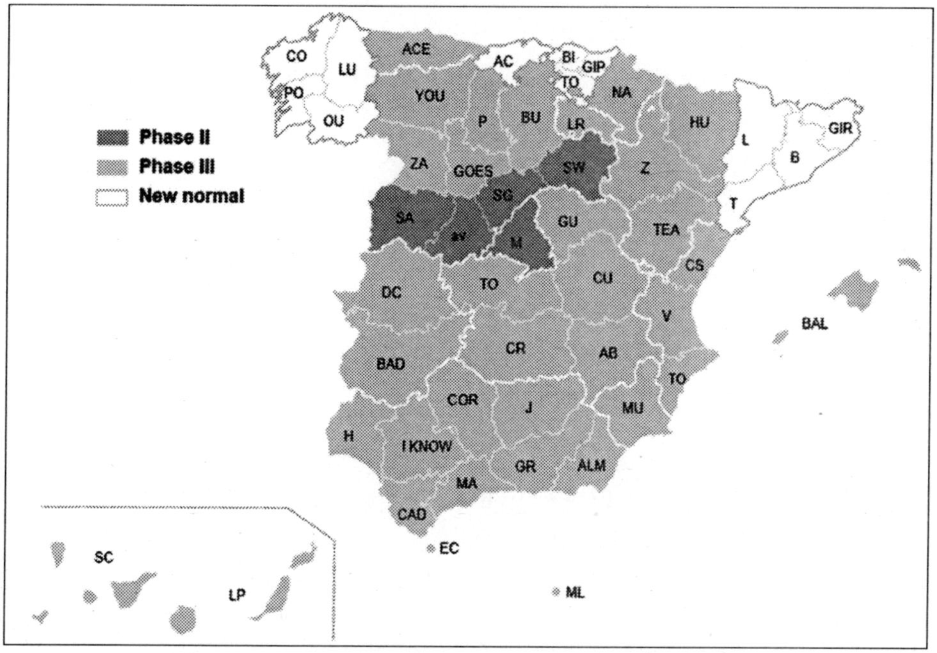

Detection and Diagnostic: Implementation and Challenges

Spain is using 3 types of techniques to detect COVID-19 cases:[22]

- *PCR standard:* it is used in the hospitals and laboratories for the identification of positive cases, the problem is that it takes several hours to get the result, but it is highly specific.
- *PCR rapid test:*[23] developed in Spain, is a real time PCR rapid test for the identification of the COVID-19.
- *Antibodies:* They rely on a paper immunochromatography, that is, a platform that has the virus proteins 'stuck' to detect antibodies or specific antibodies to detect the virus proteins. Its operation is similar to that of pregnancy tests.[24,25,26]

It is important to note that not all the autonomous communities have the same infrastructure to face the pandemic and the same is true when it comes to detection. Even during the early part of the outbreak when the central government recommended to them to have at least one laboratory with detection capacity, this requirement was not easy to meet and, of course, this situation conditioned the response capacity.

Additionally, with the degree of autonomy some of the communities took the WHO recommendation and tested as much as possible while others did less.[27]

The country suffered a set-back when some Chinese rapid tests were defective. They were bought from an unauthorized local supplier named Shenzhen Bioeasy Biotechnology (not included in the list provided by the Chinese government).[28]

Looking to the future, under Horizon 2020, and led by the researcher Laura M. Lechuga, from the Spanish Superior Council of Scientific Research (CSIC), there is the ConVaT European project. This endeavor from the Catalan Institute of Nanoscience and Nanotechnology (ICN2) consists of the development of 'a microchip that allows the detection and qualification of molecules or viruses in a single step, without the need for previous or subsequent amplification. These characteristics indicate that the analysis can be performed in less than 30 minutes'.[29]

Treatment of the COVID-19 Infection and Prevention

The Ministry of Health has developed a protocol for the management and treatment of patients with COVID-19 infection that is continuously updated.[30] Some of the available treatments are newly developed molecules and others are new uses of drugs as authorized in other indications. A large amount of information is constantly generated from all the practitioners and healthcare centers involved in the response, which is analyzed as it becomes available to the agencies.

The drugs and treatments used so far are Remdesivir, Lopinavir/Ritonavir (LPV/r), Cloroquina/Hidroxicloroquina, Tocilizumab (TCZ), Sarilumab, Ruxolitinib (RXT), Siltuximab (STX), Baricitinib (BAR), Anakinra (ANK), and Interferon Beta-1B (IFNb) and Interferon Alpha-2B.[31]

The Puerta de Hierro Majadahonda University Hospital coordinates a controlled clinical trial studying the efficacy and safety of plasma from patients cured of SARS-CoV-2 infection in the treatment of hospitalized patients in the acute phase of COVID-19 disease (ConPlas-19 Study). The study includes more than 20 hospital centers throughout the National Health System of Spain and more than 300 patients.[32]

As part of the prevention strategy, beyond that of social distancing measures, the government started to look for options for local vaccine production once it is discovered[33]. Until the 11 June 2020, the WHO has included 4 Spanish vaccines in its list of initiatives that public centers and companies are investigating globally to find a product against the virus.[34] Enumerated below is the current development:

- At the Poxvirus and Vaccines Group at the National Biotechnology Center of the Higher Council for Scientific Research (CNB-CSIC), and under the coordination of Luis Enjuanes, are working in two approaches to produce a vaccine. One is a vaccine with an attenuated virus by genetic engineering, and the other is a vaccine in which some genes that are important to induce the immune response will be selected and then incorporated into another vector, which is the one that will produce the immune response in an organism.[35]

- Another development is an innovative SARS CoV-2 mRNA/MVA vaccine. The group is led by Felipe García, from the AIDS and HIV infection research group (IDIBAPS, Clinic Barcelona). To do this, the researchers will use computational methods to identify the parts of the virus that elicit the largest response from the immune system and will design the vaccine with these regions in mind to achieve long-term immunity against the virus.[36] The work will be performed together with Belgium.[37]
- The Project led by Antoni Torres, from the Applied Research in respiratory infections and critically ill, will analyze immunoglobulin G (IgG) antibodies from patients who have recovered from COVID-19, to identify their epitopes[38] to the surface protein S of SARS-CoV-2 are directed. This study will allow the subsequent production of specific antibodies against SARS-CoV-2 to block the infection.[39]

There are many Spanish initiatives regarding the development of antivirals as a potential treatment to the COVID-19 infection, 58 of them are already under clinical trial.[40]

The Way Forward

When the State of Emergency gradually ends, the new normality[41] will start, with gradual openings phase-wise. In many provinces, it will be on 21 June, in others much later.

It will be mandatory to wear masks when outside (a fine of 100 Euro would be imposed) unless the person has a health condition or is practicing any sport; maintaining a social distance of 1.5 meters is necessary, and that will condition the capacity of the indoors commercial activities. But it will be possible to travel again. There are many other details about what will be possible to do and under which conditions.[42]

According to the new normality decree, COVID-19 becomes an urgent declaration disease and the autonomous communities will have to provide information when emergencies for public health occur, provide the data for epidemiological monitoring and surveillance, and ensure a sufficient number of professionals for the prevention and control of the disease and its early diagnosis.[43]

Conclusion

By the time this chapter was finished, Spain was ranked 6 among the countries with the highest number of cases, having 296,351 positive cases and 28,355 deaths.[44]

A broad analysis of the number of new cases and deaths due to COVID-19 in the context of the measures taken by the Spanish Government show a positive correlation, but an open-source scientific analysis was not possible to be performed as the quality of the available data was not good. For the same day, there were multiple inconsistent values for the number of new cases as well as for the accumulated ones. The same happened with many variables under study.

The Government has specified its forecasts for the Spanish economy after the emergence of the coronavirus. GDP will contract sharply this year due to the fall in domestic demand and the state of emergency up to 9.2 percent, although it will recover by 6.8 already in 2021.[45] Nevertheless, the impact will not be the same in all the provinces since the type and magnitude of the economic activity varies to a great degree among them, and as a consequence some will recover fast than others.[46]

Even when it is possible to state that the central government was able to cope with the diseases, the loss of lives was extremely high. The economy also had to bear the brunt of the disease.

The coronavirus crisis revealed the deficiencies in the health system as a whole when it comes to lack of financing as well as well trained personnel. But also evidenced the differences between the autonomous communities, that will be much more evident in the following months, when they to do everything possible to get out of the crisis, in the context of the new normality restrictions.

The New Normality plan intends to prepare the society -for how long?- to face the challenges posed by a world post-pandemic but is a series of arrangements that do not take into consideration the uniqueness of the Spanish people, who are hard workers, and enjoy outdoor life and is almost not addressed in the plans. The psychological aspects are critical for the survival of society.

This is an open question for the future to answer, a society that loses its essence in order to survive, is it not paying a price too high? Would it be sustainable in the long run?

* * *

Acknowledgment: *I would like to thank Inma Bueno from IBATECH for her help on gathering information.*

NOTES

1. The Spanish Constitution, available at http://www.lamoncloa.gob.es/IDIOMAS/9/Espana/LeyFundamental/index.htm, accessed on 07 June 2020
2. Las Comunidades Autónomas de España (Spain' Autonomous Communities), available at https://comunidadesautonomas.org/, accessed on 07 June 2020.
3. El Gobierno confirma el primer caso de coronavirus en España (The Government confirms the first coronavirus case in Spain), available at https://www.elplural.com/sociedad/gobierno-confirma-caso-coronavirus-espana_232391102, accessed on 07 June 2020.
4. Coronavirus: infectados en España y la evolución del brote desde el origen (Coronavirus: infected people in Spain and the evolution of the outbreak since its origin), Coronavirus: infectados en España y la evolución del brote desde el origen, accessed on 7 June 2020.
5. El mapa del coronavirus en España: 27.136 muertos y más de 243.000 contagiados (The coronavirus map in Spain: 27,136 dead and more than 243,000 infected), available at https://www.rtve.es/noticias/20200614/mapa-del-coronavirus-espana/2004681.shtml accessed on 14 June 2020.
6. COVID-19 Statistics, available at https://cnecovid.isciii.es/covid19/#ccaa, accessed 13 June 2020.
7. F. Díez-Fuertes, María Iglesias-Caballero, Sara Monzón, Pilar Jiménez, Sarai Varona, Isabel Cuesta, Ángel Zaballos, Michael M Thomson, Mercedes Jiménez, Javier García Pérez, Francisco Pozo, Mayte Pérez-Olmeda, José Alcamí, Inmaculada Casas. Phylodynamics of SARS-CoV-2 transmission in Spain. bioRxiv 2020.04.20.050039; available at https://doi.org/10.1101/2020.04.20.050039, accessed on 7 June 2020.
8. F. Díez-Fuertes op.cit.
9. Qué medidas se tomaron y cuándo: así ha sido la evolución de la pandemia del coronavirus desde el primer día hasta hoy (What measures Were Taken and When: This has been the evolution of the coronavirus pandemic from the first day until today), available at https://www.eldiario.es/sociedad/medidas-tomaron-evolucion-pandemia-coronavirus_0_1012099616.html accessed on 09 June 2020.
10. Cronología del Coronavirus en España: 136 días de crisis (Coronavirus chronology in Spain: 136 days of crisis), available at https://www.marca.com/tiramillas/2020/04/08/5e8dcfa3e2704e9b948b458b.html accessed on 13 June 2020.
11. WHO, WHO Director-General's opening remarks at the media briefing on COVID-19 - 11 March 2020, available at https://www.who.int/dg/speeches/detail/who-director-general-s-opening-remarks-at-the-media-briefing-on-covid-19--11-march-2020, accessed on 13 June 2020.
12. Consejo Interterritorial del Sistema Nacional de Salud (Inter-territorial Council of the National Health System) available at https://www.mscbs.gob.es/organizacion/consejoInterterri/home.htm, accessed on 13 June 2020.
13. 'In a very schematic way, the content of this decree can be synthesized in six points: limitation of free movement of people (except for essential activities how to buy food or pharmaceutical products); the authorities may requisite goods necessary for compliance with the decree; suspension of teaching activity face-to-face in all educational centers; suspension of the opening to the public of leisure and cultural establishments, hotels and restaurants, and local and retail establishments (with some exceptions); transportation restriction traveler audiences at least 50%; and taking measures to ensure the food supply'. FERNÁNDEZ RODRÍGUEZ, José

Julio. Cuestiones constitucionales sobre el estado de alarma en España y la pandemia del COVID-19. Documento de Opinión IEEE 43/2020, available at http://www.ieee.es/Galerias/fichero/docs_opinion/2020/DIEEEO43_2020JOSFER_alarma.pdf, accessed on 13 June 2020.

14. Pedro Sánchez anuncia el plan de desescalada del Gobierno (Pedro Sánchez announces the government's de-escalation plan), available at https://www.marca.com/tiramillas/2020/04/28/5ea8104522601d75188b45ef.html, accessed on 13 June 2020.
15. Raul Sanchez and AnaOrdaz, 'Data: The Speed of the Coronavirus Curve in Each Autonomous Community: This is How Cases Grow in Spain,' available at https://www.eldiario.es/sociedad/evolucion-curva-coronavirus-Espana-comunidades-21-mayo_0_1008949744.html, (elaborated with Ministry of health data) accessed on 9 June 2020.
16. Geographical Distribution, available at https://cnecovid.isciii.es/covid19/#grupos-de-poblaci%C3%B3n, accessed on 9 June 2020.
17. Raul Sanchez and Ana Ordaz, 'The Coronavirus in Data: Maps and Graphs of the Evolution of Cases in Spain and the World,' available at https://www.eldiario.es/sociedad/mapa-evolucion-coronavirus-expansion-Espana-11-junio_0_1005099739.html, accessed on 9 June 2020.
18. El secreto letal de España: no teníamos "la mejor Sanidad del mundo" (The lethal secret of Spain: we did not have "the best healthcare in the world"), The lethal secret of Spain: we did not have "the best healthcare in the world" accessed on 14 June 2020.
19. La gestión de las comunidades ante la crisis del coronavirus gana apoyos frente a los fiascos de Moncloa (The management of the communities in the face of the coronavirus crisis gains support against the Moncloa fiascos) available at https://www.abc.es/sociedad/abci-gestion-comunidades-ante-crisis-coronavirus-gana-apoyos-frente-fiascos-moncloa-202004240207_noticia.html, accessed on 13 June 2020.
20. Ministerio de Sanidad. El Consejo de Ministros aprueba el Plan de Transición hacia una Nueva Normalidad, available at https://www.mscbs.gob.es/gabinete/notasPrensa.do?id=4884, accessed on 11 June 2020.
21. Transition Map to New Normal, available at https://www.lamoncloa.gob.es/covid-19/Paginas/mapa-fases-desescalada.aspx
22. Así son los tres tipos de test para detectar el coronavirus, available at https://elpais.com/sociedad/2020-03-23/tres-tipos-de-test-para-detectar-el-coronavirus.html, accessed on 9 June 2020.
23. CerTest VIASURE SARS-CoV-2 Real Time PCR Detection Kit, available at https://www.abacusdx.com/infectious-disease/diagnosis-for-coronavirus-covid-19-2/, accessed on 13 June 2020.
24. PCR y test rápidos para el diagnóstico del coronavirus ¿cómo funcionan y en qué se diferencian?, available at https://www.mscbs.gob.es/gabinete/notasPrensa.do?id=4824, accessed on 9 June 2020.
25. 'Adiós a los test de anticuerpos' (Goodbye to antibody tests?), available at https://elpais.com/sociedad/2020-05-19/adios-a-los-test-de-anticuerpos.html, accessed on 14 June 2020.
26. Abbott anuncia que ya está disponible en España su test de detección de anticuerpos (Abbott announces that its antibody detection test is now available in Spain) accessed on 14 June 2020.
27. Sin medios contra el coronavirus: cómo España intentó huir a ciegas del "tsunami" (Without means against the coronavirus: how Spain tried to flee blindly from the "tsunami"), available at https://civio.es/medicamentalia/2020/04/08/coronavirus-sars-cov-2-pruebas-pcr-espana/, accessed on 14 June 2020.
28. El Gobierno aclara que los test fallidos fueron comprados a un proveedor nacional (The Government clarifies that the failed tests were purchased from a national supplier), available at

https://www.marca.com/tiramillas/actualidad/2020/03/26/5e7ca27fca47419d238b460e.html, accessed on 14 June 2020.

29. 'CoNVat', el proyecto europeo que lidera España para detectar el coronavirus ('CoNVat', the European project led by Spain to detect the coronavirus), available at https://gacetamedica.com/investigacion/convat-el-proyecto-europeo-que-lidera-espana-para-detectar-el-coronavirus/, accessed on 14 June 2020.
30. Ministerio de Sanidad Español, Documentos técnicos para profesionales, available at https://www.mscbs.gob.es/profesionales/saludPublica/ccayes/alertasActual/nCov-China/documentos.htm, accessed on 14 June 2020.
31. Agencia Española de Medicamentos y Productos Sanitarios, available at https://www.aemps.gob.es/la-aemps/ultima-informacion-de-la-aemps-acerca-del-covid%E2%80%9119/tratamientos-disponibles-para-el-manejo-de-la-infeccion-respiratoria-por-sars-cov-2/, accessed on 14 June 2020.
32. El plasma de pacientes COVID-19 es seguro y eficaz en el 76% de los casos (Plasma from COVID-19 patients is safe and effective in 76% of cases), available at https://www.abc.es/salud/enfermedades/abci-plasma-convaleciente-covid-19-seguro-y-eficaz-76-por-ciento-pacientes-202006021855_noticia.html, accessed on 14 June 2020.
33. El Gobierno trabaja con compañías para garantizar que la vacuna del COVID-19 pueda ser fabricada en España (The Government works with companies to guarantee that the COVID-19 vaccine can be manufactured in Spain), available at https://www.infosalus.com/asistencia/noticia-gobierno-trabaja-companias-garantizar-vacuna-covid-19-pueda-ser-fabricada-espana-20200514132133.html, accessed on 14 June 2020.
34. La OMS incluye otras dos vacunas españolas en la I+D global del COVID-19 (The WHO includes two other Spanish vaccines in the global R&D of COVID-19), available at https://cincodias.elpais.com/cincodias/2020/06/10/companias/1591813843_575727.html, accessed on 14 June 2020.
35. España prepara su vacuna contra el coronavirus (Spain prepares its coronavirus vaccine), available at https://gacetamedica.com/investigacion/espana-prepara-su-vacuna-contra-el-coronavirus/, accessed on 14 June 2020.
36. Nuestra investigación en COVID: Desarrollo de una vacuna innovadora contra el SARS CoV-2 (Our research at COVID: Development of an innovative vaccine against SARS CoV-2), available at https://www.clinicbarcelona.org/noticias/nuestra-investigacion-en-covid-desarrollo-de-una-vacuna-innovadora-contra-el-sars-cov-2 accessed on 14 June 2020.
37. Coronavirus: la vacuna 'made in Spain' que inocula ARN mensajero (Coronavirus: the 'made in Spain' vaccine that inoculates messenger RNA), available at https://www.redaccionmedica.com/secciones/sanidad-hoy/coronavirus-la-vacuna-made-in-spain-que-inocula-arn-mensajero-1248 accessed on 14 June 2020.
38. Encyclopedia Britannica, Epitope definition, available at https://www.britannica.com/science/epitope, accessed on 14 June 2020.
39. Salud financia dos proyectos de investigación sobre SARS-CoV2 y COVID-19 del Hospital Clínic-IDIBAPS (Health funds two research projects on SARS-CoV2 and COVID-19 of the Hospital Clínic-IDIBAPS), available at https://www.clinicbarcelona.org/noticias/salud-financia-dos-proyectos-de-investigacion-sobre-sars-cov2-y-covid-19-del-hospital-clinic-idibaps accessed on 14 June 2020.
40. Dentro del laboratorio español que estudia un antiviral contra el coronavirus (Within the Spanish laboratory studying an antiviral against the coronavirus), available at https://hipertextual.com/

2020/05/lucha-antiviral-coronavirus accessed on 14 June 2020.

41. Plan para la Transición hacia una nueva normalidad (Plan for the Transition towards a new normality), available at https://www.mscbs.gob.es/profesionales/saludPublica/ccayes/alertasActual/nCov-China/planDesescalada.htm accessed on 14 June 2020.
42. Así será la nueva normalidad en España: preguntas y respuestas (This will be the new normality in Spain: questions and answers), available at https://www.elperiodico.com/es/sociedad/20200611/nueva-normalidad-espana-preguntas-7995547 accessed on 14 June 2020.
43. La letra pequeña del decreto de la 'nueva normalidad' en España (The fine print of the decree of the 'new normality' in Spain), available at https://www.elcorreo.com/sociedad/salud/letra-pequena-decreto-20200610095719-nt.html accessed on 14 June 2020.
44. El mapa del coronavirus en España: 27.136 muertos y más de 243.000 contagiados (The coronavirus map in Spain: 27,136 dead and more than 243,000 infected), available at https://www.rtve.es/noticias/20200614/mapa-del-coronavirus-espana/2004681.shtml accessed on 14 June 2020.
45. El impacto económico del coronavirus en España: 140.000 millones (The economic impact of the coronavirus in Spain: 140,000 million), available at https://www.economiadigital.es/finanzas-y-macro/el-impacto-economico-del-coronavirus-en-espana-140-000-millones_20058816_102.html accessed on 14 June 2020.
46. La España a dos velocidades por la crisis del coronavirus (Spain at two speeds because of the coronavirus crisis), available at https://www.elconfidencial.com/economia/2020-04-25/crisis-coronavirus-espana-dos-velocidades-provincias_2561520/ accessed on 14 June 2020.

11

Italy's COVID-19 Crisis: An Overview

Chiara De Cuia

Italy was the first European country to experience an overwhelming COVID-19 outbreak and, after two months of national efforts, the country has gradually resumed social and commercial activities. Positive cases, individuals needing intensive care, and daily death numbers are declining, but caution, social-distancing, patience, and perseverance will still need to guide Italians to avoid a new wave of contagion.

COVID-19 has affected the whole country (some regions more, some less) requiring national effort and sacrifice. With some exceptions, Italians have demonstrated a remarkable degree of endurance, solidarity, sense of duty, and responsibility. But as people start populating the streets again, uncertainty looms. This chapter aims to shed light on Italy's response to the COVID-19 crisis, what went wrong, and the way forward, addressing the country's mistakes and shortcomings, the social, political, and economic elements of the emergency, and the pre-existing systemic weaknesses exacerbated by the crisis.

COVID-19 in Italy: A Short Timeline and Adopted Measures

On 21 February, the first cases of COVID-19 not directly linked to China were discovered in the Italian towns of Codogno, in the region of Lombardy, and Vò, in Veneto. Before then, the only registered cases of COVID-19 in Italy had been two Chinese tourists visiting Italy and an Italian citizen who had repatriated from Wuhan, China.[1]

The Italian government declared the state of emergency on 31 January 2020,[2] one day after the World Health Organization (WHO) declared COVID-19 a Public Health Emergency of International Concern and two days after the Chinese couple visiting Italy was hospitalized in Rome.[3] However, the outbreak began only three weeks later, initially in a way that seemed possible for it to be contained within those few towns, and then rapidly taking over Italy's northern regions (Lombardy, Veneto, Piedmont, and Emilia-Romagna), and spreading across the rest of the country.

From 21 February, the number of positive cases grew dramatically (reaching a peak at the end of March) and with that the number of individuals needing hospitalization and intensive care, rapidly stressing healthcare structures in the affected areas. By the end-June, 34,767 COVID-19 deaths were registered in the country,[4] one of the highest figures worldwide.[5]

After declaring the state of emergency, the government suspended incoming flights from China – a move that was criticized by the Chinese government[6] and the efficacy of which is unclear, since COVID-19 had already been introduced in Italy. The government, together with the *Dipartimento della Protezione Civile* (Department of Civil Protection), also enhanced monitoring and screening activities in airports and ports.

Following the first detected cases, the regional presidents of Lombardy[7] and Veneto[8] issued the first coronavirus-related ordinances – in Italy, regional presidents have authority in case of health emergencies, and they are equipped with powers to issue emergency ordinances. Initially aimed at the small towns where the outbreaks occurred, the cautionary and restrictive measures were then extended to the whole regions, affecting the bustling city of Milan, the engine of Italy's economy, and terminating the historic Venice carnival festivities two days in advance.

On 23 February, the central government issued a decree establishing circumscribed red zones in the affected towns of Lombardy and Veneto.[9] As the situation elsewhere worsened, with new cases detected outside the red zones, the government issued further decrees, progressively implementing stricter measures nationwide: schools of all levels moved to online teaching on 4 March;[10] all of Lombardy and 14 provinces (within the regions of Emilia-Romagna, Piedmont, Veneto e Marche) were declared red zones on 8 March;[11] nationwide "stay at home" orders and strict measures were issued on 9 March;[12] non-essential commercial activities closed on 11 March;[13] and all non-essential industrial production was halted on 21 March.[14]

While the government initially sought to begin the reopening phase on 3

April, the daily numbers of registered deaths and positive cases were still high and growing,[15] prompting the government to postpone the date, first to 13 April, and then to 3 May.

The 26 April governmental decree finally described the gradual reopening of the country in multiple phases.[16] From May 4, factories and construction sites got up and running again (after six weeks of inactivity), take-away from bars and restaurants were once again allowed, and parks were reopened to the public.[17] On 16 May, new opening directives were announced:[18] on 18 May, stores and museums were allowed to reopen, and bars, restaurants, and personal care activities like hairdressers and religious services resumed. On 3 June, inter-regional travel was allowed again, and Italy opened its borders to Europe.[19]

The reopening phase has been characterized by trends like the decrease in the number of COVID-19 deaths per day, of the number of new positive cases recorded, and of the number of individuals needing hospital care. While occasional, small, circumscribed hotspots are still registered, the *Servizio Sanitario Nazionale* – Italy's national health system – has been able to detect and control them.[20] Nevertheless, as the Italian Health Minister Roberto Speranza noted, the pandemic is not over: caution, social-distancing, patience, and perseverance will still need to guide Italians.

Italy's Pandemic Plan

Italy's first pandemic plan was drafted in 2002[21] and subsequently updated[22] following the WHO's global influenza preparedness plan, published in 2005 in response to the 2003 outbreak of the Avian Influenza A/H5N1 and its global pandemic threat.[23] Published in 2006, Italy's updated plan incorporates the WHO's six pandemic phases, identifying key measures to face such emergencies, highlighting the importance of communication and information, and delineating the chain of command and responsibilities for each phase and activity.[24] Each region subsequently adopted a regional plan based on the national one.

Reading through the plan, it is possible to recognize many of the measures adopted during the COVID-19 pandemic, but it is also evident that many others were not put in place. Given that the pandemic did not originate in Italy, the question that is pervading the international community is whether there was a timely communication of information from China, where COVID-19 originated, or whether this was stalled, impacting the role of the WHO in collecting and sharing information, providing monitoring guidance, and determining the pandemic risk and spread of the disease.[25] While *time* is crucial for effective prevention and containment, so is crisis management: Italy's response to COVID-19 has been an exemplar in some ways, leading the way with measures that were subsequently replicated by other governments, but it has not been immune to mistakes and shortcomings.

Italy's Response to COVID-19

Italy's response to COVID-19 has been shaped by several elements: how authority and responsibility are divided between the Italian government and regions; the Italian civil security system headed by the National Civil Protection Department which, during states of emergency, directs and coordinates activities nationally; and a set of institutions such as the national health system and the Italian law enforcement and armed forces.

This year marked the 50th anniversary of the establishment of Italy's regions: originally envisaged under Title V of the Constitution of the Italian Republic, written by the Italian Constituent Assembly after World War II (after Italians chose the Republic over monarchy), regions only came to be in 1970 and progressively became fully operational, especially with the 2001 reform that granted regions financial and organizational autonomy.

The pandemic, however, has raised new questions on the relationship between the national government and the regions, especially during a national emergency. As the President of the Republic Sergio Mattarella noted during the celebration of this anniversary, there is still room to improve this relationship to avoid conflicts and redundancies that may create paralyzing inefficiencies or dangerous social divisions.[26] In this statement, the President was implicitly referencing the case of Alzano and Nembro, two towns in the area of Bergamo (Lombardy), the hardest hit in Italy because of the failure to implement red zones. Ongoing investigations will determine whether the responsibility fell upon the national government or Lombardy's authorities: the region claims it was waiting for the national government to act, while the government stated that the region had full powers to declare a red zone.

The government had, in fact, established the first red zones in the towns of Codogno and Vò, and then subsequently extended it to the whole region of Lombardy and other 14 cities. While governmental decrees legally supersede regional ordinances, regions had the power to tighten local rules if needed since regional presidents have the legal authority to act in cases of health emergencies.[27] Other regions, in fact, established red zones in several towns that became local hotbeds, often linked to people returning to their region of origin from Lombardy.[28]

In addition to the issue of regional and governmental authority, regional strategies seem to also have made a difference.

COVID-19 was not a homogenous experience for the whole country: 70% of the total registered cases are concentrated in the aforementioned northern regions,[29] while the south was largely spared the unmanageable figures that stressed the north's healthcare system (which was, nationally, the best equipped to face such an emergency)[30] thanks, in part, to the measures taken which included the restriction of inter-regional travel. COVID-19 has, in fact, tested Italy's regionally based national health system, highlighting its weaknesses – including personnel shortage,[31] the general decline in the number of hospital beds during the past decade,[32] and the lack of coordination between the regional governments and the local medical nodes, namely family doctors, local clinics, and nursing homes.[33] To face the emergency, retired doctors were called back, young graduates were speedily enabled as doctors and nurses, and makeshift hospitals were set up.[34] But these weaknesses also meant that those doctors on the frontlines, the ones who had the first contact with positive patients – especially family doctors – were initially left without direction or the protection to carry out their work due to a nationwide shortage of supplies.[35]

Among the four hardest hit northern regions – namely Lombardy, Piedmont, Emilia-Romagna, and Veneto – Lombardy and Veneto, the first regions affected by COVID-19, followed two different approaches to contrast the spread of the disease. Lombardy followed a "hospital-centric" approach, where diagnosis and care were provided at hospitals, exposing the structures, hospital personnel, and other patients to the risk of contagion, and followed the national recommendation of testing only symptomatic individuals.[36] Over 200 doctors (family and hospital doctors), nurses, pharmacists, and care-workers died in the fight against COVID-19 in Italy,[37] many of whom worked in Lombardy.[38]

Veneto, by contrast, adopted a more proactive, community-based approach[39] that favoured widespread testing based on contact-tracing, remote or at-home diagnosis and follow-up, and the coordination of local hospitals to designate COVID-only hospitals and structures to limit the contagion to personnel and other patients. This system also allowed for the economization of the short supply of protective equipment.[40] It is important to note that the initial situations in Lombardy and Veneto differed in many ways, likely affecting the response approach: for example, Lombardy was overwhelmed by an *explosion* of cases, perhaps due to the presence of the virus prior to February, and the region's population density is higher compared to that of Veneto, affecting the rate of contagion.[41] As the country recovers, it will be important to study and analyse the different approaches adopted across all regions to identify shortcomings and best-practices.

Finally, nursing homes – which host the most vulnerable section of Italy's society – became hotbeds of contagion across the territory:[42] over 70% of COVID-19 victims were over 70 years old, many of whom were in nursing homes.[43] Investigations are shedding light on nursing home deaths, and the disastrous decisions to use some of these structures as COVID-19 wards due to the shortage of hospital beds.[44]

While the government has been responsible for the legislative aspects of crisis management, the national Civil Protection Department – still acting through the Council of Ministers, Italy's executive organ – has directed and coordinated national efforts. The Civil Protection Department ensures joint management and coordination of emergency activities, including monitoring activities, information and data gathering.[45] It works closely with different bodies such as law enforcement and military forces, voluntary forces like the Italian Red Cross, as well as its own force, local administrations and authorities (from regions, provinces, and municipalities), and all entities whose participation is required to manage a given emergency.[46] During the COVID-19 crisis, the Civil Protection Department (with its network of local offices) has been responsible for holding daily press conferences with updates on the national situation, collecting and publicly sharing numbers and data. The Civil Protection Department has also served as the hub for the collection and national distribution of medical supplies, its volunteers have manned regional hotlines to keep emergency lines free, and it has supported Italy's national health system by setting up field hospitals and triage areas, and coordinating the transportation of patients in need of intensive care to available hospitals. These, however, are just some examples of the wide range of activities carried out by the Civil Protection Department.

Finally, Italian law enforcement and military forces have also played a crucial role during the emergency. Italian Police forces and the Carabinieri have manned checkpoints around the red zones, patrolled cities, and enforced the measures contained in the decrees, but they have also engaged in many spontaneous acts in service of the population, from bringing chocolate Easter eggs to children in hospitals or foster care, to providing support to the elderly. The Italian military has been crucial in repatriating citizens from China, making its medical personnel, hospitals, and structures available to support the national healthcare system, producing respirators, disinfectants and face masks,[47] supporting public safety activities and check-point control, and offering logistical support like the transfer of patients and equipment nationwide.[48]

Italy's Fractious Politics

Politics is a critical element in the management of national emergencies – for better or for worse – as we are witnessing worldwide.

In a country where fractious politics has been a constant feature for decades, the government was able to muster general support from political opponents for the sake of national unity at the height of the crisis but was not immune to criticism. However, as the health emergency is giving way to what will likely be Italy's next economic crisis, criticism has evolved into finger-pointing and threats of new elections from opponents, and from within the fragile coalition government: but political unity is fundamental for recovery as well. The government has been accused of initially underestimating the threat and for its slow adoption of more restrictive measures. It has also been under pressure for the delivery of the promised social and economic safety nets,[49] during its negotiations with the European Union (EU),[50] and was criticized for mismanaging communication efforts throughout the crisis.

Because Italy was the first European country to experience an overwhelming outbreak, the Italian government was faced with making decisions entailing short-term and long-term consequences, especially economic ones, requiring both caution and proportionality: an example was the decision to halt non-essential and non-strategic production which was taken on 21 March, four weeks after the first measures were implemented in Lombardy and three weeks after the whole country was subject to "stay at home" orders.[51] Given Italy's weak pre-coronavirus economic situation, such decisions were not easy ones to take.

In addition to the economic consequences of Italy's industrial and commercial pause, there have been social repercussions as unemployment grows, business-owners incur debts, families plunge into poverty, and pre-existing inequalities only grow deeper, especially for those whose livelihoods depend on the shadow economy,[52] which has been forced to halt as well. Even one of Italy's most important societal equalizers, its (underfunded) public-school system, has been dramatically affected. As schools moved to online teaching, thousands of students were not able to access online education: students without means like Personal Computers, tablets, or access to the internet were left out,[53] and teachers lacking the same means or digital competence were not able to teach online classes.[54] This is only a symptom of Italy's wider digitalization problem: the 2020 Digital Economy and Society Index that monitors Europe's overall digital performance and tracks a country's digital competitiveness, ranked Italy 25 out of 28 member states (the United Kingdom is still included), well below the European average.[55]

In the meantime, frustration grows as the promised social safety nets for Italian workers and businesses are slow to arrive, often tied down by bureaucracy or pre-existing weaknesses of the Italian system rather than by governmental decisions, and have, so far, not been enough.[56]

While the Italian government has strived to adopt a transparent approach and to enhance communication to inform the public, the result has sometimes been a little different: the daily briefing on national trends led by the Department of Civil Protection has been crucial in helping Italians understand the extent of the crisis, and Prime Minister Giuseppe Conte, who has received credit for his performance during the crisis, increasing his approval ratings,[57] personally owned the government's decisions, talking to Italians and announcing the introduction of new measures on streamed social media press conferences. However, his press conferences have sometimes been streamed late at night, somewhat undermining the intended widespread reach. A controversial moment during these press conferences was when the Prime Minister publicly called out centre-right opposition leaders Matteo Salvini and Giorgia Meloni for peddling false information on the European Stability Mechanism (an element in the negotiations with the EU),[58] a move that was not well-received among the opposition and their supporters.

Finally, unofficial statements of measures being considered but not introduced have often been shared publicly by the media, unnecessarily stirring reactions and, ultimately, Italy's systemic use of *officialese* has made the hyper-bureaucratic decrees hard to decipher, leaving Italians with more questions than answers in what were already uncertain times. [59]

A Friend in Need... Italy and the EU

Italy's relationship with the EU can be best described as a love-hate relationship. While Italy is a founding member of the European communities – the bases of the European project – Italy has often found itself at odds with the EU in times of crisis, from the eurozone crisis to the migrant crisis of 2015-16, and now during a global pandemic.[60]

Italy was the first Western and first European country to face a dramatic COVID-19 outbreak. Regrettably, European solidarity was slow to kick in: when Italy asked its European partners for medical supplies, the plea was initially met with export blocks.[61] As the President of the European Council noted, at first "Europe looked at Italy and the way the virus was developing with incredulity, perhaps even detachment."[62] It was only once the virus spread to other European member states, that European solidarity started to kick in: for example, France donated 1 million masks and 20,000 protective suits; Germany delivered 7.5 tons of medical equipment to Italy, including ventilators and face masks and, together with Austria, treated critically ill patients from Italy; and Poland sent a team of doctors and paramedics.[63] While the help received hasn't been too little it was, perhaps, too late in terms of optics. Optics were also important when the president of the European Central Bank (ECB) Christine Lagarde, stated "We are not here to close spreads," responding to calls for the ECB to ease borrowing costs for highly indebted eurozone countries like Italy.[64] However, despite these initial bumps which prompted anti-European feelings and fed into Italy's Eurosceptic narratives, the European Commission has put forward an ambitious proposal for a major recovery plan worth 750 billion Euros, aimed at supporting the recovery of member states and investing in the future of the EU.[65]

The initial tensions between Italy and the EU also provided an opportunity for China to play a role in the country and wider region. Through the so-called "face mask diplomacy" and information operations on social media, China exploited these political tensions and the void in global leadership created by the crisis to shape and manipulate global perceptions of China and its role in the COVID-19 pandemic by sowing confusion on the origin of the outbreak and deflecting the blame.[66] In Italy and other European countries, China portrayed itself as a reliable partner of the first resort while attempting to discredit the EU as confirmed by a European External Action Service report[67] and the High Representative of the European Union, Josep Borrell who highlighted the "need to defend Europe against its detractors [...] with facts" in the current global battle of narratives.[68]

What Lies Ahead?

Many sacrifices were made, from staying indoors on beautiful spring days or not seeing a loved one for an extended period of time, to the long hours worked by doctors and nurses to guarantee care.[69] Much has been lost too, from jobs and livelihoods to the lives of thousands of Italians.

Italians are now eager to get moving despite the many uncertainties laying ahead and the looming economic crisis. Patience and caution will still be needed because the road back to *normal* will likely be long and socially, economically, and politically bumpy. In the meantime, the government has adopted a law decree,[70] which has been nicknamed *rilancio* – comeback – mirroring the country's mood. Officially published on 19 May,[71] the decree – a de facto recovery plan – was supposed to be introduced in April, but given the magnitude of the plan, worth 55 billion euros which will increase Italy's deficit (complementing the 25 billion euros that the government had approved to face the emergency back in March),[72] lengthy negotiations stalled its deliberation within the Council of Ministers. With over 250 articles, the decree aims at laying the foundations for Italy's recovery with temporary measures and introducing changes that may help address some of the pre-existing systemic weaknesses.

Measures include fiscal discounts, grants, and emergency income and allowances to support businesses, workers, families, and hard-hit sectors such as tourism. Significant investments will be made to empower the national health system, building on the lessons learned to build readiness for future health emergencies: local health networks will be strengthened to enhance assistance, prevention and monitoring, intensive care hospital beds will be increased, and additional personnel will be hired.[73] The school system will also receive funds to prepare its infrastructure to safely welcome back students and invest in digitalization.[74] The decree also aims to reduce irregular, off-the-books employment for domestic workers and seasonal agricultural laborers. Finally, acknowledging the hurdles posed by hyper-bureaucratization that have hindered initial payments, the decree aims to simplify and streamline some bureaucratic processes and procedures, to ensure timely disbursement of the much-needed benefits and liquidity.

The decree and its measures will not be the panacea to Italy's post- COVID-19 situation, but it definitely is a first, important step. Some measures will bring temporary relief, some might bring about long-term changes, and additional measures will be needed. The opposition forces have voiced criticism,[75] and it will be up to them to improve the decree in Parliament through amendments, which the Prime Minister has openly invited them to do.[76]

The aim, however, is to not only make a comeback but re-launch Italy. In April, Prime Minister Conte established a committee of social and economic experts to push forward recommendations and objectives for post- COVID-19 Italy based on digitalization and innovation, environmental sustainability, gender parity and inclusion.[77]

Along these lines, Prime Minister Conte also convened the *Stati Generali*. Labelled as a political stunt by the centre-right opposition forces who have refused to participate, the *Stati Generali* is a week-long national consultation with political leaders and representatives from all sides, Italy's economic and social actors, EU representatives, economists, intellectuals, Nobel prize winners, and CEOs of Italy's main industrial and financial firms.[78] Loosely inspired by the pre-1789 French *États généraux*, the aim is to set a road map for the recovery plan that best utilizes all resources allocated by national and European measures to improve and strengthen Italy and not merely reinstate the status quo.[79]

As they say, in every crisis there are opportunities, and the challenge will be seizing them through hard work, patience and, most importantly, political unity and political will.

* * *

A shorter version of this essay was published in the CBW Magazine Vol. 13, No. 1, Jan-June 2020.

NOTES

1. Giovanni Battistuzzi, 'Il Coronavirus in Italia. La mappa del contagio', *Il Foglio*, 30 March 2020, available at https://www.ilfoglio.it/salute/2020/02/24/news/il-coronavirus-in-italia-la-mappa-del-contagio-303522/, accessed on 15 May 2020.
2. 'Delibera del Consiglio dei Ministri 31 gennaio 2020', *Gazzetta Ufficiale Della Repubblica Italiana*, 31 January 2020, available at https://www.gazzettaufficiale.it/eli/id/2020/02/01/20A00737/sg, accessed 20 May 2020.
3. 'Coronavirus (COVID-19) Outbreak', *World Health Organization*, available at https://www.who.int/westernpacific/emergencies/covid-19, accessed on 20 May 2020.
4. Federico Barbara, Alice Calvi, Luca Galimberti, et al., 'Coronavirus in Italy: Updated Map and Case Count', *Il Sole 24 Ore*, available at https://lab24.ilsole24ore.com/coronavirus/en/, last accessed on 14 June 2020.
5. 'WHO Coronavirus Disease (COVID-19) Dashboard', *World Health Organization*, last updated on 14 June 2020, available at https://covid19.who.int/?gclid=EAIaIQobCh MIjafJ04H86QIVFeDtCh1kpQi8EAAYASAAEgLq6_D_BwE, accessed on 13 May 2020.
6. 'Coronavirus, tensione fra Italia e Cina per lo stop dei voli. Di Maio: «Il blocco resta»', *Il Messaggero*, 7 February 2020, available at https://www.ilmessaggero.it/mondo/coronavirus_blocco_voli_italia_cina_ultime_notizie-5036130.html, accessed on 5 May 2020.
7. 'Ordinanza 21 Febbraio, Regione Lombardia,' *Regione Lombardia*, 21 February 2020, available at https://regione.lombardia.it/wps/wcm/connect/fe581599-e646-43e2-a676-e66404ebb50b/Ordinanza-21-2-2020.pdf?MOD=AJPERES&CACHEID=ROOTWORKSPACE-fe581599-e646-43e2-a676-e66404ebb50b-n1P9S4M
8. https://www.regione.veneto.it/documents/10136/2648298/Ordinanza+n.+1+23.02.2020.pdf/fc933772-8be1-4d34-b5d8-6da58daeeaea, accessed on 4 May 2020.
9. 'Decreto del Presidente del Consiglio dei Ministri 23 febbraio 2020', *Gazzetta Ufficiale Della Repubblica Italiana*, 23 February 2020, available at https://www.gazzettaufficiale.it/eli/id/2020/02/23/20A01228/sg, accessed on 5 May 2020.
10. 'Coronavirus, firmato il Dpcm 4 marzo 2020', *Governo Italiano Presidenza del Consiglio dei Ministri*, 4 March 2020, available at http://www.governo.it/it/articolo/coronavirus-firmato-il-dpcm-4-marzo-2020/14241, accessed on 4 May 2020.
11. 'Decreto del Presidente del Consiglio Dei Ministri 8 marzo 2020', *Gazzetta Ufficiale Della Repubblica Italiana*, 8 March 2020, available at https://www.gazzettaufficiale.it/eli/id/2020/03/08/20A01522/sg, accessed on 5 May 2020.

12. 'Decreto del Presidente del Consiglio Dei Ministri 9 marzo 2020', *Gazzetta Ufficiale Della Repubblica Italiana*, 9 March 2020, availabe at https://www.gazzettaufficiale.it/eli/id/2020/03/09/20A01558/sg, accessed on 5 May 2020.
13. 'Coronavirus, Conte firma il Dpcm 11 marzo 2020', *Governo Italiano, Presidenza del Consiglio dei Ministri*, 11 March 2020, available at http://www.governo.it/node/14299, accessed on 6 May 2020.
14. 'Coronavirus, firmato il Dpcm 22 marzo 2020', *Governo Italiano, Presidenza del Consiglio dei Ministri*, 22 March 2020, available at http://www.governo.it/node/14363, accessed on 5 May 2020.
15. Federico Barbara, Alice Calvi, Luca Galimberti, et al., 'Coronavirus in Italy: Updated map and Case count', Il Sole 24 Ore, available at https://lab24.ilsole24ore.com/coronavirus/en/, last accessed on 14 June 2020.
16. 'Decreto del Presidente del Consiglio Dei Ministri 26 aprile 2020', *Gazzetta Ufficiale Della Repubblica Italiana*, 26 April 2020, available at https://www.gazzettaufficiale.it/eli/id/2020/04/27/20A02352/sg, accessed on 4 May 2020.
17. 'Fase 2: dalle fabbriche ai negozi, ai bar ecco il calendario della ripartenza dal 4 maggio al 1 giugno - I documenti', *Il Sole 24 Ore*, 24 April 2020, available at https://www.ilsole24ore.com/art/fase-2-ecco-calendario-ripartenza-27-aprile-18-maggio-ADjmMJM, accessed on 5 May 2020.
18. 'Conferenza stampa del Presidente Conte', *Palazzo Chigi*, *YouTube Video*, 16 May 2020, available at https://www.youtube.com/watch?v=9JztWZNiUKM, accessed on 18 May 2020.
19. 'Le notizie di sabato sul coronavirus in Italia', *Il Post*, 30 May 2020, available at https://www.ilpost.it/2020/05/30/notizie-coronavirus-sabato-30-maggio/, accessed on 1 June 2020.
20. 'Covid-19, analisi dell'andamento epidemiologico e aggiornamento tecnico-scientifico del 22 maggio', *Canale1 AGTW*, *YouTube Video*, 22 May 2020, available at https://youtu.be/Y1Ckq7tAKVE, accessed on 25 May 2020.
21. 'Piano italiano multifase d'emergenza per una pandemia Influenzale (Pag. 57)', *Gazzetta Ufficiale Della Repubblica Italiana*, 26 March 2002, available at https://www.gazzettaufficiale.it/eli/gu/2002/03/26/72/sg/pdf, accessed on 5 June 2020.
22. 'Piano Nazionale di Preparazione e Risposta ad una Pandemia Influenzale', *Ministero della Salute*, 2006, available at http://www.salute.gov.it/imgs/C_17_pubblicazioni_501_allegato.pdf, accessed on 4 June 2020.
23. 'WHO global influenza preparedness plan. The role of WHO and recommendations for national measures before and during pandemics', *World Health Organization*, 2005, available at https://www.who.int/csr/resources/publications/influenza/WHO_CDS_CSR_GIP_2005_5.pdf, accessed on 6 June 2020.
24. 'National Plan for Preparedness and Response to an Influenza Pandemic, *Ministero della Salute*, 2006, available at http://www.salute.gov.it/imgs/C_17_pubblicazioni_501_allegato.pdf, accessed on 4 June 2020.
25. 'WHO global influenza preparedness plan. The role of WHO and recommendations for national measures before and during pandemics', World Health Organization, 2005, available at https://www.who.int/csr/resources/publications/influenza/WHO_CDS_CSR_GIP_2005_5.pdf, accessed on 6 June 2020.
26. '50 anni dalle prime elezioni regionali: dichiarazione del Presidente Mattarella', *Conferenza delle Regioni e delle Province Autonome*, 7 June 2020, available at http://www.regioni.it/home/50-anni-regioni-2513/#:~:text=Roma%2C%2016%20maggio%202020%20(comunicato, Speciale%2 C%20 diventava%20finalmente%20una%20realt%C3%A0, accessed on 8 June 2020.

27. 'Legge 23 dicembre 1978, n. 833', *Gazzetta Ufficiale Della Repubblica Italiana*, 23 December 1978, available at https://www.gazzettaufficiale.it/eli/id/1978/12/28/078U0833/sg, accessed on 8 June 2020.
28. Carlotta De Leo, 'Chi poteva decidere le zone rosse per il Coronavirus in Italia?', *Corriere della Sera*, 30 May 2020, available at https://www.corriere.it/cronache/20_maggio_30/chi-poteva-decidere-zone-rosse-il-coronavirus-italia-bc61cee0-a258-11ea-bc2b-bdd292787b00.shtml, accessed on 5 June 2020.
29. Federico Barbara, Alice Calvi, Luca Galimberti, et al., 'Coronavirus in Italy: updated map and case count', *Il Sole 24 Ore*, available at https://lab24.ilsole24ore.com/coronavirus/en/, last accessed on 14 June 2020.
30. Marzio Bartoloni, 'Sanità:le cure migliori in Veneto, Emilia e Toscana, ma il Sud avanza', *Il Sole 24 Ore*, 8 January 2020, available at https://www.ilsole24ore.com/art/sanita-le-cure-migliori-veneto-emilia-e-toscana-ma-sud-avanza-ACc2fTAB, accessed on 4 June 2020.
31. 'Misure per il personale del SSN e professioni sanitarie' *Camera dei Deputati*, 21 April 2020, available at https://www.camera.it/temiap/documentazione/temi/pdf/1209271.pdf?_15881633 82501, accessed on 3 May 2020.
32. 'La riduzione di ospedali e posti letto negli ultimi 10 anni', *AGI Agenzia Italia*, 14 March 2020, available at https://www.agi.it/fact-checking/news/2020-03-14/coronavirus-rianimazione-posti-letto-7500889/, accessed on 3 May 2020.
33. Davide Maria De Luca, Elena Zacchetti, Stefano Vizio, Luca Misculin, 'Two months that shook Lombardy', *Il Post*, 7 May 2020, available at https://www.ilpost.it/2020/05/07/two-months-that-shook-lombardy-to-the-core-coronavirus/, accessed on 13 May 2020.
34. 'Covid-19, in Gazzetta ufficiale il decreto per il potenziamento del Ssn', *Ministero della Salute*, 10 March 2020, available at http://www.salute.gov.it/portale/nuovocoronavirus/dettaglioNotizieNuovoCoronavirus.jsp?lingua=italiano&id=4188, accessed on 12 May 2020.
35. Michele Bocci, 'Coronavirus, morti 150 camici bianchi. "Noi, medici di famiglia prima linea contro l'epidemia', *La Repubblica*, 25 April 2020, available at https://www.repubblica.it/cronaca/2020/04/25/news/coronavirus_morti_150_medici-254860106/, accessed on 5 May 2020.
36. Ernesto Diffidenti, 'Quanti se ne fanno? Quanto costano? Chi paga? Tutto quel che c'è da sapere sul test del tampone', *Il Sole 24 Ore*, 16 March 2020, available at https://www.ilsole24ore.com/art/quanti-se-ne-fanno-quanto-costano-chi-paga-tutto-quel-che-c-e-sapere-test-tampone-ADYu6fD, accessed on 4 May 2020.
37. Michele Bocci, 'Coronavirus, morti 150 camici bianchi. "Noi, medici di famiglia prima linea contro l'epidemia', *La Repubblica*, 25 April 2020, available at https://www.repubblica.it/cronaca/2020/04/25/news/coronavirus_morti_150_medici-254860106/, accessed on 5 May 2020.
38. 'Covid-19: morti 163 medici e 40 infermieri. Operatori sanitari la categoria più colpita', *L'Eco di Bergamo*, 16 May 2020, available at https://www.ecodibergamo.it/stories/bergamo-citta/covid-19-morti-163-medici-e-40-infermierioperatori-sanitari-la-categoria-piu-co_1354386_11/, accessed on 20 May 2020.
39. Nancy Binkin, Federica Michieletto, Francesca Russo, Stefania Salmaso, 'Veneto e Lombardia a confronto nella strategia contro il covid-19', *Internazionale*, 23 April 2020, available at https://www.internazionale.it/notizie/nancy-binkin/2020/04/23/covid-veneto-lombardia-strategie, accessed on 3 June 2020.
40. Ibid.
41. Ibid.
42. Nicoletta Cottone, 'Coronavirus, ecco dove sono le 106 zone rosse d'Italia: 70 solo in Emilia

Romagna', *Il Sole 24 Ore*, 24 April 2020, available at https://www.ilsole24ore.com/art/coronavirus-ecco-dove-sono-106-zone-rosse-d-italia-70-solo-emilia-romagna-ADXjebM, accessed on 5 May 2020.

43. 'Characteristics of SARS-CoV-2 patients dying in Italy Report based on available data on May 7th, 2020', *Istituto Superiore di Sanità*, 7 May 2020, available at https://www.epicentro.iss.it/en/coronavirus/bollettino/Report-COVID-2019_7_may_2020.pdf, accessed on 12 May 2020.
44. 'Anziani morti nelle Rsa lombarde, Fontana: "L'utilizzo di quelle case di riposo per i malati Covid è responsabilità dell'Ats"', *La Repubblica*, 17 April 2020, available at https://milano.repubblica.it/cronaca/2020/04/17/news/anziani_morti_nelle_rsa_lombarde_fontana_l_utilizzo_delle_case_di_riposo_per_i_malati_covid_e_responsabilita_dell_ats_-254256674/, accessed on 12 May 2020.
45. Federica Di Camillo, Alessandro Marrone, Stefano Silvestri, Paola Tessari, Alessandro R. Ungaro, 'The Italian Civil Security System," *Istituto Affari Internazionali*, February 2014, available at https://www.iai.it/sites/default/files/iairp_11.pdf, accessed 4 May 2020.
46. 'D.P.C.M., Organizzazione e funzionamento di Sistema presso la Sala Situazione Italia del Dipartimento della protezione civile', *Protezione Civile*, 3 December 2008, available at http://www.protezionecivile.gov.it/documents/20182/0/dpcm_3_dic_2008_sala.pdf/c3712084-756c-4de6-bde7-799c26719a1f, accessed on 6 May 2020.
47. Michela Della Maggesa, 'Mascherine, respiratori e disinfettanti. Ecco cosa farà l'industria della Difesa', *Formiche*, 18 March 2020, available at https://formiche.net/2020/03/mascherine-piani-difesa/, accessed on 5 May 2020.
48. 'Coronavirus: il contributo delle Forze Armate', *Ministero Della Difesa*, available at https://www.difesa.it/SMD_/Avvenimenti/Coronavirus_Forze_Armate_operazioni_per_rientro_italiani_da_Wuhan_Cina/Pagine/Coronavirus_il_contributo_delle_Forze_Armate.aspx, accessed 15 May 2020.
49. 'Il via libera al Mes «ultralight» riaccende lo scontro M5S-Pd, tensioni nel Governo', *Il Sole 24 Ore*, 8 May 2020, available at https://www.ilsole24ore.com/art/il-via-libera-mes-ultralight-riaccende-scontro-maggioranza-pd-e-m5s-ADas4NP, accessed on 12 May 2020.
50. Roberto Castaldi, 'Conte still 'cautious' on ESM but up to Italian parliament to decide activation', *Euractiv*, 9 May 2020, available at, https://www.euractiv.com/section/economy-jobs/news/conte-still-cautious-on-esm-but-up-to-italian-parliament-to-decide-activation/, accessed on 13 May 2020.
51. 'Ulteriori disposizioni attuative del decreto-legge 23 febbraio 2020, n. 6, recante misure urgenti in materia di contenimento e gestione dell'emergenza epidemiologica da COVID-19, applicabili sull'intero territorio nazionale. (20A01807)', *Ministero Della Salute*, 22 March 2020, available at http://www.trovanorme.salute.gov.it/norme/dettaglioAtto?id=73729, accessed on 5 May 2020.
52. 'L'Economia Non Osservata Nei Conti Nazionali | Anni 2014-2017', *Istituto Nazionale di Statistica*, 15 October 2020, available at https://www.istat.it/it/files/2019/10/Economia-non-osservata-nei-conti-nazionali-2017.pdf, accessed on 5 May 2020.
53. 'Italia sotto sforzo. Diario della transizione 2020', *Centro Studi Investimenti Sociali*, 9 June 2020, available at https://images.agi.it/pdf/agi/agi/2020/06/09/093133436-fa073eb1-d556-446f-87d6-2eecb90b0d76.pdf, accessed on 12 June 2020.
54. 'Italia sotto sforzo. Diario della transizione 2020', *Centro Studi Investimenti Sociali*, 9 June 2020, available at https://images.agi.it/pdf/agi/agi/2020/06/09/093133436-fa073eb1-d556-446f-87d6-2eecb90b0d76.pdf, accessed on 12 June 2020.
55. 'Digital Economy and Society Index (DESI) 2020 Questions and Answers', *European*

Commission, 11 June 2020, available at https://ec.europa.eu/commission/presscorner/detail/en/qanda_20_1022, accessed on 12 June 2020.

56. Andrea Carli, 'Cura Italia: tutte le misure per famiglie, lavoratori, imprese e sanità', *Il Sole 24 Ore*, 25 March 2020, available at https://www.ilsole24ore.com/art/misure-famiglie-lavoratori-imprese-e-sanita-ecco-pacchetto-cura-italia-ADSNcqF, accessed on 7 May 2020.
57. Hannah Roberts, 'Conte's coronavirus honeymoon comes to a close', *Politico*, 5 May 2020, available at https://www.politico.eu/article/contes-coronavirus-honeymoon-comes-to-a-close/, accessed on 10 May 2020.
58. 'Coronavirus, Conte furioso con Salvini e Meloni: "Mes non approvato la scorsa notte ma nel 2012"', *La Repubblica, YouTube Video*, 10 April 2020, available at https://www.youtube.com/watch?v=VPWIx1_ndrU, accessed on 30 May 2020.
59. 'Meloni all'attacco della Azzolina: Una ministra ridicola', *Oggi Scuola*, 6 May 2020, available at https://www.oggiscuola.com/web/2020/05/06/meloni-allattacco-della-azzolina-una-ministra-ridicola/, accessed on 12 May 2020.
60. Ben Hall, Miles Johnson, Martin Arnold, 'Italy wonders where Europe's solidarity is as coronavirus strains show', *Financial Times*, 13 March 2020, available at https://www.ft.com/content/d3bc25ea-652c-11ea-b3f3-fe4680ea68b5, accessed on 6 May 2020.
61. Ibid.
62. '"Strengthening Italy strengthens Europe, too" - Remarks by President Charles Michel to the 'Stati Generali dell'economia', *European Council*, 13 June 2020, available at https://www.consilium.europa.eu/en/press/press-releases/2020/06/13/strengthening-italy-strengthens-europe-too-remarks-by-president-charles-michel-to-the-stati-generali-dell-economia/, accessed on 13 June 2020.
63. 'Coronavirus: European Solidarity in action', *European Commission*, 9 June 2020, available at https://ec.europa.eu/info/live-work-travel-eu/health/coronavirus-response/coronavirus-european-solidarity-action_en#euindustrystepsintoprotecteuropeancitizens, accessed on 10 June 2020.
64. Paul Taylor, 'Lagarde's corona blunder. ECB chief flunks on her strongest suit – communication', *Politico*, 13 March 2020, available at https://www.politico.eu/article/christine-lagarde-corona-blunder-ecb/, accessed on 5 June 2020.
65. 'Europe's moment: Repair and prepare for the next generation', *European Commission*, 27 May 2020, available at https://ec.europa.eu/commission/presscorner/detail/en/ip_20_940, accessed on 4 June 2020.
66. Chiara De Cuia, 'Face Masks and Cheap Fakes: China's Italian Twitter Campaign', *NextGen 5.0*, June 2020, available at https://www.nextgen50.org/insecurity/analysis/Face-Masks-and-Cheap-Fakes%3A-China%E2%80%99s-Italian-Twitter-Campaign, accessed on 12 June 2020.
67. 'EEAS Special Report Update: Short Assessment of Narratives and Disinformation Around the Covid-19/Coronavirus Pandemic (Updated 2 – 22 April)', *EUvsDisinfo*, 24 April 2020, available at https://euvsdisinfo.eu/eeas-special-report-update-2-22-april/, accessed on 27 May 2020.
68. 'EU HRVP Josep Borrell: The Coronavirus pandemic and the new world it is creating', *Delegation of the European Union to China*, 24 March 2020, available at https://eeas.europa.eu/delegations/china/76401/eu-hrvp-josep-borrell-coronavirus-pandemic-and-new-world-it-creating_en, accessed on 27 May 2020.
69. Patrice Taddonio 'Covering Coronavirus: Cremona, Italy', *The FRONTLINE Dispatch, PBS*, 23 March 2020, available at https://www.pbs.org/wgbh/frontline/article/italy-doctors-offer-dire-coronavirus-warning-for-america/, accessed on 25 May 2020.

70. 'Decreto Rilancio, Gualtieri: 'Misure per reggere il colpo, Italia ce la farà, ripartiremo', *ANSA*, 17 May 2020, available at https://www.ansa.it/sito/notizie/politica/2020/05/13/dl-rilancio-cdm-alle-14_0ffce2b2-dec8-4a26-8e08-46dd7d0f91c3.html, accessed on 25 May 2020.
71. 'Decreto-Legge 19 maggio 2020, n. 34', *Gazzetta Ufficiale Della Repubblica Italiana*, 19 May 2020, available at https://www.gazzettaufficiale.it/static/20200519_128_SO_021.pdf, accessed on 26 May 2020.
72. 'Fisco, scuola, sanità, lavoro: dove vanno i 25 miliardi di aiuti per il coronavirus', *Il Sole 24 Ore*, 17 March 2020, available at https://www.ilsole24ore.com/art/fisco-scuola-sanita-lavoro-dove-vanno-25-miliardi-aiuti-il-coronavirus-AD7u8oD, accessed on 2 May 2020.
73. 'Decreto rilancio, Speranza: 'Tre miliardi e 250 milioni per il Ssn', *Ministero Della Salute*, 14 May 2020, available at http://www.salute.gov.it/portale/news/p3_2_1_1_1.jsp?lingua=italiano&menu=notizie&p=dalministero&id=4749, accessed on 28 May 2020.
74. Riccardo Liberatore, '«Quei bambini che si vergognano perché non hanno internet e non possono seguire le lezioni online» – L'intervista,' *Open*, 7 May 2020, available at https://www.open.online/2020/05/07/bambini-vergogna-internet-lezioni-online-intervista/, accessed on 18 May 2020.
75. 'Dl rilancio, critiche dalle opposizioni. Salvini: Bellanova pianga per gli italiani' *Sky tg24*, 14 May 2020, available at https://tg24.sky.it/politica/2020/05/14/dl-rilancio-salvini-bellanova-piange, accessed on 18 May 2020.
76. 'Decreto Rilancio, conferenza stampa a Palazzo Chigi', *Governo Italiano, Presidenza del Consiglio dei Ministri*, 13 May 2020, available at http://www.governo.it/it/articolo/decreto-rilancio-conferenza-stampa-palazzo-chigi/14600, accessed on 17 May 2020.
77. Comitato di esperti in materia economica e sociale, 'Iniziative per il rilancio. "Italia 2020-2022." Rapporto per il Presidente del Consiglio dei Ministri', *Governo Italiano, Presidenza del Consiglio dei Ministri*, 9 June 2020, available at http://www.governo.it/sites/new.governo.it/files/comitato_rapporto.pdf, accessed on 10 June 2020.
78. 'Coronavirus, cosa sono gli Stati generali voluti da Conte per il rilancio dell'Italia', *Sky tg24*, 11 June 2020, available at https://tg24.sky.it/economia/2020/06/11/stati-generali-cosa-sono, accessed on 12 June 2020.
79. 'Stati Generali dell'Economia: la conferenza stampa del premier Conte', *Corriere della Sera, Facebook Live*, 13 June 2020, available at https://www.facebook.com/watch/live/?v=376969909933881&ref=watch_permalink, accessed on 13 June 2020.

12

Sweden Reacts to COVID-19

Kanchana Ramanujam

Sweden is a Scandinavian country with a population of 10 million and a low density of population of 23.5 people per square kilometre. As for the age demography, one in four Swedes is younger than 20, and one in five is 65 years or older. In 2019, Sweden had a per capita GDP of 51,960 USD. It generally invests more than 3 percent of its GDP (Gross Domestic Product) in Research and Development (R&D).[1] The top five trading partners of Sweden as of 2020 are Germany, Norway, Netherlands, Denmark, and China.[2] The top exports of Sweden in 2018 were cars, refined petroleum, packaged medicaments, vehicle parts, and broadcasting equipment, while the imports in the same time-frame were cars, crude petroleum, refined petroleum, vehicle parts, and broadcasting equipment.[3] The northern part of Sweden is located in the cold, polar zone of the Arctic, and the southern areas in the temperate climatic zone.[4] Sweden follows a parliamentary democracy form of governance.[5] Its healthcare is largely tax-funded, ensuring that everyone has equal access to healthcare services. In 2018, health and medical care constituted around 11 percent of Sweden's GDP. The bulk of health and medical costs are paid for by regional and municipal taxes. Contributions from the national government are another source of funding, while patient fees cover only a small percentage of costs. There are also many digital healthcare solutions, such as patient-doctor apps. Sweden has one of Europe's largest elderly populations, which puts pressure on its healthcare system. Government spending on health, medical, and social care amounted to 78.4 billion SEK in 2018 – one of the larger expenses for the government.[6]

Figure 1: Sweden Map and Satellite Image

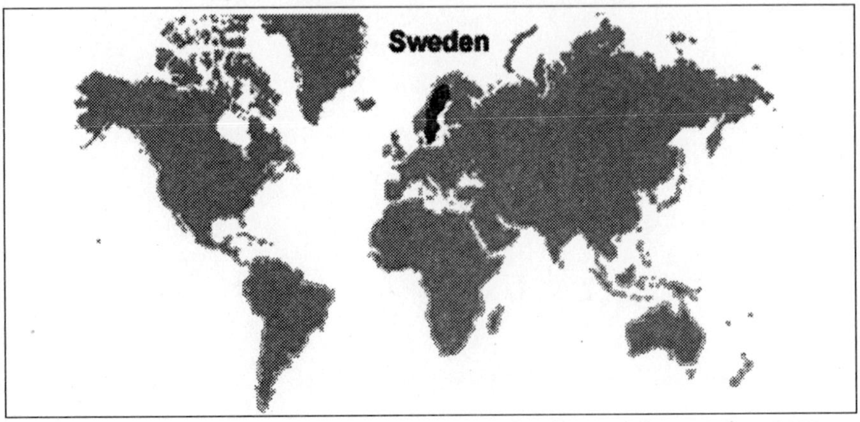

Source: https://geology.com/world/sweden-satellite-image.shtml, accessed on 19 June 2020.

The Emergence of the Virus in Sweden

The first case of Coronavirus disease 2019 (COVID-2019) in Sweden was detected on 31 January 2020, after a woman in Jönköping county tested positive for the virus. She had experienced respiratory problems upon returning from a trip to Wuhan on 24 January.[7] On 11 March, Sweden confirmed its first death related to COVID-19 when an elderly patient succumbed to the disease.[8]

Sweden adopted an unconventional, scientific, and trust-based approach in response to the pandemic, based on the following five aspects:[9]

(i) The pivotal role of expert agencies and international bodies despite the government being in charge.
(ii) Prioritising the protection of the elderly and risk groups.
(iii) Social distancing and incentives to stay at home.
(iv) Aim for endurable strategies and public trust.
(v) Flexible adjustment to developments on the ground.

A Different Approach Based on the Constitution

What sets the Swedish approach apart from other international responses is an expert agency, the Public Health Agency, being in virtual control of the entire response to the pandemic, and the focus on voluntary adherence to guidelines with no enforced lockdowns. This approach is in harmony with the Swedish Constitution which guarantees full freedom of movement for Swedes during peacetime conditions. While this freedom is not absolute, there is no exception for an eventuality like a pandemic. The freedom of assembly and freedom to demonstrate may be limited in the event of an 'epidemic'. Hence, a nation-wide lockdown owing to a 'pandemic' was perhaps not seen as the best option. The Constitution also, quite uniquely, guarantees the independence of public agencies. The Public Health Agency of Sweden (*Folkhälsomyndigheten*) is run by experts in the field, not by political appointees, and the state epidemiologist–Anders Tegnell–is leading Sweden's response against COVID-19. Besides, the Constitutional empowerment of local self-government decentralises the response to such emergencies, greatly improving efficiency.[10]

A Strategy that did not Require an Exit-Plan

What dictated Sweden's approach to the pandemic was the understanding that a long-term, sustainable model of living with the virus needed to be devised. The aim has been to keep the transmission rate as low as possible on the basis of a sustainable strategy that did not require an exit plan (as opposed to countries that went in for lockdown and then had to devise plans for opening up). The COVID-19 virus had already reached every major European country, there was uncertainty over when the vaccine would be discovered, and the virus was expected to be around for a long time; hence, rather than enforce restrictions, Sweden decided to keep going, taking its citizens into confidence. When its Scandinavian neighbours such as Denmark, Norway, and Finland resorted to drastic measures like lockdowns, Sweden issued voluntary, 'trust-based' measures for responsible behaviour. To ensure responsible behaviour, Sweden has issued the following advice for its citizens:

- Stay at home if you have symptoms.
- Wash your hands frequently with soap and water for at least 20 seconds.
- Keep your distance from other people, both indoors and outdoors.
- Be careful when visiting people who are aged more than 70 or belong to an at-risk group.
- If you are aged 70 or over, it is particularly important to limit social contacts and avoid places where people gather.
- Avoid large social gatherings.

In addition, advice on safe socialising and hygiene, and guidelines to be followed when one or one's family member is ill have been made available. Interestingly, the Public Health Agency of Sweden has not made face-masks mandatory, stating that good hand-hygiene and social distancing would suffice. In the section on advice on face masks, it has been stated that "According to the Public Health Agency of Sweden, face masks are not needed in everyday life. It is better to keep a distance from other people and maintain good hand hygiene." The World Health Organization (WHO) writes that "face masks can create a false sense of security in people who wear them, which can result in wearers forgetting important safety measures such as good hand hygiene and keeping a physical distance from others. According to the WHO, face masks that are not approved for medical use risk increasing the spread of infection if they are not used properly. One example is if you touch the face mask with your hands, thereby picking up the virus or transferring your own virus to your hands."[11] Since the WHO acknowledges that there is no direct, scientific evidence to support the widespread use of masks and that masks are required only where social distancing cannot be practised, Sweden has not made masks mandatory.[12] Sweden has also changed its sick-pay rules as a response to the pandemic. While Swedish laws guarantee sick-pay from the second day of illness, for one-and-a-half months from 11 March 2020, workers got sickness benefits from the day they took leave on account of illness. The bill for the same was footed by the State and not the employers.[13]

Identifying those over 70 years of age as particularly vulnerable, Sweden has issued special guidelines for them focussing on social distancing. They have been advised to seek assistance from the municipality for food shopping and performing errands. To quote from the advisory – 'Advanced age is the foremost risk factor for developing severe symptoms in case of infection with COVID-19. Therefore, if you are older than 70 years, you are encouraged to do the following:

- Limit close contact with others.
- Avoid places where large numbers of people gather, for example, shops or public transport.
- Maintain contact with your nearest and dearest via telephone or computer.
- Walk outdoors.
- Ask for assistance with food shopping and performing errands. Contact your municipality if you do not have anyone who can help you. The Swedish eHealth Agency (eHälsomyndigheten) provides information about which rules apply for collecting prescribed medicines from pharmacies on someone else's behalf.'[14]

Additionally, the government has also placed a national ban on visiting all of the country's retirement homes (since 1 April 2020), a ban on public gatherings and events, and entry to Sweden. All these bans come with reasonable exemptions. It is also pertinent to note that schools (for below 16 years of age), public transport, private events, and visits to shops are exempt from the ban on public gatherings and events. As restaurants, cafés, and pubs remain functional, they have been issued rules on avoiding crowding of people in queues, at tables, buffets, or bar counters. The 'new rules for restaurants, cafés and pubs' issued by Sweden are given as under:

- crowding of people in queues, at tables, buffets or bar counters must not occur. Visitors should be able to maintain a distance between each other;
- visitors must eat and drink while sitting at a table. Staff should carry out the orders;
- if it is possible to allow the guests to order and pick up food and drink themselves then this is allowed as long as it does not lead to crowding or queues;
- takeaway can be handed over as usual as long as it can take place without crowding of people;
- restaurants and après-ski activities at ski resorts are subject to the rules for restaurants and pubs issued by the Public Health Agency.[15]

Starting 13 June 2020, Swedes who showed no symptoms of the disease were allowed to travel domestically and take the public transport while observing social distancing.[16] From 30 June 2020, the Swedish Ministry of Foreign Affairs will remove the advisory against non-essential travel to ten countries: Belgium, France, Greece, Iceland, Italy, Croatia, Luxembourg, Portugal, Switzerland, and Spain. However, the travel advisory against non-essential travel to other countries would remain.[17]

Herd Immunity not the Central Thrust

Many commentators have pointed to Sweden's approach as being centred on the concept of 'herd immunity'. What is herd immunity? When the majority of a population is immune to an infectious disease, it offers indirect protection to others who are not immune. It happens because the chain of infection gets disrupted, stopping/slowing the spread of the disease. This is called herd immunity. As is evident, herd immunity is of relevance only to contagious diseases. Rinderpest and Smallpox are two diseases that have been eradicated using herd immunity and vaccination.

There are two ways to achieve herd immunity – either the majority of the population gets infected or is administered a vaccine. Diseases like Polio and Chickenpox, which were earlier very common, have now become rare as vaccines have helped in establishing herd immunity. Depending on the contagiousness of the disease, 70-90 percent of the population needs immunity to achieve it. Some studies suggest that at least 70 percent of the population to be immune to establish herd protection against COVID-19.[18]

Herd immunity is a critical means of protecting those who cannot be vaccinated or cannot develop immunity after vaccination because of medical conditions. For example, infants and immunocompromised patients cannot be administered many vaccines. Additionally, vaccine contraindications may also prevent its use in certain people. These people could be protected if people around them are immune.

Anders Tegnell has denied herd immunity being the focus of Sweden's strategy. Tegnell has stated that while herd immunity will benefit Sweden in the long-run, it is not the central thrust of Sweden's strategy. Had the case been so, Sweden would not have put in place any measures to combat COVID-19 and just allowed the disease to spread.[19]

Statistics and the Situation

According to reports published on 26 May 2020, half of Sweden's COVID-19 deaths have been in nursing homes or other elderly care facilities. As such, a mandatory lockdown could not have impacted the statistics significantly. Sweden's dismal statistics notwithstanding, fewer people are being admitted to intensive care units (ICU), and there has been a drop in the number of cases and deaths in nursing homes.[20]

As of 30 June 2020, Sweden has recorded 5,310 deaths and the death statistics (as also the infection statistics) show a definite downward trend (see Figure 1). The Reproduction Rate (R rate[21]) of the disease stands at 0.84, meaning that the virus is coming under control.[22] However, the contagion rate in Sweden is the highest in the Nordic region and it has one of the worst COVID-19 mortality rates in the world. The high contagion rate notwithstanding, the trends in immunity have been low. While this remains unexplained, Tegnell has also pointed to the time-lag in the collection of samples and the reporting of results.[23]

Figure 2: Confirmed Daily COVID-19 Deaths in Sweden

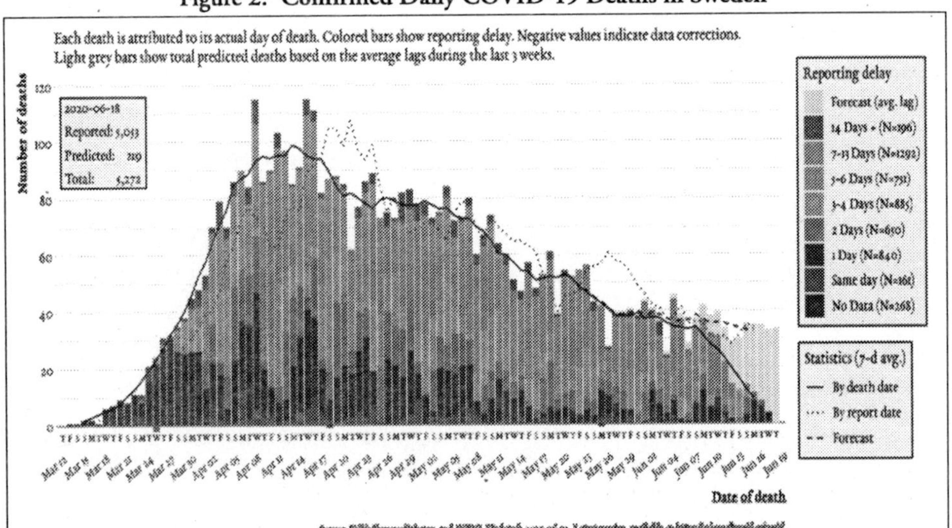

Source: https://adamaltmejd.se/covid/, accessed on 20 June 2020.

25 percent of the Swedish population is of recent non-Swedish descent and immigrants from Somalia, Iraq, Syria, and Afghanistan are grossly overrepresented in the COVID-19 death statistics. The reasons are believed to be the housing density in immigrant suburbs and a lack of information in the languages of the immigrants.[24]

Is Sweden Better Placed to Deal with the Pandemic?

While other countries have given a forceful reaction to the pandemic, Sweden has focussed on adapting to the situation. This will not only cushion the economic impact of COVID-19 on Sweden but also make Swedes more prepared for a second wave of the virus expected in Autumn. In fact, being able to avoid multiple lockdowns would have even helped Swedes escape its impact on mental health as well. The lessons learnt initially, especially from the deaths in the elderly homes, improvements in the contact tracing system and the healthcare, and immunity built up in the population would further add to Sweden's preparedness.

It has to be borne in mind that cultural/demographic factors were force-multipliers in Sweden's approach to the pandemic. These are:

- There is a strong bond of trust amongst Swedes and between Swedes and the government. This means that even recommendations are taken as seriously as rules.
- There is a difference in the family structures in Sweden where almost half of Swedish households consist of a single person. The elderly tend to live alone or in state-supported homes as there is no tradition of living with grandparents.[25]
- Sweden has a very low density of population.

The Swedish Model: Jury is Still Out!

While many media outlets and even experts have been critical of Sweden's approach, it is too early to write-off the 'Swedish model'. It would be wrong to cite statistics to criticise the Swedish model until a reasonable time has lapsed. The very fact that Sweden's healthcare system is functional and has not exceeded the maximum capacity is reflective of the relative success of the strategy. It is also pertinent to mention that despite the lockdown, the rest of Europe has not been able to contain the spread of the virus significantly.[26] Only a long-term perspective can decide whether the Swedish approach is a success or a failure (or something in between).

NOTES

1. *Quick Facts about Sweden, Sweden Sverige,* available at https://sweden.se/quick-facts/, accessed 18 June 2020.
2. Imports from Our 30 Largest Trade Partners, *Statistics Sweden,* available at https://www.scb.se/en/finding-statistics/statistics-by-subject-area/trade-in-goods-and-services/foreign-trade/foreign-trade--exports-and-imports-of-goods/pong/tables-and-graphs/imports-from-our-30-largest-trade-partners/, accessed 18 June 2020.
3. Sweden (SWE) Exports, Imports, and Trade Partners, *OEC world,* available at https://oec.world/en/profile/country/swe/#:~:text=In%202018%2C%20Sweden's%20exports%20per,Broadcasting%20Equipment%20(%243.74B), accessed 18 June 2020.
4. Climate in Sweden, *Worlddata.info,* available at https://www.worlddata.info/europe/sweden/climate.php, accessed 18 June 2020.
5. 'The Swedish System of Government,' *Sweden Sverige,* available at https://sweden.se/society/the-swedish-system-of-government/, accessed 18 June 2020.
6. 'Healthcare in Sweden,' *Sweden Sverige,* available at https://sweden.se/society/health-care-in-sweden/, accessed 18 June 2020.
7. Lee Roden, 'First Case of Corona Virus in Sweden Confirmed,' *Sveriges radio.se,* January 2020, available at https://sverigesradio.se/sida/artikel.aspx?programid=2054&artikel=7398979, accessed 20 June 2020.
8. 'Sweden Confirms First Death of Coronavirus Patient,' *The local.se,* 11 March 2020, available at https://www.thelocal.se/20200311/sweden-confirms-first-death-of-coronavirus-patient, accessed 20 June 2020.
9. Lina Hallengren, 'Sweden's Response to COVID-19,'Ministry of Health and Social Affairs, available at https://apps.who.int/gb/COVID-19/pdf_files/23_04/Sweden.pdf,accessed 20 June 2020.
10. Lars Jonung, 'Sweden's Constitution Decides its Exceptional COVID-19 Policy,' *VOX CEPR Policy Portal,* 18 June 2020,available at https://voxeu.org/article/sweden-s-constitution-decides-its-exceptional-covid-19-policy, accessed 20 June 2020.
11. Slow Down the Spread of COVID-19, *Krisinformation.se,* 20 May 2020, available at https://www.krisinformation.se/en/hazards-and-risks/disasters-and-incidents/2020/official-information-on-the-new-coronavirus/sa-minskar-vi-smittspridningen, accessed 20 June 2020.
12. Catherine Edwards, 'Why is Sweden Still not Asking People to Wear Face Masks?' *The local.se,* 8 June 2020, available at https://www.thelocal.se/20200608/why-isnt-sweden-asking-people-to-wear-face-masks, accessed 18 June 2020.
13. 'Sweden Changes Sick Pay Rules to Help Fight Coronavirus,' *The local.se,* 2020, 11 March 2020, available at https://www.thelocal.se/20200311/sweden-changes-sick-pay-rules-to-help-fight-coronavirus, accessed 20 June 2020.
14. Advice to those over 70 Years Old, *Krisinformation.se,* 20 May 2020, available at https://www.krisinformation.se/en/hazards-and-risks/disasters-and-incidents/2020/official-information-on-the-new-coronavirus/du-som-ar-over-70-ar, accessed 20 June 2020.
15. Restrictions and Prohibitions, *Krisinformation.se,* 12 June 2020, available at https://www.krisinformation.se/en/hazards-and-risks/disasters-and-incidents/2020/official-information-on-the-new-coronavirus/restriktioner-och-forbud, accessed 20 June 2020.
16. Domestic Travel and Public Transport, *Krisinformation.se,* 5 June 2020,available at https://www.krisinformation.se/en/hazards-and-risks/disasters-and-incidents/2020/official-information-

on-the-new-coronavirus/domestic-travel-and-public-transport, accessed 20 June 2020.

17. 'Changes in Travel Advisories for Ten Countries,' *Krisinformation.se*, 17 June 2020, available at https://www.krisinformation.se/en/news/2020/june/ud-lifting-travel-advice-for-ten-countries-on-30-june/, accessed 20 June 2020.
18. G. D'Souza and D. Dowdy, 'What is Herd Immunity And How Can We Achieve it with COVID-19?,' *Johns Hopkins Bloomberg School of Public Health*, 2020, available at https://www.jhsph.edu/covid-19/articles/achieving-herd-immunity-with-covid19.html, accessed 26 June 2020.
19. Kim Hjelmgaard, 'Swedish Official Anders Tegnell Says 'Herd Immunity' in Sweden Might be a Few Weeks Away,' *USA Today*,28 April 2020, available at https://www.usatoday.com/story/news/world/2020/04/28/coronavirus-covid-19-sweden-anders-tegnell-herd-immunity/3031536001/,accessed 20 June 2020.
20. Dave Russell, 'COVID-19 Deaths Top 4,000 But Overall Situation In Sweden "Getting Better,"' *Radio Sweden*, 26 March 2020, available at https://sverigesradio.se/sida/artikel.aspx?programid=2054&artikel=7481310,accessed 20 June 2020.
21. It is the number of people that one infected person, on average, will pass the virus on to.
22. Holly Ellyatt, 'Change of Plan? Here's What Sweden Will do if There's a 'Second Wave' of the Coronavirus,' *CNBC*,18 June 2020, available at https://www.cnbc.com/2020/06/17/swedens-plan-if-theres-a-second-wave-of-coronavirus.html, accessed 20 June 2020.
23. 'Sweden Proves 'Surprisingly Slow' in Achieving Herd Immunity, '*The Indian Express*, 2020,17 June 2020, available at https://indianexpress.com/article/world/sweden-proves-surprisingly-slow-in-achieving-herd-immunity6463515/,accessed 20 June 2020.
24. Hans Bergstrom, 'Grim Truth of the 'Swedish Model,' *The Japan Times*,20 April 2020, available at https://www.japantimes.co.jp/opinion/2020/04/20/commentary/world-commentary/grim-truth-swedish-model/#.Xu9c_5ozbIW,accessed 20 June 2020.
25. Paul Waldie, 'Why is Sweden Staying Open Amid the Coronavirus Pandemic?', *The Globe and Mail*, 2 April 2020, available at https://www.theglobeandmail.com/world/article-why-is-sweden-staying-open-amid-the-coronavirus-pandemic/,accessed 20 June 2020.
26. Marta Paterlini, 'Closing Borders is Ridiculous: The Epidemiologist Behind Sweden's Controversial Coronavirus Strategy,' *Nature*, 21 April 2020, available at https://www.nature.com/articles/d41586-020-01098-x, accessed 20 June 2020.

13

The UK Experience Three Months into the Pandemic

Paul Rogers

The lockdown in the UK (United Kingdom) started in late March and there was subsequently criticism of the government on a number of counts that it had been consistently slow and often inefficient in responding to the pandemic. Elements of this included delays in bringing in lockdown procedures even when other European countries had done so and calls to act faster were being made by many in the UK scientific community, delays in organising a track-trace-test programme, persistent shortages of personal protection equipment (PPE) for health and care workers and far too little attention given to the spread of COVID-19 in care homes.

Much of the criticism has its roots in what is seen as the slow pace of government actions from late January to early March and concerns the period from the first of the government's COBRA (Cabinet Office Briefing Room A) emergency meetings on 27 January onwards. There is, though, evidence that the government should have been aware of the risk of a disastrous pandemic and taken stronger action at an earlier stage. The failures during the pandemic may well be primary themes of the public inquiry that will most certainly follow the end of the pandemic, whenever that will be, and there is much evidence still to emerge as the controversy continues. While this is inevitable, the issues of preparedness and early warnings remain fundamental to understanding the predicament of the country just over three months into the pandemic.

This chapter first draws attention to the claims of the government that the UK was exceptionally well-prepared to respond to a pandemic, contrasts that with what was known of physical preparations and then explores the early evidence that a crisis was evolving. There appear to have been many failures and it can already be argued that these will have made the pandemic, the loss of life, the hardship and the long-term damage to the economy far worse than should have been the case. Moreover, while this chapter is concerned primarily with the UK, the analysis is applicable to many other states, not least in Western Europe as well as the United States. Although some states believed that they had biological security response systems, many of them were ill-prepared for the pandemic even if others acted very quickly and effectively, especially in East Asia. The UK may have been a particularly bad example, but it was not the only one. Even so, analysing the behaviour of a state with one of the worst records to date may be of particular value in the future as an example from which to learn.

Preparedness

In August 2018 the Government published the UK National Biological Security Strategy which emphasised the need to respond to the spread of serious diseases.[1] The first of its kind for the UK, the 46-page strategy was widely regarded as a good example of science-based planning and highlighted the importance of strong public communications as part of swift action in the event of a crisis. Three extracts illustrate the tenor of the report.

> First: "*The UK is globally renowned for the quality of our preparedness planning, and we have world-leading capabilities to address significant biological risks. Across local and national Government and the Devolved Administrations, and through our work internationally, the UK invests hundreds of millions of pounds a year in protecting against and preparing for disease outbreaks and biological incidents.*"
>
> Second, relating specifically to pandemic risks, the Foreword states: "*Significant outbreaks of disease are among the highest impact risks faced by any society – threatening lives and causing disruption to public services and the economy*" and "*As a global leader in the biological sciences, we have an opportunity to demonstrate our expertise and be at the forefront of work to meet these challenges.*"
>
> Third, it concludes: "*We cannot predict all the ways in which this risk landscape will evolve in the future, but it is by breaking down barriers, working in a co-ordinated way across and beyond Government, and thinking globally*

that we will be best prepared to meet the threat of significant disease outbreaks (however they occur)."

At the time of the strategy's publication, the government could, therefore, say, at least in theory, that it was doing its duty, and this was an opinion shared by the World Economic Forum's (WEF) league table of preparedness for large-scale disease outbreaks, itself using data from the Global Health Security Index. That assessment ranked 195 countries and placed the UK in the second position, arguably confirming the UK Government's view. The ten best-prepared countries were, in order, the USA, the UK, the Netherlands, Australia, Canada, Thailand, Sweden, Denmark, South Korea and Finland.[2]

As will be discussed later, most of the countries in the list have so far been relatively effective in responding to the pandemic, but the first two, the USA and the UK, have not, and this may be a reflection of parallel factors, other than medical issues, operating at a national level. While the WEF assessment appears with the benefit of hindsight to be seriously wrong in relation to these two states, it needs to be recognised that "preparedness" can be assessed primarily on what a government says it is doing and what its overall strategy is. It is, therefore, to an extent, theoretical. In this respect, the Strategy does go further and points out that the 2015 National Security Risk Assessment (NSRA), did identify a major human health crisis such as pandemic influenza as a Tier One risk. It also made it clear that not all biological risks can be prevented, crises will occur, and adequate resources must, therefore, be available.[3]

In the context of what has happened since, theory and practice turned out to be very different, as illustrated by warnings from public health officials following exercises undertaken to test the actual levels of readiness. One major planning exercise had assumed a new and dangerous flu pandemic, which according to the *Daily Telegraph* "dramatically exposed the gaps in Britain's pandemic response but its 'terrifying' findings have yet to be published".[4] Afterwards, the NHS England Board was told in October 2016 "NHS England prepared for and participated in *Exercise Cygnus*, a three-day exercise looking at the impact of a pandemic influenza outbreak, and the significant impacts on health delivery a widespread pandemic in the UK would trigger". *Exercise Cygnus* showed that NHS resources would be critically overstretched in such a pandemic.[5]

Before this, the government created several other blueprints for how the UK should respond in the event of an influenza-type pandemic. From 2011-2014, there were three strategies written: the "Influenza Pandemic Preparedness Strategy", the "Health and Social Care Influenza Pandemic Preparedness and Response" and the "Pandemic Influenza Response Plan". Yet the evaluation of *Cygnus* suggests that there was little practical implementation of these plans.

To make matters worse, as recently as last year the 2019 annual *National Security Risk Assessment* specifically dealt with the risk of a flu-type pandemic and urged the government to prepare fully. As *The Guardian* reported:

> "The detailed document warned that even a mild pandemic could cost tens of thousands of lives, and set out the must-have 'capability requirements' to mitigate the risks to the country, as well as the potential damage of not doing so."[6]

It emphasised the need to stockpile appropriate equipment to establish disease surveillance and contact tracing and even draw up plans to handle excess deaths.

According to the report, the 600-page Cabinet Office report set out reasonable worst-case scenarios (RWCS) that now make for uncomfortable reading:

- "A pandemic would play out in up to "three waves", with each wave expected to last 15 weeks … "with the peak weeks occurring at weeks 6 and 7 in each wave".
- 50% of the population would be infected and experience symptoms of pandemic influenza during the one or more waves. The actual number of people infected would be higher than this, as there would be a number of asymptomatic cases.
- A pandemic of moderate virulence could lead to 65,600 deaths.
- The potential cost to the UK could be £2.35 Trillion.
- Even after the end of the pandemic, it is likely that it would take months or even years for health and social care services to recover.
- There would be significant public outrage over any perceived poor handling of the government's preparations and response to the emergency."

Part of the explanation for why the government was slow to respond to the COVID-19 outbreak may lie in a report that a key sub-committee of the National Security Council was first mothballed by Prime Minister Theresa May because of the pressure of government work over Brexit and subsequently scrapped by Mr Boris Johnson when he took over the July last year. This was the Threats, Hazards, Resilience and Contingency Committee (THRCC) that included fifteen Cabinet Ministers among its members. According to one report, "a former Cabinet minister who was a member of THRCC until it was axed said it could have ensured the Government reacted more quickly to coronavirus, adding "Once the pandemic took hold in Italy...alarm bells would have been ringing."[7]

Overall, and in view of what is now known, it does appear that government claims of world-leadership in biosecurity were far from accurate, as became clear from an early stage in the pandemic's development.

Warning Indicators

Although the initial belief was that COVID-19 did not make it into Western Europe until well into January of this year, there are indications that cases were emerging earlier. In late December, one French patient who was taken into hospital on 27 December subsequently tested positive for COVID-19. In China itself, the authorities in Wuhan and later in Beijing tried for many weeks to suppress reports of a new disease condition. They did eventually report to the World Health Organisation (WHO) that the first infection was recorded on 8 December, but government sources subsequently indicated that an earlier case was recorded on 17 November.

Precisely when the COVID-19 virus made the "jump" from animal to human host is still not known but it is the subject of considerable research. For example, one method, phylogenetic analysis, tentatively indicates that the transfer for animals to humans could have occurred sometime between September and December last year.[8]

Separately, it was reported on 9 April by one of the main US news channels, *ABC*, that US intelligence sources first got indications of a disease outbreak in Wuhan of unknown origin in November as a result of work by a little-known element of the US intelligence system, the *National Center for Medical Intelligence* (NCMI).[9] The Center's work is focused on the health of military personnel working overseas and this extends to people based at a number of sites throughout South East and East Asia, and according to *ABC*:

> "Concerns about what is now known to be the novel coronavirus pandemic were detailed in a November intelligence report by the military's National Center for Medical Intelligence (NCMI), according to two officials familiar with the document's contents".

The report was the result of analysis of wire and computer intercepts, coupled with satellite images. It raised alarms because an out-of-control disease would pose a serious threat to U.S. forces in Asia – forces that depend on the NCMI's work. And it paints a picture of an American government that could have ramped up mitigation and containment efforts far earlier to prepare for a crisis poised to come home.

"Analysts concluded it could be a cataclysmic event," one of the sources said of the NCMI's report. "It was then briefed multiple times to" the Defense Intelligence Agency, the Pentagon's Joint Staff and the White House. Wednesday night, the Pentagon issued a statement denying the "product/assessment" existed.

The Pentagon denial was couched in carefully chosen words and might have dampened interest in the report but a week later, on 16 April, the *Times of Israel* reported on a Channel 12 News report that the Israel Defence Force (IDF) had been alerted to the Wuhan outbreak by the US intelligence community, also in November.[10] US intelligence agencies alerted Israel to the coronavirus outbreak in China already in November, Israeli television reported Thursday.

According to Israel's Channel 12 News, the US intelligence community became aware of the emerging disease in Wuhan in the second week of that month and drew up a classified document. Information on the disease outbreak was not in the public domain at that stage – and was known only apparently to the Chinese government.

US intelligence informed the Trump administration, "which did not deem it of interest," but the report said the Americans also decided to update allies with the classified document: NATO and Israel, specifically the Israeli Defence Force. The network said Israeli military officials later in November discussed the possibility of the spread of the virus to the region and how it would affect Israel and neighbouring countries. The intelligence also reached Israel's decision makers and the Health Ministry, where "nothing was done," according to the report.

There is some independent open source support for the view that COVID-19 was active in Wuhan in the autumn in an analysis of commercial satellite data conducted by the Computational Epidemiology Laboratory at Boston Children's Hospital that showed marked spikes in activity at the five major hospitals in the city and indications of a possible link with a spike in respiratory infections.[11]

The Critical Week: 30 December to 5 January

At the time of writing, it is not known whether any NATO allies took up the matter and passed on assessments to governments and according to the UK government the first communication to the health minister, Mr Matt Hancock, was not until 3 January. He spoke to ministry officials on 6 January, received advice from the UK Health Security Team and spoke to the Prime Minister, Mr Johnson, on 7 January after he had returned from a 10-day Caribbean holiday. Mr Hancock later updated parliament on 23 January when, according to a government statement, the risk level of a pandemic was "Very Low" and remained at that level through to 29 January when it was raised to "Low", two days before the first reported case in the UK.

This contrasts markedly with developments elsewhere, especially over the period 30 December to 5 January, and not least in territories neighbouring China. Taiwan, for example, was already treating the issue as a potentially substantial risk. According to its London representative,

> "Learning harsh lessons from the SARS crisis in 2003, the government of Taiwan acted swiftly and established a central command centre in order to respond to the outbreak. Taiwan's health minister held press conferences almost every day to provide updates and information. Tests on travellers from Wuhan, the Chinese city where the outbreak started, began in December."[12]

Hong Kong was also fully engaged at an early stage. By the time Mr Hancock in London had spoken to officials on 6 January and spoken to Mr Johnson on 7 January the Hong Kong authorities were already treating the risk of a major new disease outbreak as a threat requiring immediate responses.

On 3 January the Government of Hong Kong issued a notice reporting that a cluster of 44 viral pneumonia cases of unknown cause in the city of Wuhan had been recorded, with 11 in a serious condition. Because of this the Centre for Health Protection had enhanced surveillance from 31 December and stated that:

> "Doctors are requested to report to the CHP if they encounter patients with fever and acute respiratory symptoms, or pneumonia symptoms; and who had visited Wuhan (regardless of whether they have visited wet markets or seafood markets there) within 14 days prior to the onset of the illness."[13]

It also announced that a dedicated web page had been set up and that additional thermal imaging had been set up at Hong Kong International Airport dedicated to checking body temperatures of arrivals from Wuhan and

> "Additional manpower has also been assigned to Hong Kong West Kowloon Station of the Guangzhou-Shenzhen-Hong Kong Express Rail Link for checking body temperature of inbound travellers. Those with relevant symptoms and travel history will be immediately referred to public hospitals for isolation, treatment and follow-up."[14]

The following day the Government issued a further notice, this time from the hospital authority announcing the activation of Serious Response Level in public hospitals with immediate effect and launched its Preparedness and Response Plan for Novel Infectious Diseases of Public Health Significance.[15] Measures were announced to enhance monitoring and infection control in public hospitals and clinics with immediate effect and frontline healthcare staff "have been reminded to pay special attention to patient's clinical information, including the presentation of fever and acute respiratory illness, or pneumonia, and travel history to Wuhan within 14 days before the onset of symptoms." In an indication of the authorities' concern:

> "The spokesperson also stressed that any suspected case will be isolated in negative pressure isolation room for treatment with urgent laboratory investigation will be arranged immediately".

The press release also laid down procedures for more stringent infection control measures, including severe restrictions on hospital visits, and also set out requirements for the use of personal protection equipment (PPE) including N95 masks, confirming that "the current stockpile is adequate for three months' consumption."

The public impact of these measures in Hong Kong itself may have been low but this is not surprising in view of the ongoing public protests and political upheavals but they demonstrated the considerable concern of health professionals at the risk of a major disease crisis.

Thus, as early as 5 January, it was evident that at least two administrations, Taiwan and Hong Kong, were greatly concerned about the Wuhan outbreak, and had certainly been aware of developments since late December, but the UK Prime Minister was not even informed of the outbreak until 7 January. This was in spite of clear government statements about the serious risk of respiratory pandemics and claims that the UK was a world leader in biosecurity strategy.

Perhaps most surprising is that even on 7 January the issue was already in the public domain in the UK. On that day, *New Scientist* published online a report from one of its writers, Jessica Hamzelou who covers biomedical sciences, that reported on the emerging story even to the extent of including a direct link to the Hong Kong Hospital Authority press release cited above.[16]

By 13 January the WHO was warning of human-to-human transmission risk, this was confirmed by China's health ministry the following day and that the virus had spread across the country.[17] On 23 January a complete lockdown of the whole of Wuhan province was enacted and on the following day, *The Lancet* published the first detailed report on the clinical features of the infection. By 19 January cases had been reported in Thailand, Japan and South Korea and by 24 January there were 835 cases in China. Only on that day did the UK government finally called a meeting of the COBRA emergency committee but this would not meet until 27 January and the Prime Minister did not attend.

Preliminary Analysis

The UK experience of the COVID-19 pandemic through to late June raises a number of specific questions as well as the major issue of why the UK government, with its stated position of world leadership in pandemic preparedness, had so far failed on a number of counts. How and when was the government informed by intelligence, diplomatic and other sources of the nature and extent of the outbreak and the early responses of governments such as Hong Kong and Taiwan? Some press reports state that the Secret Intelligence Service (MI6) kept the government fully informed of developments, although neither source nor specific dates were given.[18] If these are accurate, though, when did the government receive such information and how did it act on it?

The UK is a key member of NATO, including staff in senior leadership roles, and is also part of the five eyes intelligence consortium along with the United States, Australia, Canada and New Zealand. If NATO was informed of the outbreak in November, as US and Israeli sources have indicated, did NATO act on it and, if so, how? Why was the UK government so slow to respond to the emerging crisis and why did the Prime Minister, as head of government, take such a back-seat role when a Tier 1 emergency was developing and was recognised as such by the Hong Kong government and others?

On the major question, the issue is how do these early failings and the continuing controversies over the speed of reaction relate to the political environment at the time which appears to have prioritised economic growth over risk to health? At the time of writing that remains an issue of the current controversy over the question of accelerating the easing of lockdown, from 4 July, to limit further damage to the economy against the risk of stimulating a second COVID-19 wave. While it seems reasonable to argue that any critique of government can be countered by the benefit of hindsight is a marvellous thing, and that governments in Hong Kong and Taiwan had experienced SARS and had the COVID-19 outbreak uncomfortably close to them, Wuhan is less than 12 hours direct flight from London and the UK claimed to be fully prepared.

On the more general economic issue, from the term of office of Prime Minister Margaret Thatcher in the 1980s, most UK governments pursued policies accentuating the private sector and privatising many elements of public service including energy, water, transport, telecommunications and parts of the National Health Service (NHS). The public health system, in particular, saw successive funding cuts relative to need, and in the NHS itself, there was a decline in the provision of hospital beds in favour of more emphasis on primary care. This all meant that with the COVID-19 emergency the government had to call on private contractors to fill many of the gaps leading to persistent problems of coordination, consistency and quality of provision.

Furthermore, in the three years prior to the COVID-19 outbreak government activities were dominated by the decision to leave the European Union ("Brexit"), with very large numbers of civil servants re-deployed to this end, leaving numerous government departments short-staffed in key areas. Matters then came to a head in December 2019 with a sudden general election which the Conservative Party won by an unexpectedly large majority. As a result, there was a strong culture of success, combined with a determination to concentrate on the formal leaving of the EU which was due at the end of January 2020.

The first clear indication of the incoming government's approach to the COVID-19 issue came in a major policy speech by the Prime Minister on 3 February following Brexit, his one mention of the pandemic being a clear reminder of the dominant importance of free trade and economic growth over health risks:

> "...we are starting to hear some bizarre autarkic rhetoric, when barriers are going up, and when there is a risk that new diseases such as coronavirus will trigger a panic and a desire for market segregation that go beyond what is medically rational to the point of doing real and unnecessary economic damage, then at that moment humanity needs some government somewhere that is willing at least to make the case powerfully for freedom of exchange, some country ready to take off its Clark Kent spectacles and leap into the phone booth and emerge with its cloak flowing as the supercharged champion, of the right of the populations of the earth to buy and sell freely among each other."[19]

Shortly after the speech the Prime Minister took a further 12-day break from Downing Street and did not attend four meetings of the COBRA emergency committee concerned with the evolving pandemic.

Conclusion

This theme of the centrality of economic growth in relation to health issues continues to be a major feature of the debate on government policy as reflected in the decision to ease the lockdown, a position that is even more strongly advocated in the United States. Meanwhile, COVID-19 is having a devastating impact on health and well-being across the world and is the greatest challenge to human security for half a century. At the time of writing (late June) there were around 10 million confirmed cases and close to half a million deaths worldwide, with clear indications of second waves in many countries including the United States, India and Iran and, globally the pandemic was accelerating rapidly.

The experience across the world has been of much suffering and grief but the longer-term consequences will also be economic, with much of the world tipping into a deep recession. The UK, for example, experienced a 20 percent decrease in GDP in March and April and has entered the deepest recession in three hundred years. There have been over 53,000 deaths from COVID-19 and excess deaths overall are already more than over 65,000. Poorer people are much more likely to die from COVID-19 and there have been disproportionate deaths among the BAME (Black and Minority Ethnic) population. Lockdown is about to be eased before the pandemic is fully under control and there are serious concerns over the high risk of a second wave through the autumn and winter. There are fears that potentially this would result in even more suffering and an eventual death toll in excess of 100,000. The UK government was confident six months ago that it was well prepared for a pandemic, yet it is abundantly clear that this was not the case, with its responses all too often being too little, too late. This has been despite the best efforts of millions of people and especially the courage of health and care workers.

* * *

Acknowledgement: *This chapter is adapted from: Paul Rogers, "Writing on the Wall? The UK and the Early Signs of COVID-19", International Security Monthly Briefing, Oxford Research Group, June 2020. Alasdair McKay, Malcolm Dando and Lee Chadwick are thanked for assistance with that report.*

NOTES

1. 'UK National Biological Security Strategy, July 2018', available at https://www.gov.uk/government/publications/biological-security-strategy, accessed on 18 June, 2020.
2. Niall McCarthy, 'These are the Top 10 Countries for Pandemic Preparedness', *World Economic Forum*, Geneva, 15 November 2019, available at https://www.weforum.org/agenda/2019/11/countries-preparedness-pandemics/, accessed on 19 June, 2020.
3. 'National Security Strategy and Strategic Defence and Security Review 2015', November 2015, available at https://assets.publishing.service.gov.uk/government/uploads/system/uploads/attachment_data/file/478936/52309_Cm_9161_NSS_SD_Review_PRINT_only.pdf, accessed on 20 June 2020.
4. 'Exercise Cygnus Uncovered: The Pandemic Warnings Buried by Government', *Daily Telegraph*, 28 March 2020, available at https://www.telegraph.co.uk/news/2020/03/28/exercise-cygnus-uncovered-pandemic-warnings-buried-government/, accessed on 20 June, 2020.
5. 'What was Exercise Cygnus and What Did it Find?', *The Guardian*, 7 May 2020, available at https://www.theguardian.com/world/2020/may/07/what-was-exercise-cygnus-and-what-did-it-find, accessed on 20 June, 2020.

6. 'Revealed: UK Ministers were Warned Last Year of Risks of Coronavirus Pandemic', *The Guardian*, 24 April, 2020, available at https://www.theguardian.com/world/2020/apr/24/revealed-uk-ministers-were-warned-last-year-of-risks-of-coronavirus-pandemic, accessed on 20 June, 2020.
7. 'Revealed: Boris Johnson Scrapped Cabinet Ministers' Pandemic Team Six Months before Coronavirus hit Britain', *Daily Mail*, 13 June 2020, available at https://www.dailymail.co.uk/news/article-8416075/Boris-Johnson-scrapped-Cabinet-Ministers-pandemic-team-six-months-coronavirus-hit-Britain.html, accessed on 20 June, 2020.
8. 'COVID-19: Genetic Network Analysis Provides "Snapshot" of Pandemic Origins', *Cambridge University Research*, available at https://www.cam.ac.uk/research/news/covid-19-genetic-network-analysis-provides-snapshot-of-pandemic-origins, accessed on 21 June, 2020.
9. 'Intelligence Report Warned of Coronavirus Crisis as Early as November: Sources', *ABC News*, 8 April 2020, available at https://www.goodmorningamerica.com/news/story/intelligence-report-warned-coronavirus-crisis-early-november-sources-70031273, accessed on 21 June, 2020.
10. 'TV; US Intelligence Alerted Israel of Corona Virus in mid-November', *Times of Israel*, 16 April 2020, available at https://www.timesofisrael.com/liveblog_entry/tv-us-intelligence-alerted-israel-of-coronavirus-in-mid-november/, accessed on 21 June, 2020.
11. 'Satellite Data Suggests Coronavirus may have Hit China earlier: Researchers', *ABC News*, 8 June 2020, available at https://abcnews.go.com/International/satellite-data-suggests-coronavirus-hit-china-earlier-researchers/story?id=71123270, accessed on 22 June 2020.
12. 'Taiwan's Response to COVID-19', *The Economist*, 26 May 2020, available at https://www.economist.com/letters/2020/03/26/letters-to-the-editor, accessed on 22 June 2020.
13. 'CHP Provides Latest Information on Cluster of Pneumonia Cases in Wuhan', *The Government of Hong Kong Special Administrative Region* 3 January 2020, available at https://www.info.gov.hk/gia/general/202001/03/P2020010300836.htm, accessed on 22 June 2020.
14. Ibid.
15. 'Serious Response Level activated in public hospitals', Hong Kong Hospital Authority Press Release, 4 January 2020, available at https://www.ha.org.hk/haho/ho/pad/200104Eng1.pdf, accessed on 22 June 2020.
16. 'Doctors Scramble to Identify Mysterious Illness Emerging in China', New *Scientist* 7 January 2020, available at https://www.newscientist.com/article/2229196-doctors-scramble-to-identify-mysterious-illness-emerging-in-china/, accessed on 22 June 2020.
17. 'WHO Warned of Transmission Risk in January, Despite Trump Claims', *The Guardian*, 9 April 2020, available at https://www.theguardian.com/world/2020/apr/09/who-cited-human-transmission-risk-in-january-despite-trump-claims, accessed on 24 June 2020.
18. 'PM Speech in Greenwich: 3 February 2020' *Prime Minister's Office*, available at https://www.gov.uk/government/speeches/pm-speech-in-greenwich-3-february-2020, accessed on 24 June, 2020.
19. See note 18.

14

The Pandemic in Russia

Nivedita Das Kundu

The outbreak of the COVID-19 Pandemic in Russia from the middle of March 2020 affected the population with unexpected disruptions in almost all spheres of life and drastically altered the lifestyle of the Russian population. The lockdown announced on 29 March 2020, to contain the infection and slow down the spread of the virus was an extraordinary decision taken by Russia's government in post-Soviet history.[1] The COVID-19 crisis reached Russia when Kremlin was busy focussing its political decisions to push for the constitutional amendments to allow Vladimir Putin to stay in power after 2024. However, as the coronavirus cases increased, the Russian government hurriedly declared lockdown measures and asked citizens to stay home and maintain social distancing.

Although, Russia's response to the coronavirus outbreak had started much earlier and it was quick in deciding to close its borders with China which is around 2,615 kilometres long. On 27 January 2020, Russia also created special coronavirus headquarters. However, on 31 January, two Russian regions announced that two Chinese tourists carried the virus, making them the first confirmed cases in Russia. Chinese tourists were temporarily banned from entering Russia from 20 February 2020. But the closing of borders created other difficulties and therefore, the border had to be partially open.[2] The Russian government was active in controlling the cases in January and February and the situation was under control as there were very few cases of infection. However, things changed fast and confirmed cases gradually spiked. In response to this increase in infections, the Russian government opted for strict quarantine measures.

Russia rapidly climbed up the global COVID-19 ladder and by May 2020, reached third place. However, these statistics are continuously fluctuating since many states are entering the peak phase or experiencing second wave of the infection. By 30 June 2020 Russia had reported more than 9300 deaths. It may be noted that even though the number of cases in Russia was increasing yet the country has a good recovery rate. More than half of Russia's COVID-19 cases are being found in big crowded cities like Moscow and St. Petersburg, making the healthcare system in these cites hard pressed and leaving the Russian healthcare workers extremely stressed.

Socio-Political Impact

The Russians had a bitter experience with the plague epidemic a few centuries back. During 1770–1772 there was a huge outbreak of plague in Russia which is known to have possibly killed around fifty to a hundred thousand people in the city of Moscow alone. Subsequently, one of the major plague pandemics began in Yunnan, China, in 1855 which had also impacted many other parts of the world. Appreciating the need to address pandemics a network of health centres was formed by the Soviet Union (USSR) in the 1920s.

Over the years these structures have evolved and at present, these facilities are useful for providing expertise in quarantines and responses to COVID-19.[3] This has also helped them to quickly develop testing facilities and increase testing capacity. The COVID-19 spread in Russia within a short time had an immediate impact on every Russian's daily routine. Though the country has a good experience in controlling infectious diseases, such as the plague. Despite these facets, the threat of pandemic has become much more dangerous than any other threat within a short period. The disruptions in normal life became evident as the educational institutions closed first, followed by the closing of various other sectors of the economy. All this led to a major crisis in the health and economic sectors.

Today, this pandemic has pushed many into poverty. Many are facing food crises and do not have the capability even to pay for basic amenities. Like many other states, Russia also has the dual task of managing the pandemic and rescuing the economy.[4] The COVID-19 has made one thing clear, that no one is safe unless the whole community is safe and maintains safety.

Understanding that the expanse of the threat is global and only a common approach can help the world to overcome the crisis. Therefore, President Putin has connected with a number of world leaders and has discussed the need for a cooperative strategy to deal with the COVID-19 crisis. The 75th Anniversary of the allied victory in the Second World War was another significant context to connect with global leaders. The US President Donald Trump offered to send ventilators to Russia, returning the favour for Russian assistance in April 2020. President Putin and Xi Jinping appreciated the two-way cooperation as Russia had sent medical equipment when the infection in China was at its peak. Thereafter, Russia has been importing PPE (Personal Protective Equipment) from China to supplement its daily production of about 9 million masks. Vietnam, which has one of the most remarkable records of dealing with COVID-19, continued assistance in this tough time.[5] Russia promised to support its neighbouring Central Asian countries of Kazakhstan, Uzbekistan and Tajikistan with medical supplies to cope up with difficulties during the pandemic.

Factors Leading to Virus Escalation in the Country

Many factors were responsible for the rapid increase in COVID-19 infections in the country. The healthcare sector faced significant shortages of PPE's making healthcare workers more vulnerable.[6] The hospitals faced problems due to the shortages of ventilators.[7] After all, the availability of PPE and ventilators was not uniform nationwide.[8] There was also a shortage of healthcare equipment in many parts of Russia beyond Moscow as well. As such the quality of the healthcare infrastructure is very uneven across the length and breadth of Russia. Beyond a few major cities, even during the pre-COVID-19 period, the healthcare system was dysfunctional.[9]

During this pandemic, many countries suffered due to an absence of clear political leadership. In the case of Russia too, it has been noted that the President's response to the pandemic was not quick and adequate. There were indications that he was not handling the situation directly and also refrained from addressing citizens regularly to explain the state's response. He preferred to stay away from the agencies which were responsible for handling the crisis and did not show much interest in how the crisis was being handled.[10] Mr. Putin's absence from the state's COVID-19 response mechanism indicates the nature of the Kremlin's response strategy. The President was probably unwilling to take on unpleasant questions about containing the virus which could upset his approval rating at a time when the government is planning to put constitutional amendments to vote.[11] Strong leadership in the face of the global pandemic is an essential element. However, it appears that the Russian leadership has different ideas.

President Putin's popularity peaked immediately after Russia annexed Crimea. However, recent reports and the author's informal interaction with a few subject experts suggest that, due to COVID-19 concerns, there has been a significant drop in the levels of his public support. Besides, the discontent among Russia's working population has also grown due to the fall in real wages, owing to the rise in taxation and inefficient delivery of essential services. All in all, the economic pain caused due to COVID-19 and the unhappiness about its handling by the Russian government seems to have damaged President Putin's popularity. This should be a cause of concern for Putin since he is to face the referendum on constitutional changes on 01 July 2020. Actually, the vote on the reforms was earlier planned for 22 April but had to be postponed after Russia experienced a surge in coronavirus infections.[12] The reforms are for a provision that would reset the clock on his term (as President) limits to zero. This would allow the 67-year-old to run for President again when his fourth term expires in 2024, and potentially to stay in power until 2036.[13]

In Russia, for the last two decades, people have relied on President Putin's direct intervention and control over major crises, however, during the COVID-19 pandemic it looks as if President Putin's intervention was limited.[14] He was found conspicuously absent during the first weeks of Russia's COVID-19 outbreak. His response to the pandemic was quite unusual for the leader of centralized state power like Russia and in general what was practiced during the last two decades of his presidency in Russia.

Pandemic Confusion and Measures

During the pandemic, the regional leaders were given a free hand to make decisions about their own region's safety and health measures. This was unusual for Russia and it was not clear if Kremlin would intervene if a regional leader's radical decisions fail. Also, it was not clear if decisions taken by the regional leaders were approved by the Kremlin or not.[15] However, one thing clear was that Putin was unwilling to take charge of the pandemic situation and therefore, the decision making process to tackle the crisis shifted to other local leaders. This created confusion in the minds of the people and they started struggling to adjust to the new normal.

On 11 May, President Putin in his address to the Nation on the pandemic called an end to Russia's "non-working period". President Putin mentioned in the televised address to the nation that the pandemic and the lockdown had a strong impact on the Russian economy, and it affected millions. Therefore, the lockdown measures that have prevented workers from going to their work formally ended on 12 May in Russia, even though the COVID-19 cases were showing an increasing trend.[16] However, many COVID-19 related health restrictions remained in place with gradual easing permitted at different junctures in various regions of the country, depending on local developments.

Russian army medical personnel who had been sent to Italy to fight COVID-19 cases were asked to return to Russia to help in combating the increasing spread of the virus within Russia.[17] During the lockdown period, it was not that the country was entirely closed. Several places in the country did not close down their industrial establishments altogether. Many manufacturing units outside the urban centres functioned as usual. As part of the lockdown measures, wages were paid by companies for furloughed workers. But some companies refused to pay their workers who did not return to work after the lockdown was called off. Nonetheless, the 'return to work' under crisis for Russian workers indicated confusing messages from the regional leaders.[18]

Owing to the lockdown and other problems during the spread of COVID-19 infection, Russia's overall industrial output shrunk by about 25 percent in April, as per some estimates. To boost the economy, Russia has unveiled a 72 billion USD recovery plan aimed at boosting employment, incomes and economic growth. The proposal contains over 500 measures for improving the economy. Putin described the plan as a "foundation" for repairing the economy and implementing "long-term structural change". This plan would be rolled out over three separate stages. The first stage is an immediate action for stabilising the economy and should be delivered by the current quarter. There is a provision for targeted tax cuts and some emergency aid for families and recently unemployed people since the lockdown was introduced. The second and third steps are aimed at rebuilding the economy and putting it on a trajectory for stable economic growth. The lockdown ended up compounding various existing problems of the Russian economy, ranging from the effects of sanctions following the annexation of Crimea in 2014 to the oil price crash this year. The government forecasts that the economy will shrink by 9.5% in the second quarter and up to 6% for the year 2020.[19]

Russia announced that around 236,000 Russian citizens had been brought back to Russia from COVID-19 affected countries. Another 30,000 Russians are waiting to return to Russia. The Russian government has extended the visa period for foreign nationals whose visas expired after 15 March till 15 September 2020.[20]

Effect of Restrictions during Pandemic

Migrant labourers mainly from neighbouring countries of Central Asia, engaged in Russia's agricultural and service sectors that need physical labour work, such as at construction sites, on farms, in factories, suffered due to COVID-19 restrictions, leading to the closure of the border and lockdown. Russia's agricultural sector is highly dependent on neighbouring Central Asian workers to harvest their seasonal crops and that got affected due to the lockdown, as thousands of migrant labourers from Central Asian countries were stopped from entering Russia. This in turn affected the food supply chains. However, to reduce the difficulty in certain seasonal agricultural sectors, students and prisoners were recruited.[21] But such options could not work in all the sectors as many sectors required skilled and dedicated workers which were difficult to get during the pandemic.

Education during Pandemic

Due to the COVID-19 pandemic, Russia's digitalization became a reality. Within a few weeks of the lockdown, digital cafes, google meet-ups, zoom meetings and other virtual remote work arrangements enabled Russians to continue with their work and educational activities from home. COVID-19 disrupted the overall education system. Schools, colleges and universities in Russia remained closed. Due to the closedown of the educational institutions, students and teachers adapted to the online education system and were obliged to follow distance learning.[22] Though online learning cannot fully replace the in-class experience, the main aim was to help students to continue their education and the learning process. There have been challenges adjusting to these changes for students and teachers both.[23] Teachers also address the queries of parents of young students who were struggling to learn how to navigate the online tools and assist their children. During online teaching, students and teachers were in continuous contact with each other. The self-isolation regime probably allowed many students to concentrate even better on their studies.[24] However, the story for medical students was different. There was a realisation by April/May that Russia needs more doctors at various temporary facilities set up for light coronavirus cases. A good number of doctors were known to have died treating the infection. Hence, a decision was taken to send the medical students in their fourth, fifth and sixth years to work in corona hospitals. It was said that those who refuse would not get their qualification and could face expulsion. Some are of the opinion that the healthcare reforms of the past have led to the departure of many doctors from the profession and particularly crises like COVID-19 have exposed the fissures in the system.[25]

Treatment during the Pandemic

The pandemic helped Russians to be more connected with their local community and the local healthcare system. In all likelihood, this pandemic will stay for long until a vaccine is invented. The Kremlin mentioned that Russian scientists and researchers are working on almost 50 different vaccine projects. A drug called Avifavir received a temporary registration certificate from the Ministry of Health of the Russian Federation for treating COVID-19 patients. Health officials registered a second drug for a treatment called Levilimab (trade name Ilsira).[26]

Russian media reports mentioned that at least seven research facilities are currently working on coronavirus vaccines. Two forms of the vaccine have been developed by the Moscow-based Gamalei National Research Center for Epidemiology and Microbiology in cooperation with the Russian Defence Ministry and they are set to begin clinical trials soon. Vaccine research and development in both liquid and powder form for injections are currently underway. Both military and civilian personnel are expected to be enrolled in the trials for such vaccines. The Russian Defence Ministry has informed that the parameters for the sample of volunteers have already been discussed with the Ministry of Health. The tests would be (or are being) conducted on two groups of volunteers who are isolated in two Moscow hospitals for observation.[27] The aim is to assess the safety and tolerability of the vaccine components. This part of the trial is intended to evaluate the vaccine's effectiveness and development of antibodies against COVID-19.

Assessment

The COVID-19 pandemic, lockdown and self-isolation have changed many things around the world and the same is found happening in Russia too. People are found spending more time in the virtual world. The pressure on the medical infrastructure is increasing. Particularly, non-COVID-19 patients are suffering a lot. The health sector is finding it difficult to manage both professional as well as administrative aspects in handling the overall load on the medical system. Conceivably, the initial reluctance of the administration to recognise the possible enormity of the threat is probably responsible for their medical system's failure in some parts of the country. Owing to the massive influx of patients the inadequacies of social support became evident and healthcare sectors are found to be increasingly overwhelmed. Even though Russia was among the first states to immediately respond to reports of the disease in China back in January 2020 and closed the borders by giving notice to the Chinese partners in advance. The COVID-19 cases in Russia increased drastically and are continuously growing. This could be because the infection could have entered the state from various other routes too.

The COVID-19 pandemic has taught Russians that access to healthcare and medication is of utmost importance for the survival of the state itself. Only time will tell if there is a necessity to change the lifestyle and control excessive urbanization. There are various challenges from education to the environment which would require apt handling in the post-COVID-19 era. All this could lead to a fundamental restructuring of societies around the ideals of local self-sufficiency, improvised medical practices and environmental sustainability. There is a realisation that managing pandemics like this requires global support. Russia cannot operate in isolation and there is a need for international collaboration. Internally, there is a requirement to address such challenges at the highest political level. The leadership has to be upfront in managing the crisis and also needs to be seen as managing the crisis. All, this could help boost the confidence of the people in the political dispensation.

Russia has been active at multilateral fora like the SCO (Shanghai Cooperation Organisation), BRICS (Brazil, Russia, India, China and South Africa) and other such forums. However, when it comes to agencies like the WHO (World Health Organisation) not much exuberance is visible and this needs to change. Thereby, the country needs to be more proactive in its dealings with multilateral organisations. Over the years President Putin has tried to project Russia's influence at the global level by leveraging military, political, economic and business ties with some key countries. All in all, handling crisis is not new for Russian polity and surely, they would come out of this crisis as will the rest of the world in a few months' time. However, the dents caused due to the crisis would take time to heal.

* * *

Author Speaks Russian language and took online interviews on COVID-19 and Russia's response to tackle the situation with native Russian citizens living in Moscow and Tver.

NOTES

1. Duclos Michel, 'Is COVID-19 a Geopolitical Game Changer?' 24 March 2020, available at https://www.institutmontaigne.org/en/blog/covid-19-geopolitical-game-changer, accessed on 10 June 2020.
2. Basit Mahmood, 'Russia is Now in the Top 5 Countries Most Affected by the Coronavirus,' 5 August 2020, available at https://www.newsweek.com/russia-covid-19-coronavirus-moscow-putin-1502737, accessed on 10 June 2020.
3. Andrew E. Kramer, 'How Bubonic Plague Has Helped Russia Fight the Coronavirus,' *The New York Times*, 15 April 2020, available at https://www.nytimes.com/2020/04/15/world/europe/coronavirus-plague-russia-soviet-union.html?auth=login-email&login=email, accessed on 22 June 2020.
4. Interview on COVID-19 with a business women and Russian citizen living and working in Moscow. Ekaterina Nazarovna, on 10 June 2020.
5. COVID-19 and Russia's Response, Gorbachev Foundation Research Report, April 2020.
6. Reports on Russian Personal Protective Equipment Shortages, *BBC*, 8 May 2020, available at

https://www.bbc.com/news/av/world-europe-52508834/coronavirus-russian-hospital-staff-working-without-masks, accessed on 15 June 2020.

7. Maria Tsvetkova, Polina Nikolskaya and Gleb Stolyarov, 'Russia's Ventilators: Plentiful, but often Old and sometimes Broken,' *Reuters*, 5 May 2020, available at https://in.reuters.com/article/health-coronavirus-russia-ventilators-in/russias-ventilators-plentiful-but-often-old-and-sometimes-broken-idINKBN22H03X, accessed on 12 June 2020.
8. 'Salient Lessons from Russia's COVID-19 outbreak,' *The Lancet*, vol 395, 6 June 2020, p. 1739, available at https://www.thelancet.com/journals/lancet/article/PIIS0140-6736(20)31280-0/fulltext, accessed on 10 June 2020.
9. Sarah Rainsford, 'Coronavirus: Russian Republic Dagestan Enduring a Catastrophe,' *BBC*, 21 May 2020, available at https://www.bbc.com/news/world-europe-52737404, accessed on 14 June 2020.
10. Fabrice Deprez, 'Russia's Confusing COVID-19 response,' *Foreign Policy Research Institute*, 7 April 2020, available at https://www.fpri.org/article/2020/04/russias-confusing-covid-19-response/, accessed on 12 June 2020.
11. Ksenia Kondratieva, 'The Fight Putin Shies Away From,' *The Hindu*, 18 April 2020, available at https://www.thehindu.com/news/international/the-fight-putin-shies-away-from/article31377245.ece, accessed on 23 June 2020.
12. P.S Raghavan, 'Russia's COVID-19 Challenges Mount,' *Ananta India Russia Review*, May 2020, vol 05, no. 5.
13. 'Russia: Putin sets July 1 for Constitutional Reform Vote', *Aljazeera*, 02 June 2020, available at https://www.aljazeera.com/news/2020/06/russia-putin-sets-july-1-constitutional-reform-vote-200601172359510.html, accessed on Jun 23, 2020
14. See Note 8.
15. See Note 8.
16. Russia TV Report, 11 May 2020.
17. 'Russian Medics 16x More Likely to Die From Coronavirus Than Foreign Colleagues: Analysis,' *The Moscow Times*, 19 May 2020, available at https://www.themoscowtimes.com/2020/05/19/russian-medics-16x-more-likely-to-die-from-coronavirus-than-foreign-colleagues-analysis-a70311, accessed on 22 June 2020.
18. Najibullah Farngis & Cizonova Lyubov, 'COVID-19: Putin Ends Russia's 'Nonworking Period'; Kazakhstan Eases Restrictions", 11 May 2020, available at https://www.rferl.org/a/covid-19-moscow-mortality-surge-death-toll-underreported/30605393.html, accessed on 12 June 2020.
19. Maria Antonov and Anna Malpas, 'Russia Unveils 'modest' $72-billion Virus Recovery Plan,' *Asia Times Financial*, 03 June 2020, available at https://www.asiatimesfinancial.com/russia-unveils-modest-72-billion-virus-recovery-plan, accessed on 23 June 23 2020.
20. 'COVID-19 & Russia,' available at https://yandex.ru.covid19/stat?utm_source+main_graph&geold=213, accessed on 12 June 2020.
21. Farngis Najibullah and Lyubov Cizonova, 'Russian Farmers Suffering as COVID-19 Pandemic Keeps Central Asian Workers At Home,' *RadioFreeEurope*, 4 June 2020, available at https://www.rferl.org/a/russian-farmers-suffering-as-covid-19-pandemic-keeps-central-asian-workers-at-home/30652482.html, accessed on 15 June 2020.
22. Interview with Nina Papova (works in Information Technology Company and lives in Moscow, Russia) to know about the go back to work implications on Russian Citizens.
23. Interview with Elizabeth Peskova, "about the epidemic haters and plans for the future."

24. Experience shared by Moscow State University Masters in Economics Student Andrei Popov on COVID-19 and online teaching and learning experiences, 5 April 2020.
25. 'Russia medical students slam 'forced labour' in coronavirus wards,' *Aljazeera*, 11 May 2020, available at https://www.aljazeera.com/news/2020/05/russia-medical-students-slam-forced-labour-coronavirus-wards-200511081858609.html, accessed on 24 June 2020
26. 'Russia to Roll out COVID-19 Drug next week,' *The Hindu*, 1 June 2020, available at https://www.thehindu.com/news/international/russia-to-roll-out-covid-19-drug-next-week/article31725174.ece, accessed on 10 June 2020.
27. Jonny Tickle, 'Light at the End of the Tunnel? Russian Scientists Test Potential COVID-19 Vaccine on 18 Volunteers,' 18 June 2020, available at https://www.rt.com/russia/492252-russian-scientists-covid19-vaccine-tested/, accessed on 20 June 2020.

Africa

15

Coronavirus Containment in Africa

Margaret W. Muturi and Eucharia U. Kenya

COVID-19 pandemic has been around the globe for more than six months. Within this period, it has caused unprecedented loss of life and devastation of livelihood across the world. According to John Hopkins COVID-19 resource center, COVID-19 cases globally have crossed 10 million.[1] Africa has had its share of the epidemic. The new coronavirus was first reported as mysterious pneumonia disease on December 2019 in Wuhan, Hubei province of China, with epidemiological links to the Huanan Seafood Market.[2] Weeks later, the Chinese Centre for Disease Control and Prevention identified a novel coronavirus as the cause of the outbreak. It was named severe acute respiratory syndrome coronavirus 2 (SARS-CoV-2).[3] As of 18 March 2020, cases were reported in approximately 195 countries, the World Health Organization (WHO) declared coronavirus disease 2019 (COVID-19) a pandemic. As of 30 June 2020 coronavirus cases in Africa were almost 383,747 and the number of fatalities were about 9691 according to Africa center of Disease Control and Prevention (Africa CDC).[4] Although cases in Africa are increasing but are lagging with respect to other countries, a situation not guaranteed since the trend has changed in the last 20 days.

Soon after the WHO described the outbreak as a pandemic, there was concern among health specialists about the ability of some African nations to meet the logistical and financial challenges posed by COVID-19. There were fears that Africa would be torn apart by the virus necessitating the WHO Director-General Tedros Ghebreyesus to issue a warning to the African continent: "The best advice for Africa is to prepare for the worst...".[5] Well, the warning could be justified taking into consideration that many countries in Africa are poor. In many states, the ratios of hospital beds, ICUs (Intensive Care Unit) and health professionals are lower to its population. The human resource is a challenge with the doctor-citizen ratio being less than 2 in 10000. Africa is highly dependent on imported therapeutic and pharmaceutical products. Each African country is a net importer of these products and approximately 94 percent of Africa's total stock of pharmaceuticals are imported.[6]

Besides, critical care capacity is inadequate, and the testing infrastructure is limited. In Kenya, for instance, at the beginning of the pandemic, there were roughly 518 ICU beds countrywide. The Central African Republic (CAR) had only eight. South Sudan had four, Uganda had only fifty-five ICU beds, while Nigeria has less than 500. Globally there has been a lack of COVID-19 supplies, and Africa would join in a competition while already disadvantaged by the lack of manufacturing industries.

The virus moved from China to the neighbouring countries, then to Europe and America. While in China, the world looked at COVID-19 as a Chinese problem. When it spread out to the Far East and Europe, it was seen as a white people problem. The delay of the coronavirus to Africa would have been a golden opportunity to prepare for the epidemic. Regrettably, myths took centre stage through social media. One of the myths was that coronavirus was not infecting the dark-skinned people since they had a stronger immune system, and the second was the virus would not survive in tropical Africa. Unfortunately, it looks like the Government and health Ministries fell prey to the myth since they did nothing to be prepared against the virus. Africa lost the opportunity that would have put her ahead of the pack. The messages meant to caution on the need for preparation were taken with mixed reactions, some of which portrayed anger in media. For example, two French doctors caused a media uproar, when they unconsciously uttered on television that, sub-Saharan Africa is occasionally where ethical boundaries are pushed when developing vaccines. In the same tone, Melinda Gates, the American Philanthropist, was quoted as saying, "I am worried.... It's going to be horrible in developing countries. We are gonna see dead bodies in streets of Africa".[7] Although she could have said this out of concern for Africa, yet the utterance was seen as discrimination and racialism by some. It appeared that while the looming spread of COVID-19 was treated with shock elsewhere, in Africa, the onslaught of COVID-19 was considered inevitable. United Nations prediction was of up to 3.3 million deaths in Africa if interventions were not put in place.[8] To a lot of people outside Africa, the blend between a COVID-19 pandemic in Africa and, genocidal violence is obvious. It draws from a radicalized history of objectifying black bodies, and a hopelessness frame in which Africans are cast as helpless victims, lacking independence and needing a savior. Indeed, there is no denial that sub-Saharan Africa is likely facing a full-blown pandemic and could be overwhelmed. On the surface, the odds are stacked against the region. COVID-19 requires treatment in ICUs at least for the small percentage that requires hospitalization and critical care. However, many sub-Saharan African countries cannot deal with an increasing number of cases because most states have weak healthcare systems. Meanwhile, many people may be suffering from other life-threatening infectious diseases like HIV (Human Immunodeficiency Virus)/AIDS (Acquired Immunodeficiency Syndrome), TB (Tuberculosis) and so on. All said and done, had the WHO timely advised Africa to close its borders, the 1.2 billion people would have escaped the virus onslaught.

The Epidemic in Africa

The first cases of COVID-19 infections on African soil finally dismissed the circulating myths about the new coronavirus and baseless expectations of the people. Coronavirus first arrived in the African continent through people returning home from hotspots in Asia, Europe and the United States. Africa's first COVID-19 case was recorded in Egypt on 14 February.[9] Since then, all the other countries have reported cases and most of them have reported deaths as well.

Nigeria, Africa's most populous nation with over 206 million people, was the first sub-Saharan country to report a confirmed case of coronavirus on 28 February, after an Italian citizen tested positive for the disease. The man arrived in Lagos from Milan on 25 February. Most of the Western African nations got the infection much earlier around late February for example in Senegal French national who arrived in Dakar, the capital, on 26 February, who tested positive two days later after showing COVID-19 symptoms.

Ethiopia, confirmed its first case of COVID-19 on 13 March while Djibouti confirmed its first case of coronavirus on 18 March from a Spanish national who was part of a 32-member Spanish Special Forces unit that arrived in the East African nation on 14 March and tested positive. Uganda confirmed the first case on 22 March, from a Ugandan who arrived from Dubai. Lesotho was the last nation in the continent to confirm coronavirus cases, from a student who arrived home from Saudi Arabia in May 2020 and currently it has less than ten cases. In Africa, the number of COVID-19 cases and impacted countries has been increasing steadily. To flatten the curve, interventions such as lockdowns began to be introduced to reduce the potential spread of infection, thus preventing fragile healthcare systems from being overburdened by rapidly increasing cases. Infections increased exponentially, spreading not only between African countries but within different localities in the hardest-hit states. It took 16 days from the first confirmed case in the African region to reach 100 cases and a further ten days to reach a thousand cases. Three days later, there were 2000 cases, and two days later, the figure of confirmed cases stood at 3000.[10]

Case Study: Kenya's Response to Coronavirus

Coronavirus has been in Kenya for the last 3 months. As of 30 June 2020, the national tally of positive coronavirus cases stood at 6,190 with a national death toll of 144.[11] This is less than 0.1 percent of the total but the cases have been rising steadily. This small percentage of infected people has already overwhelmed the health system and now, the government is currently looking into ways of relieving the health system. However, the testing capacity of COVID-19 is not optimum due to the continued shortage of test kits. With low capacity, there is a high possibility that infections are far higher than reported; taking into consideration that community transmission has begun.

Initially Kenya felt safe because the disease was thought to have occurred far away. However, towards the end of February at the height of the coronavirus outbreak in China, a passenger plane from China landed in Nairobi.[12] It created a significant media and public backlash to the government for allowing entry to the passengers from a coronavirus infected country without any form of screening or isolation. This incident was an indicator of the public's awareness and rising anxiety about the deadly virus. The tension reached fever pitch when on 13 March 2020, the first case was reported in Kenya's Nairobi County, where a 27-year-old Kenyan woman who travelled from the US through London, was confirmed positive for the said virus.[13] That afternoon, there was an unexpected presidential address to the nation that confirmed the news. A few people who had come into contact with the first case were traced and isolated, and two days later, two people who had come into contact with the initial patient also tested positive for the virus. The announcement created a lot of anxiety and uncertainty, and the general populace became more aware of each other and the surfaces around them, afraid that the unseen enemy was lurking within their vicinity.

The Presidential address in response to the confirmed cases outlined several measures to curb COVID-19. Travel from countries with cases of Coronavirus was halted and only Kenyan Citizens and foreigners with valid residence permits were allowed to enter the country provided they either self-quarantine or go to a government-designated quarantine facility; all schools and institutions of higher learning were to be closed in 7 days; people were advised to work from home – exemption was given to essential services ; cashless transactions over cash were recommended and all social groupings including religious gatherings were banned. A toll-free number was also set up to report suspected coronavirus cases. Many people felt that the measures taken were draconian, but they adhered to them because of the fear of the new virus.

Within two days, a fourth case had been diagnosed. The cases increased daily, and by 25 March, the first recovery was confirmed, and three more cases were recorded, bringing the total confirmed cases to 28.[14] Before the end of March, the infection had spread to four other counties namely Mombasa, Kilifi and Kwale and Kajiado. The first fatality was also recorded.[15]

Cases continued to be announced daily and on 6 April a cessation of movement was implemented in an area encompassing the nation's capital and designated as the Nairobi Metropolitan Area for a containment period of 21 days.[16] Other counties that were seen as epicentres for the virus and affected by the cessation are namely, Mombasa and Kilifi and Kwale county where the cessation of movement was implemented at the beginning of April 2020. The government also imposed a nation-wide curfew between 7 pm and 5 am which under the strict supervision of police.

The initial control measures did not hinder the spread of the virus within the community, and many counties confirmed infected cases. In response, the government increased mass testing, but it was met with unexpected challenges. A vast majority of the people refused to come out for testing for fear of being forced into quarantine.[17] The infected individuals and their contacts were subjected to mandatory quarantine in government facilities, which they were, expected to foot the bill. Experts criticize the government for militarizing public health control measures, resulting in resistance by the people. Some of the infected persons attempted to escape, and others indeed managed to escape from the quarantine facilities posing a severe risk of fueling community transmission. Some of those facilities were accused of poor conditions where the sanitary facilities were shared, and masks were not provided, posing fear of getting the virus from the quarantine centres in case one was not infected. Some were unwilling to be tested, due to the stigma attached to the infection and the disease, COVID-19. They dreaded to be shunned by family and community if found positive, something that had been happening to COVID-19 survivors.

When the COVID-19 epidemic strikes everyone is at risk of infection, but health workers are most vulnerable since they are at the frontline. Although high rates of infection and death amongst medical staff in other countries like Spain and Italy has not been witnessed in this part of the world. However, increased infections and fatality among health staff reduce the capacity of the healthcare system when at its highest demand. In Kenya, the infection rates have been low probably due to the few numbers of infections compared to other countries. However, the number of medical personnel is not adequate, but the government has already laid down strategies on how to enroll more personnel. Personal Protective Equipment (PPE) for health professionals were not available initially, but the government has moved to close the gap by having local companies manufacture the same. Through the support of the African Center of Disease Control and Prevention, the medical staff have been trained and the available medical supplies have been availed.[18] However, the government is expected to do more because these efforts are not adequate.

Creating awareness among vulnerable communities took time at the beginning of the epidemic. However, the Ministry of education is aware that it is an effective way to battle the spread of COVID-19. The government supplemented the efforts in prevention campaigns by volunteers and Non-Governmental Organization (NGOs) in low-income communities, especially those in the cities of Nairobi and Mombasa. So far, these efforts are producing fruits, since the people in the slums are practicing the public health measures to keep corona at bay. However, these efforts are threatened by the loss of jobs coupled with the prolonged period of lockdown resulting in most of them facing starvation. The community has joined hands to help and support those in need.[19] There is a need for governments to balance among the two requirements of protecting the vulnerable from hunger and the virus.

The control measures, including practicing good hygiene and social distancing, according to WHO guidelines as well as recognized best practice has been emphasized across the nation. Hand washing places have been created in many areas despite the perennial shortage of water. There are efforts to distribute water and sanitizers as well. Mass testing has been going on despite the shortage of testing kits. Community testing target areas in the states and institutions where confirmed cases of infection have been identified. For example, after two employees in one of the government institutions at the port died of coronavirus, the whole institution was tested where a large number of workers were found to have been exposed to the virus.[20] The infected people were quarantined in government facilities and those showing symptoms were hospitalized.

With contact tracing, it is expected that more people would be tested. All these efforts among others are just a drop in the ocean, considering the population at risk and the enormous amount of resources required. Besides, the vulnerable groups are diverse, including people with disabilities, people living with HIV and other underlying conditions, those in prisons, refugee camps and hard to reach areas. There is a need for calculated efforts by the government to protect these groups. For example, messages on COVID-19 should be translated to sign language for the deaf.

The country's government should be accountable to the people. They should ensure that the information shared is not only accurate, but also culturally acceptable, gender-responsive, available in local languages, and accessible. A long-term plan needs to be put in place focusing on anticipated future challenges, that will arise post lockdown, and mitigate against them.

Kenyans, like other African regions, was not spared from the myths. Information overload, misinformation from different sources and the lack of understanding about Coronavirus drowned expert opinions early in the epidemic. Deep-seated stereotypes plus fake news flooded the social media within a short time. Myths such as COVID-19 was synthesized as a bio-weapon in a laboratory in Wuhan; scientists have found a cure for the disease, and that black Africans are immune to the disease which later evolved to think that young people were resistant-were rapidly spread.[21] Additionally, there were people who thought that mosquito bites can cause infection or the goods from China could cause the infection. None of which is true.[22] Since the virus came from outside the country from travelers, it was seen as a disease for the affluent, those who could afford to travel overseas. Those in the rural areas called it a city disease since the epicenters were in the cities. However, Kenya has made progress because the Ministry of Health with the support of the mainstream media have continually passed the expert information to all the people. Furthermore, there has been misinterpretation of the WHO-issued guidelines on the use of an alcohol-based sanitizer occurred, with some people opting to drink alcohol instead. Further, false "remedies" such as boiling onions with lemon or taking tea without sugar to cure the disease were also widely circulated in forums as therapeutic options.

Some myths that were part of international conversations and headlines, including the consumption of bleach as a curative option and the role of 5G technology in the spread of the disease were also subjects of discussion.[23] Time and an intensive public campaign on providing scientific facts about the disease have since proved these lingering myths to be wrong while others became subjects of international geopolitics.

COVID-19 pandemic has affected Kenyans in so many ways. One of the most worrying facets is that all health facilities have been reporting significantly fewer patients. Following checks across the country, it was found that both inpatient and outpatient traffic has reduced by more than half in some counties, amid fears over the health conditions of patients with chronic diseases like cancer, asthma, and diabetes.[24]

Some of the hospitals are laying off staff while others are on half-pay. This does not mean that people are not getting sick. While research needs to be done to identify the cause, it is evident that people are afraid of going to the facilities to avoid contracting coronavirus from other patients, contaminated surfaces, and healthcare workers. The sick could also be self-medicating at home.

Coronavirus has not only affected human health but also the economy. COVID-19 severely interrupted usual business operations with people being advised to stay and work from home, people receiving pay cuts and others being laid off. The situation has been principally terrible for people engaged in the informal sector, which accounts for about 80% of jobs in Kenya.[25] The government set aside measures to cushion this segment from the economic shocks. These measures include reduction in various taxes, as well as budgets. However, it remains to be seen if these measures will be adequate to stimulate Kenya's economy. Additionally, the government partnered with Google to ensure 4G internet connectivity throughout the country using high altitude balloons. There have been mixed sentiments as 4G connectivity may not be a priority in the midst of a health crisis. However, this was an opportunity to shift to digital economy post COVID-19. 4G connectivity could transform all operations. For instance, digitalised agriculture could facilitate online platform to obtain agricultural inputs as direct access to markets for their produce. It would be possible to access healthcare solutions via online platforms that would also make it possible to achieve universal healthcare. The digital innovations in Kenya have already seen a slight upward trend and gives hope in uncertain times. Hence, it strengthens the argument for Kenya to completely embrace a changeover to a digital economy in the post COVID-19 era.

The pandemic has disrupted the education of nearly 15 million students in Kenya. The first case to be confirmed led to the abrupt closure of all learning institutions, including colleges and universities in March 2020. Students were subjected to home learning with the hope that the school would open up when new sessions starts in May. Lecture halls in Universities remain quiet, a few laboratories operate but with minimal staff. The administrators of various institutions wrestle with digital content delivery and options to resume physical classes safely. The dominant alternative model for teaching has been tethered to internet access and broadcast stations. The government fronted use of the e-learning to deliver content in all the institutions of learning. However, this has just exposed the country's inadequacy of the prerequisites. It was not practical for institutions that have no digital learning platform and the teachers that have no knowledge of the digital platforms. Worse still was a large number of students without access to technology and those who live in places without an internet connection. Where the duo was not a challenge, it was an uphill task for primary school parents who had to take on the unfamiliar role of a teacher.

The institutions of higher learning are facing severe financial shortages except for a few private universities that had already adopted online teaching to complete the semester.[26] Currently, most universities are training staff on the use of online platform like Zoom. Many staff are now developing online content to meet the requirement of teaching in the post-COVID era. Besides, they should improve the quality and relevance of the teaching. Universities in the west have been putting courses online for the last decade but local Universities have lagged in this area. However, many institutions that had established online teaching are learning the hard way that merely delivering course materials through digital platforms is not the best way to teach students. Online education is still going on for the privileged in primary and secondary schools. The telecommunication companies offer students free mobile bundles as their contribution support during this season. However, providing digital connectivity has remained an uphill task for the government.

The COVID-19 crisis has adversely affected global communities and economies. The pandemic will certainly change our world forever. Despite the challenge it has presented both by amplifying familiar risks and creating new ones, it has also created unprecedented opportunities. In Kenya for example the stiff competition on resources globally to combat the pandemic has caused the country to look on to its inside capabilities. The government has mobilized the ministry of Trade and Industry to manufacture the required items for coronavirus control. As a result, within the first few weeks of infection, there were several companies making sanitizers to complement the government efforts. In the last 3 months, the capacity to produce PPEs and masks has been built in the textile industry.[27] There is no more shortage of these items and now the industries are expanding capacity to supply for export. The universities have come up with local designs for ventilators which through government support are in advanced stages of assembly and production.[28] The collaboration of research Institutes and Universities is focused on coming up with drugs to combat the virus, and Point of Contact Rapid Test (PoCT) kit in response to COVID-19 pandemic.

Measures to Combat the Virus

The fight against the virus started when cases were confirmed in various countries. The response was marred by unpreparedness on the side of most governments and panic and confusion in the populace. Most of the countries had inadequate hospital staff, lacked protective equipment, and ventilators were scarce. Most health professionals did not know how to handle COVID-19 patients. No wonder some closed doors of the only available health facility when a suspected patient showed up. The actions caused anxiety and apprehension among people.

Nevertheless, there was a hurry to implement mitigation measures to lessen the transmission of the coronavirus within most African nations. Senegal was the first to implement these measures. These measures included flight restrictions, border closures, banning of public gatherings, dusk to dawn curfews, partial and total lockdown.[29] These actions were followed by instituting public health measures; hand-washing/sanitizing, no handshaking and hugging, touching the face elbow sneezing, wearing masks and social distancing.

These coronavirus control measures have found challenges such as inadequate water, insufficient infrastructures in low-resource settings along with costs, financing and regulatory aspects. However, some of the countries were lax. The examples are Tanzania and Burundi. Tanzania did not lockdown, and citizens were encouraged to carry out their business as usual. The Tanzanian government's approach to fighting the COVID-19 pandemic remains opaque and unknown to the general public. COVID-19 information remains a contentious subject not only to Tanzania citizens but also globally; exhibiting sharp opinions between those who feel that the situation in the country is fine and those blaming the government of underestimating the magnitude of the pandemic.[30] There is a concern that the economy has been prioritized above public health, thus risking the lives of Tanzanians. However, life moves on normally in Tanzania. Burundi is another African country that did not take any course of action to curb the spread of infection. Everything went on as usual including the May 2020 presidential election amidst COVID-19. Although much is not known about the events in the country, but the president's wife is currently hospitalized in a neighbouring country as a result of coronavirus infection.[31] The president himself died in early June, and the report blamed a heart disease.

As of June, Africa recorded over 383,747 COVID-19 cases with more than

9,000 deaths. Although this appears to be small relative to the global burden, the sad truth is that it is the tip of the iceberg. This is because of the low testing capacity in most African countries. According to the Africa Center for Disease Control, testing capacity ranges from 10 tests per 100,000 people in Ethiopia to 280 per 100,000 in South Africa. This is pale in comparison to the rate of testing in Western countries such as the United States, New Zealand and even Lithuania. the events in the country. During the AIDS pandemic, lifesaving diagnostics and drugs were given to the African countries only after they were made available elsewhere in the world. The delay is one of the factors that contributed to an epidemic of greater magnitude than anywhere else in the world. In the face of COVID-19, this problem recurred again only this time the situation is much worse. Africa could not compete in acquiring the much-needed diagnostics, as countries with the technology have restricted exports and preferentially sell to wealthier buyers.

Currently, the pandemic is growing quickly due to increasing community transmission. The WHO on 11 June 2020 indicated that it took 98 days for the continent to get to 10000 infections and only 18 days to get 200000 which translates to 3 percent of the world's total infections. Within the same period, 5500 deaths have been confirmed across the content.[32] Millions of people in the continent live in refugee camps. They have been displaced from their homes as a result of conflict, yet significant infections have not been reported in those camps. As of the time of writing this chapter, ten countries in the African region were driving the epidemic, accounting for 75 percent of all the cases in Africa. South Africa (SA) is the worst hit country, with West Cape Province having the highest daily cases. Nigeria comes third after, SA and followed by Egypt with 14000 cases. The conflict in the north of the country due to Boko Haram and ethnic fighting is expected to impact negatively the epidemic. The cases in Senegal are approximately 5000 and there is a fear of increased case as the country moves to ease the lockdown measures.

Challenges of Combating the Coronavirus

In the beginning, the epidemic was confined mainly in capital cities, where the patient zero appeared. Most of the international airports in Africa are located primarily in capital cities, serving as the entry point. In many countries, the cases have spread in multiple regions, causing concern to the local and international leadership. For example, Addis Ababa is so far considered the hotbed of COVID-19 infections in the country.

Implementation of measures to control the spread of the disease is not a walk in the park for many residents of the African continent. It is important to note that in Sub Saharan Africa has experienced massive rural to urban migration in recent years resulting in the formation and expansion of informal urban settlements (slums). Therefore, about 62% of the urban population in this region is slum dwellers, particularly at-risk of infection.[33] These people are daily wage workers who live hand to mouth. These measures are a luxury for many of these people who cannot afford it. In fact, the economic hardship faced by many of those working for daily wages in the informal labour market has made the imposition of a lockdown difficult and painful if not unbearable. This is an unprecedented challenge that many of these countries are struggling along with the fight against the virus.

Social distancing is an uncomfortable aspect for the Africans. To many, the requests to socially distant themselves from others feel abnormal. It is unimaginable not to shake hands when greeting people - even if you bump into them for the tenth time in a day, one is expected to shake hands says a Sudanese in Khartoum. However, the less disadvantaged in the suburbs of Khartoum like any other African city are the most vulnerable. The resident places here are small, overcrowded, or too close for social distancing. Adults and children sell their goodies in streets and at traffic lights, and they cannot afford social distancing.[34]

Water crises were ranked above both infectious diseases and food crises in the World Economic Forum's latest Global Risks Report. It is a daily occurrence in the informal settlements. In Ethiopia's capital city, Addis Ababa, with about 4.8 million residents, suffers perennial interruptions to the water supply. At the height of the corona pandemic, the latest outage caused havoc, exposing the inequality created by insufficient and unpredictable access to clean water.[35] Lack of sustainable access to clean water makes it difficult to wash hands which is a necessity to keep the virus away. It is not a problem unique to Africa. As the world celebrated the "World Water Day 2020", it was noted that globally 2.2 billion do not have access to clean water.[36]

The virus is currently spreading rapidly raising concern that the continent is about to tip into massive escalation. Healthcare systems are already underfunded and poorly equipped. Conflict, climate change and natural disasters have driven some 18 million people across the continent into poorly serviced and crowded camps for refugees and the internally displaced where social distancing, or even hand washing, is impossible.[37] Poverty turns lockdowns into a death sentence. And in countries where trust in government is poor, rumors and misinformation thrive in the place of leadership. An overwhelming long-term humanitarian crisis across the region is unavoidable. It is feared that if the virus hits the continent's overcrowded cities, its underserved refugee camps, or populations already suffering from the multiple health burdens of malnutrition, HIV, malaria, tuberculosis and cholera could easily overwhelm the already weak health systems. Besides, if those cases skyrocket just as wealthy nations start to recover from their own outbreaks, it may be even harder to rouse the international assistance that the continent would need for survival.

An African Remedy for Combating Coronavirus

The novel coronavirus has neither treatment nor vaccine. Finding a cure is of high priority to reduce the casualties from the virus and give hope to the world. Africa has a share of these efforts. The herbal tonic, marketed as COVID-Organics, was promoted as a cure for coronavirus by the Madagascar president in the initial days of COVID-19 in Africa. The drink was launched as COVID-Organics and sold after being tested on fewer than 20 people over three weeks. COVID-Organics produced from the artemisia plant is the source of an ingredient used in malaria treatment. However, the WHO has discouraged its use, indicating that proof of any cure for the herbal tonic was absent.[38] In Africa, the practice of traditional healing and magic is part of life, and 80% of people in African countries use these medicines.[39] Having this understanding, it is absurd to prevent people to treat themselves in the way they know, while there is no alternative treatment in place. However, the African Union, Africa Center of disease control and prevention is working with Madagascar to obtain technical data regarding the safety and efficiency of the herbal product for the reported prevention and treatment of COVID-19.

Will Africa Survive COVID-19 without Significant Damage?

There is a group of experts that believes that Africa will not be affected severely by COVID-19 as the other continents of the world. The argument is that Africa will survive the massive deaths caused by coronavirus. The theories in favour of this argument are related to social and health factors. First among them is that people living in Africa are continually exposed to various microbes from early childhood. Besides, a myriad of infectious diseases such as HIV, Ebola, malaria, tuberculosis and many others are endemic in Africa.[40] Although exposure to these infections causes high mortality and morbidity, it may also prepare the immune system to fight off new infectious agents such as coronavirus. Coronavirus is comparatively a mild infection compared to these endemic infections. Beside many countries already have existing infrastructure to deal with endemic infectious agents. Lots of lessons learned in addressing previous epidemics are being used as a foundation to respond to COVID-19. The theory has some weight, but it is yet to be confirmed especially now that the epidemic in African has not reached the peak and the number of infections continues to rise.

Secondly, there is continuing debate within the scientific community regarding the link between compulsory Bacillus Calmette–Guérin (BCG) child vaccination policies in sub-Saharan Africa and mortality of COVID-19 virus patients.[41] Additional epidemiological investigations in multiple different locations comparing the effects of COVID-19 against national policies on BCG are needed to ascertain the association.

Third, African communities are more cohesive and social gatherings are of great importance. For example, weekly attendance in a religious service is highest in Africa with rates as high as 82% in Uganda and Ethiopia.[42] Funeral ceremony gatherings are of great significance and are attended by many people who tend to ignore lockdown regulation.

In addition, it is now certain that the virus is mainly killing the elderly and those with an underlying medical condition. Research on the COVID-19 virus shows, that the elderly have decreased immune strength that predisposes them to infections.[43] Global North's most vulnerable population is in the Nursing homes living together, an excellent environment for quick transmission of the virus, making the nursing homes a focus of control. In Africa, the elderly lives with their families which may safeguard them against the spread of COVID-19, but this is something that is yet to be confirmed. Africa has a young population with a median age of 20 years compared to Europe and North America with an ageing population where mainly the median age is above forty-five. Therefore, the argument is that communities in Africa are better placed to absorb the blows from infections such as COVID-19. Africa was among the last regions in the world to get the virus, perhaps due to reduced global travel as compared to other regions. The continent benefited and continues to benefit from the knowledge and experiences from regions that had the virus earlier. Finally, the rapid large-scale public health and social measures implementation enabled the protection of the most vulnerable populations and allowed time for countries to ramp up critical healthcare and diagnostic services. It prevented the overwhelming of the already weak health systems, giving time for farmiliarizing and understanding the disease. The epidemic is continuing to bite, and only time will tell whether these hypotheses are true or false. For now, we only remain hopeful that most sub-Saharan African countries will come out of the COVID-19 storm without significant injury.

Economics

In a speech Dr Matshidiso Moeti, WHO's Regional Director for Africa said "COVID-19 has the potential not only to cause thousands of deaths but also to unleash economic and social devastation. Its spread beyond major cities means the opening of a new front in our fight against this virus," "This requires a decentralized response, tailored to the local context. Communities need to be empowered and provincial, and district levels of government need to ensure they have the resources and expertise to respond to outbreaks locally."[44]

The WHO has been working with governments across Africa to scale up their capacities in critical response areas such as coordination, surveillance, testing, isolation, case management, contact tracing, infection prevention and control, risk communication and community engagement, and laboratory capacity. From their evaluation, Ghana, Kenya, Ethiopia, Egypt, Morocco, Tunisia and Nigeria have expanded national testing to multiple laboratories and testing centres, allowing for decentralized testing.[45] Coronavirus has adversely affected the economy. The growth of the economy is expected to drop from 3.2% to 1.8%. The continent has suffered disruptions of global supply chains leading to a drop in value creation. Many countries depend on tourism that has temporarily halted leading to loss of revenue and jobs. Other countries like Nigeria depend on oil exports. Increases in Health expenditure and increased revenue losses could lead to unsustainable debt for most of the poor nations.

Conclusion

Since the early 1918 influenza pandemic, the number and variety of epidemics and pandemics have been rising over the past 30 years. Researchers have determined that an average, one new infectious disease jumps from animals to humans every four months.[46] Additionally, they predict that the next pandemic is only a matter of time and would be even worse than COVID-19.

Globalization has made the world more vulnerable to the collective and economic impacts of infectious-disease outbreaks. Increasing trade, travel globally has dictated the need for unified systems for fighting epidemics. It is now apparent that an epidemic anywhere in the globe is a threat to the whole world. It calls for collective responsibility at all levels of regional, political, social and economic spheres. The economic damage caused by epidemics and pandemics when they occur is vast and unprecedented. These effects have no social or geographic boundaries thus they require soberness and alertness as the government admits that the need for response and control is dire. COVID-19 pandemic has not only amplified the world unpreparedness for biological threats but also the defective supply chains for items for intervention and control.

Most of the epicentres of the virus are the cities. In Kenya, on 27 May 2020, Nairobi County was leading with 85 coronavirus cases, followed by Mombasa with 24. Since then the two cities have become the epicentre for the virus. Nairobi and Mombasa, the leading portals of entry into the country have had the highest numbers of infections.[47] The current scenarios highlight the need for the cities to be more prepared for pandemics in the future. Soon after the COVID-19 overwhelmed Wuhan in early 2020, the pandemic's centre of gravity shifted cities in the west Seoul, Milan, Madrid and New York. Around the world, cities are the first place of infection and the source of the virus that spread to other parts of the country. It was distressing to see the level unpreparedness in cities that shook the governments. Most of these cities were struggling to respond and control the virus effectively. Almost all the major cities in Africa have been hit by the pandemic; however, they have not adequately controlled the infection. Transmission continues to take place from cities to the countryside, which stands as an evidence of lack or inadequate preparedness on the part of the government and the cities. Nevertheless, cities continue to remain the main centres of response and control. The governments of African nations should come up with a robust national coordinate response mechanism with particular attention to the cities. Although similar strategies were laid down during the recent Ebola epidemic, they were not sufficient since the epidemic was only seen to affect the western and central African countries.

Africa CDC was launched by the African union in 2017 to strengthen the capacity and capability of Africa's public health institutions as well as partnerships to detect and respond quickly and effectively to disease threats and outbreaks.[48] This institution is timely and could transform Africa's response and control to the pandemic. It is envisaged that this development will yield dividends beyond the diagnostics for coronavirus and will create a platform for African countries to respond to future emerging diseases. The epidemic has exposed the immense need to improve health security worldwide in order to achieve the goals of the international Global Health Security Agenda. Responses to past outbreaks created partnerships among civil society to complement the official response. However, these partnerships have been challenged by the COVID-19 pandemic. Now there is a need to rethink the strategy. A change in the way the global community responds to epidemics and pandemics is inevitable. The challenge lies in an all-round and inclusive infrastructure focusing on preparedness and development of the necessary trust-based relationships.

NOTES

1. COVID-19 Dashboard by the Center for Systems Science and Engineering (CSSE) at Johns Hopkins University (JHU), available at https://coronavirus.jhu.edu/map.html, accessed on 1 June 2020.
2. Liangjun Chen, Weiyong Liu, Qi Zhang, and et al., 'RNA based mNGS Approach Identifies a Novel Human Coronavirus from Two Individual Pneumonia Cases in 2019 Wuhan Outbreak,' *Emerg Microbes Infect*, vol. 9, February 2020, pp. 313-319.
3. A.E. Gorbalenya, S.C. Baker, R.S. Baric, *et al.*, 'The Species Severe Acute Respiratory Syndrome-related Coronavirus: Classifying 2019-nCoV and Naming it SARS-CoV-2,' *Nature Microbiology*, vol. 5, no. 4, 2020, pp. 536–544.
4. Coronavirus Disease 2019, Africa CDC, available at https://africacdc.org/covid-19/, accessed on 2 June 2020.
5. Samira Sawlani, 'COVID-19: Africa Told to Prepare for Worst. What's the Response?' *Aljazeera*, 19 March 2020, available at https://www.aljazeera.com/news/2020/03/covid-19-africa-told-prepare-worst-response-200319085112877.html, accessed on 3 June 2020.
6. Healthcare and Economic Growth, UNECA, 2019, available at https://www.uneca.org/sites/default/files/uploaded-documents/ABHF2019/healthreport_executive_summary.pdf, accessed on 4 June 2020.
7. ' "I see dead bodies on African streets soon" Melinda Gates predicts,' *News Break*, 13 April 2020, available at https://www.newsbreak.com/news/0Ojx8dOD/i-see-dead-bodies-on-african-streets-soon-melinda-gates-predicts, accessed on 3 June 2020.
8. COVID-19 in Africa: Protecting Lives and Economies, UNECA, April 2020, available at https://www.uneca.org/sites/default/files/PublicationFiles/eca_covid_report_en_rev16april_5web.pdf, accessed on 3 June 2020.
9. 'Africa Identifies First Case of Coronavirus Disease: Statement by the Director of Africa CDC,' *Africa CDC*, 15 February 2020, available at https://africacdc.org/news-item/africa-identifies-first-case-of-coronavirus-disease-statement-by-the-director-of-africa-cdc/, accessed on 5 June 2020.
10. Mapping the Coronavirus Pandemic in Africa, *The Elephant*, available at https://www.theelephant.info/mapping-the-coronavirus-pandemic-in-africa, accessed on 5 June 2020.
11. Kenya Records 213 Positive Cases of COVIS-19 Nairobi, Ministry of Health (MoH), 18 June 2020, available at https://www.health.go.ke/kenya-records-213-positive-cases-of-covid-19-nairobi-thursday-june-18-2020/, accessed on 10 June 2020.
12. Eyder Peralta, 'Kenya Criticized For Letting China Flights Land Amid Coronavirus Scare,' *NPR News*, 3 March 2020, available at https://www.npr.org/2020/03/03/811504574/kenya-criticized-for-letting-china-flights-land-amid-coronavirus-scare, accessed on 10 June 2020.
13. Kenya Coronavirus Cases Rise to Four, Ministry of Health (MoH), 2020, available at https://www.health.go.ke/kenya-coronavirus-cases-rise-to-four-cs-health/, accessed on 10 June 2020.
14. 'Kenya Announces First Coronavirus Recovery,' *Daily Nation*, accessed on 05 June 2020.
15. Claire Munde, 'First Kenyan dies of COVID-19 - CS Kagwe,' *The Star*, accessed on 05 June 2020.
16. Govt Announces Extra Measures to Prevent Spread of Coronavirus Nairobi, Ministry of Health, 6 April 2020, accessed on 07 May 2020.
17. Hilary Kimuyu, 'Mass testing: Kawangware Residents Refuse to be Tested for COVID-19,' *Nairobi News*, 1 May 2020, available at https://nairobinews.nation.co.ke/general/mass-testing-kawangware-residents-refuse-to-be-tested-for-covid-19, accessed on 05 June 2020.

18. More than 600 Confirmed Cases of COVID-19 in Africa, Africa CDC, 19 March 2020.
19. April Zhu, 'Briefing: Five ideas on how to ease the impact of COVID-19 Lockdowns in Kenya,' *The New Humanitarian*, 6 April 2020, available at https://www.thenewhumanitarian.org/news/2020/04/06/kenya-coronavirus-lockdowns, accessed on 08 June 2020.
20. COVID-19 Mombasa Port Situation Statement by the Acting Managing Director Eng. Rashid Salim, KPA Press News, available at https://www.kpa.co.ke/Pages/COVID-19-MOMBASA-PORT-SITUATION-STATEMENT-BY-THE-ACTING-MANAGING-DIRECTOR-ENG.-RASHID-SALIM.aspx, accessed on 05 June 2020.
21. Peter Kirira, 'Battle Against COVID-19: Debunking the Myths & Providing Solutions through Research,' *MKU*, 11 April 2020, available at http://mku.ac.ke/ebulletin/2020/04/11/battle-against-covid-19-debunking-the-myths-providing-solutions-through-research/, accessed on 08 June 2020.
22. James Kahongeh, 'Explainer: Nine Common Coronavirus Myths,' *Daily Nation*, available at https://www.nation.co.ke/kenya/news/explainers/explainer-nine-common-coronavirus-myths-279554, accessed on 08 June 2020.
23. 'A Bioweapon or Effects of 5G? 7 Conspiracy Theories Around Coronavirus that will Shock You,' *ET Times*, 28 February 2020, available at https://economictimes.indiatimes.com/magazines/panache/is-covid-19-a-bioweapon-five-conspiracy-theories-around-coronavirus-that-will-shock-you/origins-in-the-seafood-market/slideshow/74388529.cms, accessed on 08 June 2020.
24. Ahmed Iyanda, 'Tension in Kenya as patients keep off hospitals amid COVID-19 fears,' *Ventures Africa*, 8 May 2020 available at http://venturesafrica.com/tension-in-kenya-as-patients-keep-off-hospitals-amid-covid-19-fears/, accessed on 10 June 2020.
25. Economic Burden of the Informal Sector, IEA, 7 December 2016, available at https://www.ieakenya.or.ke/number_of_the_week/economic-burden-of-the-informal-sector, accessed on 10 June 2020.
26. Gilbert Nganga, Maina Waruru and Gilbert Nakweya, 'Universities Face Multiple Challenges in Wake of COVID-19 Closures,' *University World News Africa Edition*, 07 April 2020, available at https://www.universityworldnews.com/post.php?story=20200407162549396, accessed on 12 June 2020.
27. Government starts Manufacturing Mask and PPE to Prevent Coronavirus Nairobi, Ministry of Health, 3 April 2020, available at https://www.securexpoeastafrica.com/news/government-starts-manufacturing-mask-and-ppe-to-prevent-coronavirus-nairobi, accessed on 12 June 2020.
28. KU Makes Ventilators, Kenyatta University, available at http://www.ku.ac.ke/component/k2/item/1655-k-u-makes-ventilators, accessed on 12 June 2020.
29. Christopher Giles and Peter Mwai, 'Coronavirus: How African Countries are Lifting Lockdowns,' *BBC News*, 12 May 2020, available at https://www.bbc.com/news/world-africa-52395976, accessed on 14 June 2020.
30. Tom Collins, 'Tanzania Risks Pariah Status in COVID-19 Response,' *African Business*, 27 May 2020, available at https://africanbusinessmagazine.com/region/east-africa/tanzania-risks-pariah-status-in-covid-19-response/, accessed on 14 June 2020.
31. Andrew Wasike, 'Burundi First Lady in Kenya for COVID-19 Treatment,' *Anadolu Agency*, 30 May 2020, available at https://www.aa.com.tr/en/africa/burundi-first-lady-in-kenya-for-covid-19-treatment/1858977, accessed on 14 June 2020.
32. United Nations News Global Perspective Human Stories Africa, *UN News*, 11 June 2020, available at https://news.un.org/en/story/2020/06/1066142, accessed on 14 June 2020.

33. UN Habitat, 2013.
34. Munzoul Assal, 'COVID-19 and the Challenges of Social Distancing in Khartoum,' *CHR. Michelsen Institute*, April 2020, available at https://www.cmi.no/publications/7250-covid-19-and-the-challenges-of-social-distancing-in-khartoum, accessed on 18 June 2020.
35. Alan Nicol, 'The Pandemic Is Laying Bare a Global Water Crisis,' *Foreign Policy*, 12 May 2020, available at https://foreignpolicy.com/2020/05/12/coronavirus-pandemic-global-water-crisis/, accessed on 18 June 2020.
36. Water: Our Common Wealth, UN, 2020, available at https://www.un.org/en/observances/water-day, accessed on 18 June 2020.
37. Aryn Baker, 'Few Doctors, Fewer Ventilators: African Countries Fear they are Defenseless Against Inevitable Spread of Coronavirus,' *Times News*, 7 April 2020, available at https://time.com/5816299/coronavirus-africa-ventilators-doctors/, accessed on 18 June 2020.
38. COVID-19: African Union in Discussions with Madagascar over Herbal Remedy, African Union press, 4 May 2020, available at https://au.int/en/pressreleases/20200504/covid19-african-union-discussions-madagascar-over-herbal-remedy, accessed on 20 June 2020.
39. Oyinlola Oyebode, Ngianga-Bakwin Kandala, Peter J Chilton and et al, 'Use of Traditional Medicine in Middle-income Countries: A WHO-SAGE Study,' *Health Policy and Planning*, vol. 31, no. 8, October 2016, pp. 984–991.
40. Neema Kaseje, 'Why Sub-Saharan Africa Needs a Unique Response to COVID-19,' *World Economic Forum*, 30 March 2020, available at https://www.weforum.org/agenda/2020/03/why-sub-saharan-africa-needs-a-unique-response-to-covid-19/, accessed on 20 June 2020.
41. Aaron Miller, Mac Josh Reandelar, Kimberly Fasciglione and et al., 'Correlation between Universal BCG Vaccination Policy and Reduced Morbidity and Mortality for COVID-19: An Epidemiological Study,' *medRxiv*, 28 March 2020.
42. See note 40.
43. Groups at Higher Risk for Severe Illness, CDC, 2020, available at https://www.cdc.gov/coronavirus/2019-ncov/need-extra-precautions/groups-at-higher-risk.html, accessed on 18 June 2020.
44. Alexa Lardieri, 'Coronavirus Cases Top 10,000, Deaths Surpass 500 in Africa,' *US News*, 8 April 2020, available at https://www.usnews.com/news/world-report/articles/2020-04-08/coronavirus-cases-top-10-000-deaths-surpass-500-in-africa, accessed on 18 June 2020.
45. WHO, 2020 COVID-19 cases in Africa top 10,000, WHO Media Centre, available at http://www.emro.who.int/media/news/covid-19-cases-in-africa-top-10-000.html, accessed on 18 June 2020.
46. Mark S. Lesney, '2019-nCoV: Just a Stop on the Zoonotic Highway,' *Mediscape Medical News*, 30 January 2020, available at https://www.medscape.com/viewarticle/924552, accessed on 18 June 2020.
47. Kenya Reports 123 Cases of Coronavirus Nairobi, MOH Kenya, 27 May 2020, available at https://www.health.go.ke/kenya-reports-123-cases-of-coronavirus-nairobi-wednesday-may-27-2020/, accessed on 18 June 2020.
48. The African Union launches Africa CDC, a Continent-wide Public Health Agency, African Union Press release, 2 February 2017, available at https://au.int/en/pressreleases/20170202/african-union-launches-africa-cdc-continent-wide-public-health-agency, accessed on 18 June 2020.

SECTION III

SCIENCE AND TECHNOLOGY

16

COVID-19 and the Search for Effective Vaccine

Mrinmayee Bhushan

Jennifer Haller, a mother of two and operations manager at a tech company became the first person outside of China to receive an experimental vaccine against severe acute respiratory syndrome coronavirus 2 (SARS-CoV-2 virus) on 16 March. Developed by Moderna, a Boston based biotech company has yet to bring the product to the market.[1] The United States' Moderna, (Haller's vaccine source) and China's Cansino Biologics are the first to launch preliminary clinical trials of vaccines against COVID-19.[2]

SARS-CoV-2

Coronaviruses, named due to the presence of spike proteins on the surface appear like a crown, have natural animal reservoirs like bats. These viruses are known to cause acute lung injury (ALI) and acute respiratory syndrome (ARDS) leading to pulmonary failure and death. These coronaviruses include the severe acute respiratory syndrome coronavirus (SARS-CoV), H5N1 influenza A, H1N1 2009 and Middle East respiratory syndrome coronavirus (MERS-CoV). The highly infectious causative agent of COVID-19 is SARS-CoV-2, also a zoonotic virus of the same family *Coronaviridae*. SARS outbreak during 2002-2004 led to the discovery of many such SARS-like bat coronaviruses. A virus named RaTG13, isolated from the bats in Yunnan province in China have 96% phylogenetic resemblance to SARS-CoV-2.[3]

Origin, Transmission, Immune Response

The SARS-CoV-2 virus is known to be a bat virus, was first noticed to infect humans in Wuhan of China's Hubei province in December 2019. Highly infectious, it quickly spread from human to human, travelling across nations, forcing the World Health Organization (WHO) to declare it as Public Health Emergency of International Concern (PHEIC).

Mode of Transmission and Immune Response

The human to human transmission occurs primarily via respiratory droplets of sneezing and coughing of an infected person and indirect transmission from infected surfaces. An RNA-virus with 50-200 nm diameter, SARS-CoV-2 virus has four structural proteins. The N (nucleocapsid) protein holds the RNA genome of the virus while the S (spike), E (envelop) and M (membrane) proteins together form the viral envelope containing genome. A unique feature of SARS-CoV-2 within beta-coronaviruses is the presence of a polybasic cleavage site, a feature known to increase the pathogenicity and transmissibility, explaining the high infectivity of the virus.

Proposed host immune responses during SARS-CoV-2 infection suggest spike proteins of the virus have a high affinity for human cell surface receptors angiotensin-converting enzyme 2 (ACE 2). Once the virus enters through aerosol of SARS-CoV-2 leads to infection of ACE2 expressing target cells such as lung (alveolar type 2) cells. It is suggested that the virus may dampen anti-viral immune responses resulting in uncontrolled viral replication. The B cells/plasma cells produce SARS-CoV-2 specific antibodies that may help neutralize viruses.

Vaccine Development

A vaccine is designed to boost our natural immune response to a specific virus by priming it to recognize unique surface epitopes of pathogens called antigens. Ideally, the immune system responds to the presence of these antigens by producing special immune cells that directly attack the pathogen, or by producing antibodies. Antibodies attach to surface antigens and attract immune cells that engulf and destroy the invading pathogenic virus.[4]

Vaccine development in general is a time-consuming (average over 10 years), funding intensive process, with multiple vaccine candidates under trials, and with a very high rate of attrition till a successful candidate is ready for a manufacturing license. As vaccine development is a costly process along with very high rates of failure; the process runs in a linear sequential manner with frequent breaks to analyse data of each milestone taking years for the development.

- Initially, the vaccines are tested in animals before any human trials to assess probable safety and efficacy.
- After the successful completion of preclinical trials (in animals), the first safety study of the vaccine candidate in humans starts at a small scale. The manufacturing of the test samples for the Phase-I human trial is done on a small scale.
- After the successful completion of the Phase-I trial, efficacy trial (Phase-2a) in humans at a bigger scale is conducted to assess the ability of the vaccine candidate to protect against the virus.
- The evaluation stage (Phase III) of the vaccine candidate to assess the efficacy is done in a large population. While manufacturing the vaccine candidates for this stage of clinical trials, process validation of scale-up and commercial scale manufacturing is also carried out.

This linear process goes on for years. However, during a pandemic like COVID-19, vaccine development needs to be done very quickly requiring a new pandemic paradigm with many vaccine developmental stages running parallel rather than in a linear sequential manner. This parallel process involves multiple stages of vaccine development running parallel and executed fast. This obviously increases the financial need and risks as well.

Challenges of Vaccine Development

In recent years there has been an urgent demand made to the scientific vaccine development community to develop vaccines at a short notice against viral epidemics like H1N1, Ebola, SARS, Zika and now SARS-CoV-2. As the influenza vaccine platform was already well-developed and the regulatory authorities were well-conversant with the strain change nuances of vaccine development, the H1N1 vaccine could be developed relatively faster. SARS, Ebola and Zika pandemics ended before their vaccine development could be completed. This left the vaccine development and manufacturing companies with huge financial losses as the federal agencies reallocated their funding to other projects. In the case of the Ebola vaccine, the vaccine development by Merck continued even after the pandemic ended and hence the investigational product was available for use during recent outbreaks in the Democratic Republic of Congo.

These experiences have stressed the need for the development of pre-emptive vaccine development platform technologies which could be adapted quickly to any new infectious pathogen. Some Vaccine development and biotech companies, the US National Institute of Allergy and Infectious Diseases (NIAID), an international nongovernmental organization the Coalition for Epidemic Preparedness Innovation (CEPI) are all supporting development of platform vaccine technologies to enable fasten the development of a vaccine against future epidemics.[5]

Genetic Evolution of the Virus

Mutations or viral variants are common features of viruses and are part of their genetic evolution. These genetic variations or mutations are errors during replications of the viral genetic material. These genetic variants need to be tracked from the vaccine development point of view and are extensively researched to understand how the virus has adapted to its human host. These genetic variations in different strains of SARS-CoV-2 virus detected in various countries may have implications for virulence, transmissibility, therapeutic and diagnostic methods as well as vaccine development strategies.

One mutation of significance is that the Spike protein (S protein) is responsible for cellular entry of the virus. According to Australia's national science agency, Commonwealth Scientific and Industrial Research Organisation (CSIRO), two-thirds of global strains and half of the sequences in Australia and India show this mutation of S protein called D614G. However, this is not alarming to Virologists as RNA viruses like SARS-CoV-2 to undergo mutations and dominant strains appear more globally. Also, higher transmissibility of a particular strain does not equate to more severe forms of the disease. As this genetic variation is part of the normal anticipated evolution of the virus while adapting to its new human host, it need not cause undue alarm.[6] As compared to SARS 2002-2003, the new SARS-CoV-2 shows very less genetic variability.

These mutations definitely increase the risk of vaccine development. Vaccine development needs huge funding and is spread over many years. Currently, vaccine developers are taking tremendous financial risks by developing many vaccine candidates, by conducting different phases of development simultaneously. So, there is a risk of successfully developing a vaccine for a COVID-19 strain that exists no more by that time. Hence, broad based vaccines using more conserved genetic targets (which do not show mutations) are more favoured amongst the vaccine targets.

COVID-19 Vaccine Development Strategies

While developing different strategies of vaccine development the scientists need to consider a way in which the immune system interacts and responds not just to the invading pathogen, but also the vaccine itself. The paradoxical effects of vaccines against viruses such as dengue, SARS are large warning signboards. Some vaccinated test animals and humans when exposed to the pathogen later presented disease with much more severe symptoms than the non-vaccinated population. One manifestation of such vaccine-primed backfiring of the immune system may be in the form of antibody-dependant enhancement (ADE) and allergic inflammatory conditions (T-cell response).

Therefore, very careful assessment of vaccine candidates under human clinical trials is necessary considering the possible risk of immune complications, before releasing these vaccines in the market for large populations.[7]

Though there are no successful vaccines available for SARS and MERS to date, the lessons learned during these vaccine development efforts offer many guiding paths for COVID-19 vaccine development. Some suggestions include the use of adjuvants, chemicals which are known to not only enhance the efficacy of vaccine but also reduce the adverse effects of vaccination. During SARS challenge studies in animals, it was observed that in the presence of adjuvants lung immunopathology was absent, which was observed when vaccinated without adjuvants. According to some scientists, the intranasal route of administration would also have better vaccination efficacy considering that the coronaviruses like SARS, MERS and COVID-19 are respiratory viruses and intranasal route of administration might invoke better cellular and antibody response to the vaccination.[8] Similarly, nucleocapsid protein (N- protein) is conserved in SARS and MERS coronaviruses and has potential as a target protein to offer potential cross-protection and long term T-cell immunity against coronaviruses.[9]

Technology Platforms

The COVID-19 pandemic has quickly spread across the world and caused several infections and deaths due to the high infectivity potential of the virus. This unprecedented scenario now is asking the vaccine development community to research and deploy sufficient, safe and effective vaccines to the global population at an equally unprecedented speed. The global need to vaccinate very diverse populations requires diverse approaches to vaccine development. This also calls for collaboration of academia, biotech and pharmaceutical companies, governments, NGOs and regulatory authorities. Ten different technology platforms have been reported to be under development to create a safe and effective vaccine against COVID-19. These molecular platforms include:

- replicating/non-replicating viral vectors,
- RNA-/DNA-based vaccines,

- live attenuated/inactivated virus,
- virus-like particles,
- protein subunits, and
- some undefined platforms.

Individually, each technology platform has a set of distinct advantages and limitations. Many of these platforms are not yet licensed vaccines. However, the experience of development for other medicinal purposes such as for oncology has a distinct advantage to quickly develop a vaccine against COVID-19 pandemic with this known approach of the technology platform. For example, novel mRNA-based or DNA-based technology platforms can be tweaked for a specific disease. Once the SARS-CoV-2 sequence was identified, within two months Moderna began the clinical trials of its mRNA based vaccine candidate mRNA-1273.

Coalition of Epidemic Preparedness Innovations (CEPI)

CEPI is an international foundation raising 2 billion USD fund for rapid research and development of COVID-19 vaccine candidates. According to CEPI, DNA- and RNA-based vaccines are more promising candidates as they can be rapidly tested, developed and can be manufactured at large scale.

The recent development of SARS-CoV-2 hACE2 transgenic mouse (HFH4-hACE2 in C3B6 mice) is very encouraging as it is expected to fast track preclinical development of vaccine and therapeutic candidates.[10] This first SARS-CoV-2 mouse model when infected shows typical interstitial pneumonia and pathology similar to COVID-19 patients.

World Health Organization (WHO) Solidarity Trial

WHO is leading a multinational COVID-19 vaccine development coalition for long term protection of healthcare providers at higher risks and new outbreaks. This Global Target Profile Team of international vaccine scientists was formed to conceptualize, design and coordinate multinational trials at sites in high-risk countries. This adaptive design of the Solidarity Trial is expected to rapidly alter parameters at all sites simultaneously according to the test results. This is expected to further compress the time frames of clinical trials of COVID-19 vaccine candidates.

The Controversy of Proposed 'Challenge Studies'

Stages of clinical development in a sequential manner need years of Phase-II/III studies. Some strategies to conduct 'challenge studies' to bypass typical Phase-III stage to fast track the development processes are often debated. Challenge studies are ethically questionable due to the unknown nature of the virus, unknown hazards to the volunteers due to disease enhancement. Even then challenge studies may be the only option to get an effective vaccine and minimize the projected enormous number of deaths due to COVID-19. Moreover, the US Health department has published a notification under Public Readiness and Emergency Preparedness Act to protect vaccine manufacturing companies and healthcare service providers against any liability issues.

Status of India in Vaccine Development

Globally, over 100 vaccine candidates being developed. India is participating in 30 such efforts including partnerships between Indian academia and industry. Pune based Serum Institute of India (SII) has collaborated with the University of Oxford to speed up the clinical trials and manufacturing of vaccines. SII and AstraZeneca have indicated that the Oxford vaccine (AZD1222) would be made available to India and other low-income countries. SII has also entered into a collaboration with US-based synthetic biology company Codagenix to co-develop and scale up manufacturing of a live attenuated vaccine against COVID-19.[11] This vaccine platform has the distinct advantage of mounting an immune response to multiple viral surface antigens at the same time and ability to mass produce the vaccine quickly. SII is the world's largest vaccine producer by volume, manufacturing 1.5 billion doses per year.[12]The other Indian firms working on vaccines for COVID-19 are Zydus Cadila, which is working on two vaccines, Biological E, Bharat Biotech, Indian Immunologicals, and Mynvax each developing one vaccine. Indian Immunologicals Limited, has collaborated with the Griffith University of Australia to develop a live attenuated SARS–CoV-2 vaccine based on a weakened version of the virus.

Global Initiatives

(a) USA

The American collaborative partnership called Accelerating COVID-19 Therapeutic Interventions and Vaccines (ACTIV) partnership is lead principally by the National Institute of Health (NIH) and Foundation for the NIH (FNIH).[13] The steering committee on this initiative includes leaders from NIH, USFDA and research and development organizations of leading biopharmaceutical organizations. The main objective of this initiative is to develop a collaborative framework for therapeutics and vaccine development by facilitating clinical trials and necessary regulatory processes. This is government-led Pan-America response by leveraging all national assets to create a framework as a response to this and future pandemics.

(b) China

Currently, there are 83 COVID-19 related research and development programs ongoing in China. This includes vaccine developments of candidates from five categories; inactivated virus vaccines, recombinant protein vaccines, live attenuated influenza vaccines, nucleic acid vaccines and adenovirus vaccines. Five vaccine candidates have been approved for clinical trials as of now. China is also part of various international collaborative vaccine development programs like the one led by WHO, CEPI and GAVI.

(c) Pharma Majors

Global pharma majors playing a leading role in vaccine development against COVID-19 include:

- Moderna Inc on the forefront of vaccine development with their mRNA-based vaccine is expected to start their last phase of human clinical trials with 30000 volunteers in July 2020.
- If Johnson and Johnson advance their human clinical trials to begin in mid-July 2020, then the firm may be able to be part of massive clinical trial program or Operation Warp Speed by the US government.
- China National Biotec Group Co is currently offering two of its vaccine candidates to employees of state intending overseas travel for work.
- China's Sinovac is planning to start its final stage of clinical study in Brazil to test it in 9000 Brazilian patients. It comes with a promise that the vaccine will be available to immunize millions of Brazilians.

BCG and COVID-19

Bacillus Calmette-Guérin (BCG) is a live attenuated strain of *Mycobacterium Bovis*. BCG vaccine has been used all over the world, including India for years against Tuberculosis. It is part of the National Vaccination policy at birth in India as well as for many other Asian, African and Latin American countries. Live vaccines like BCG is known to induce metabolic and epigenetic effects that prime the innate immune response to future infections. BCG vaccine, in addition to its role in protecting against tuberculosis infection, is known to have non-specific effects on the immune system resulting in protection against a wide range of other infections. Similarly, the BCG vaccine has been effective in other similar viruses such as BCG-led reduction of viremia in yellow fever patients. This led to a conjecture that the BCG vaccine may provide protection against COVID-19 too.

If any BCG-like vaccine is found to be able to provide non-specific protection against COVID-19, that will provide great relief to healthcare providers globally till the disease-specific vaccine is developed.[14] However, this hypothesis needs to be proven during the randomized clinical trials underway in Australia, Netherlands, Germany and the US. Otherwise, the sudden surge in demand for BCG vaccines already in short supply would put immense pressure on supply chains in high-risk zones for tuberculosis and giving rise to a false sense of security to COVID-19 patients. Hence, it is advisable to follow the WHO recommendation to await the results of these clinical trials of BCG vaccine for COVID-19. ICMR (Indian Council of Medical Research) in India too is planning a clinical study for the same purpose and will await the results of this trial before recommending the vaccine for COVID-19.

Ensuring Global Access

The need for COVID-19 vaccines is global irrespective of the economic status of the nation. There is a need for fair access to people who are at greater risk. There is a risk of economically stronger nations negotiating large advance orders for vaccines the way it happened in 2009 during the H1N1 pandemic. The risk of poor countries getting elbowed out is very real.

Global Vaccine Alliance GAVI has committed to secure global response to COVID-19 to ensure faster development, manufacturing and distribution of the COVID-19 vaccine in an effective and fair manner. GAVI has raised 8.8 billion USD from 32 governments, 12 corporations, foundations to immunize and to support the global fight against COVID-19.[15] India's Prime Minister Mr. Narendra Modi too pledged 15 million USD to GAVI for the fight against COVID-19.

The WHO has initiated a multinational coalition of scientists to develop vaccines for rapid response to new outbreaks and to provide long-term protection for the high-risk population.

The Unpredictable Future

Despite all these efforts on a global scale, there is a fair possibility that none of the probable vaccine candidates may succeed in the clinical development path. Then what? This thought gives sleepless nights to many people. The evolutionary development of viruses has been extensively studied. It has been established that the virus evolution occurs very fast, and with this, it may lose its virulence. This may result in the gradual decline of the severity of symptoms.

In the case of COVID-19, this pattern is visible. With effective social distancing, awareness, maintenance of hygienic conditions, the severity of COVID-19 is reducing even before herd immunity sets in. This obviously does not imply lowering the guard, but there is also no reason to lose hope if no vaccine is successfully developed.

Today Jennifer Haller is a happy volunteer as she felt she could contribute to the global fight against COVID-19. The first human clinical trial for safety by Moderna has shown promising results with a well-tolerated vaccine and no side effects of the vaccine. Some of the volunteers started showing positive results, that is, antibodies production against the virus. The final testing stage Phase-III clinical trials are expected to begin in July 2020 with thirty thousand volunteers.[16] If all goes well, the Moderna team has indicated an ambitious timeline for commercial manufacturing of the vaccine by the end of 2020.

* * *

Attached Appendix to outline the latest Vaccine development status.

NOTES

1. Jon Cohen, 'With Record-setting Speed, Vaccine makers take their First Shots at the New Coronavirus,' *AAAS*, 31 Match 2020, available at https://www.sciencemag.org/news/2020/03/record-setting-speed-vaccine-makers-take-their-first-shots-new-coronavirus accessed on 25 May 2020.
2. Jon Cohen, 'Vaccine Designers Take First Shots at COVID-19,' *Science*, vol. 368, no. 6486, pp. 14-16, available at https://science.sciencemag.org/content/368/6486/14?utm_campaign=toc_sci-mag_2020-04-02&et_rid=35101294&et_cid=3270773, accessed on 25 May 2020.
3. Peng Zhou, Xing Lou Yang and et al, 'A Pneumonia Outbreak Associated with a New Coronavirus of Probable Bat Origin,' *Nature*, vol. 579, February 2020, pp. 270–273.
4. Lynne Peeples, 'News Feature: Avoiding Pitfalls in the Pursuit of a COVID-19 vaccine,' *Proceedings of the National Academy of Sciences*, vol. 117, no. 15, April 2020, pp. 8218-2221.
5. Nicole Laurie, Melanie Saville, Richard Hatchett and et al, 'Developing COVID-19 Vaccines at Pandemic Speed,' *The New England Journal of Medicine*, vol. 382, May 2020, pp. 1969-1973.
6. Pooja B. Jaiswal, 'Mutant Menace,' *The Week*, 31 May 2020, available at https://www.theweek.in/theweek/current/2020/05/22/mutant-menace.html, accessed on 31 May 2020.
7. See note 4.
8. Eriko Padron-Regalado, 'Vaccines for SARS-CoV-2: Lessons from Other Coronavirus Strains,' *Infectious diseases and Therapy*, vol 9, no. 2, 2020, pp.1-20.
9. Ping Zhao, Jie Cao, Lan Juan Zhao and et al, 'Immune Responses Against SARS-coronavirus Nucleocapsid Protein Induced by DNA Vaccine,' *Virology*, vol. 331, 2005, pp. 128–135.
10. Ren-Di Jiang, Mei-Qin Liu, Ying Chen and et al, 'Pathogenesis of SARS-CoV-2 in Transgenic Mice Expressing Human Angiotensin-converting Enzyme 2, *Cell*, May 2020.
11. 'US/Indian Collaboration on Vaccine Against COVID-19,' *The PharmaLetter*, February 2020,

available at https://www.thepharmaletter.com/article/us-indian-collaboration-on-vaccine-against-covid-19, accessed on 01 June 2020.

12. Rory Horner, 'Any Attempt to Develop a COVID-19 Vaccine Can't Afford to Overlook India and China's Role,' *Scroll.in*, 25 May 2020, available at https://scroll.in/article/962906/any-attempt-to-develop-a-covid-19-vaccine-cant-afford-to-overlook-india-and-chinas-role, accessed on 2 June 2020.
13. 'NIH to Launch Public-private Partnership to Speed COVID-19 Vaccine and Treatment Options,' *National Institutes of Health (NIH)*, 17 April 2020, available at https://www.nih.gov/news-events/news-releases/nih-launch-public-private-partnership-speed-covid-19-vaccine-treatment-options, accessed on 2 June 2020.
14. Nigel Curtis, Annie Sparrow, Tedros A Ghebreyesus and et al, 'Considering BCG Vaccination to Reduce the Impact of COVID-19,' *The Lancet*, vol. 395, no. 10236, April 2020, pp. 1545–1546.
15. 'World Leaders make Historic Commitments to Provide Equal Access to Vaccines for All,' *GAVI-The Vaccine Alliance*, 4 June 2020, available at https://www.gavi.org/news/media-room/world-leaders-make-historic-commitments-provide-equal-access-vaccines-all, accessed on 8 June 2020.
16. 'Moderna Inc to Begin Final Testing Stage of Coronavirus Vaccine on 30,000 Volunteers in July,' *Wion*, 11 June 2020, available at https://www.wionews.com/world/moderna-inc-to-begin-final-testing-stage-of-coronavirus-vaccine-on-30000-volunteers-in-july-305148, accessed on 20 June 2020.

17

Leveraging Technology in the Fight Against COVID-19

Ajey Lele and Kritika Roy

The 2020 COVID-19 outbreak has killed many people and infected billions while forcing nations to close their borders and disrupting the work-as-usual routines. This pandemic has exposed the human fragility along with the downside of the interconnected world. However, humans have always been resilient survivors. We are fighting back with all the tools we have, including some of the most sophisticated technology that is paving the way for new normals. Different technological solutions are being adopted and adapted to mitigate the effects of COVID-19. Many of these adaptations are in line with the idea of breaking the infection chain and decreasing the rate of transmission. Be it remotely operating workspaces, contact tracing apps or self-dispensing sanitisers, thanks to technological advancements, we are more prepared than any era in history to respond to a pandemic.

During the time of the SARS (Severe Acute Respiratory Syndrome) outbreak in 2002, it took scientists more than a year to decode the genome of the virus, however, the Coronavirus genome was identified within a month.[1] Had it not been for effective and advanced technology solutions, we would have been staring at an unmanageable crisis. Countries have adopted a multi-faceted approach to fighting COVID-19.

The chapter highlights how COVID-19 has facilitated agile innovation at unprecedented speed so as to cater to the needs of different sectors in these unprecedented times. Furthermore, the chapter dwells into the employment of different technologies like AI (Artificial Intelligence), supercomputers, space technology and cyber technology to subdue the spread of the outbreak and augment human capability till an efficacious cure for the disease is in place. The chapter also explores the concept of mathematical modelling, simulations and table-top exercises and its likely impact on the mitigation strategy of the pandemic. The chapter underscores the challenges of the sudden surge in internet usage and also the changes in the energy use patterns during the pandemic. Additionally, the chapter sheds light on the challenges in the full deployment of these advanced technologies in the fight against coronavirus.

COVID-19 Facilitating Technological Innovations

Innovation can be seen as the refinement or development of an original invention into usable techniques or products.[2] The current pandemic has not only brought forth a new sense of urgency to innovation efforts but has also been challenging the tech innovators to break new ground to reimagine a world with COVID-19. From hands-free door openers that can be 3D-printed to building a DIY (Do It Yourself) basic ventilator, sensors, to a wristband that buzzes if you are planning to touch your face, a wealth of new prototypes are demonstrating what human ingenuity is capable of, in the face of adversity.[3]

Considering the tremendous economic shock and burden the current pandemic has caused due to the lockdown imposed across the world to control the spread. Thus, the major agenda of innovation has been to address health and safety risks while accommodating an appropriate level of economic activity once lockdown restrictions begin to ease. In fact, many of these innovations are quick and easy to implement and may as well be akin to the Indian term "jugaad" (a frugal innovation mindset to find hacks to problems with limited resources[4]). For instance, plexiglass shields installed at the airport checkout counters or grocery counters. At the same time, there has been a development of more radical and risk-mitigating technologies like drone programmes to sanitise localities and deliver parcels, smart helmets to identify individuals with fever within a five-meter radius, temperature-detection technologies, wearables, and apps to identify customers in near real-time who are at high risk of carrying the virus.[5]

Universally, it had been observed that during the period of crisis a lot of innovations and improvisations do take place and may end up living beyond the time. For instance, technologies like cryptography, radar, battlefield communications and the internet that were the products of World War II are still very much in use and are constantly getting improvised.[6] Pandemic is presenting a unique opportunity to institutionalise blueprints for deep-tech innovation out of which many of these innovations may end up becoming a fixture of life, like various apps being used for screening individuals' health, face to face meetings for a longer duration of time could be replaced by video conferences or companies may continue with work from home model. Indeed, Twitter recently announced permanent work from home for staffers.[7] This is a very major administrative step. Only, time would tell us its efficacy. What today is disruptive technology could become the norm in the after-corona era.[8] It is important to realise that in most cases, technology would end up dictating the lifestyle changes.

At present, the use of various technologies is mostly aimed at saving lives and protecting citizens. The lack of equipment and other paraphernalia in the required numbers have allowed people to innovate to overcome such deficiency. Some procedures adopted for this purpose are almost ground-breaking and demonstrate that emergency like these forces human to think differently and teaches to make the best utilisation of available resources. In India, the Indian Institute of Technology (IIT), has given a myriad of cost-effective innovations including low-cost ventilators, affordable COVID-19 test kits, specialised digital stethoscopes, disposable bamboo furniture for makeshift isolation wards and infection proof fabric for hospitals bedsheets (to prevent Hospital Acquired Infections) and uniform, to aid the fight against COVID-19.[9] Such innovative ways of using medical equipment/medicines/ protection techniques may also impact future policymaking.

Beyond innovation at the local level, the scientific community is found depending on a few available technologies/techniques to address these crises. A few years back, some of the so-called disruptive technologies had shown potential while dealing with medical emergencies like SARS, Ebola, Zika, etc. Technologies like supercomputing, cloud computing, AI, robotics, autonomous sensing systems and various IT (Information Technology) based applications have evolved over a period of time. Such technologies are put in use to address some of the COVID-19 related challenges. Interestingly, the use of such technologies particularly some of the applications put in use for contact-tracing are giving rise to the debates on privacy and data protection.

Figure 1: Ways Emerging Technologies Tackle the Coronavirus Pandemic

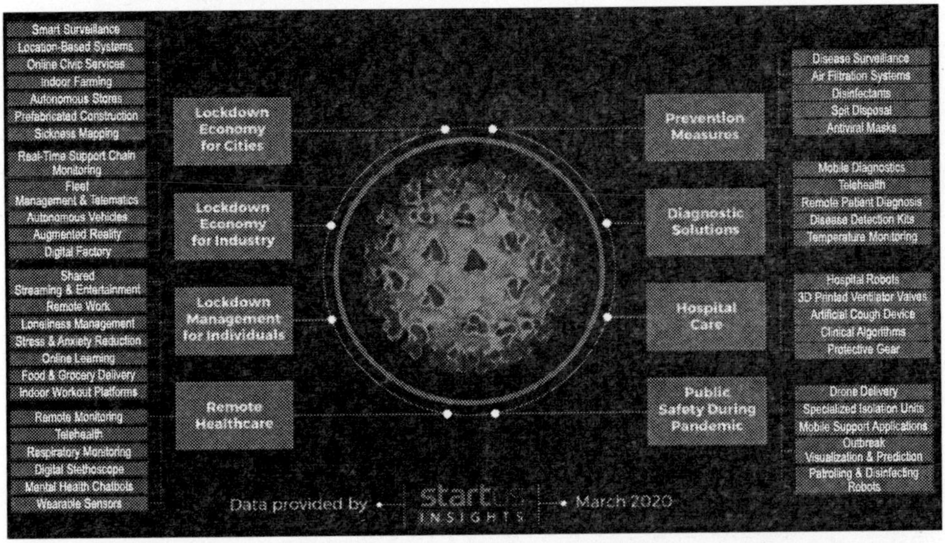

Source: startUS Insights, March 2020, available at https://3vmbig1fuckj48k8rq1n7zug-wpengine.netdna-ssl.com/wp-content/uploads/2020/03/COVID-19-Meta-Article-v2_StartUS-Insights-noresize.png, accessed on 24 June 2020.

COVID-19 and Artificial Intelligence (AI)

AI is a "simulation of human intelligence processes by machines, especially computer systems. These processes include learning (the acquisition of information and rules for using the information), reasoning (using the rules to reach approximate or denite conclusions) and self-correction."[10] The most commonly known applications have been speech/voice recognition, pattern recognition and predictive analysis.

The science of AI is still evolving. However, the level of AI technology available currently has the potential to undertake pattern analysis to know more about a particular patient and also about the disease spread in general. It has emerged as a potentially powerful tool to recognize (diagnose), predict, and explain (treat) COVID-19 infections, and help manage socio-economic impacts. AI and machine learning technologies are assisting researchers to predict the virus, its structure and its spreading methods. Since the initial report of COVID-19 in Wuhan, China has been leaning on AI and data science to track and fight the pandemic. This has also paved the way for technology sector leaders like Huawei, Alibaba, Baidu to multiply its healthcare initiatives.[11] The US (United States of America) administration has already announced a collaborative project with tech companies and academics to make maximum research available to the AI researchers so that they could dig deeper through the mountain of information and bring forth solutions for scientists working on COVID-19.[12]

Enumerated below are the contributions of AI against the COVID-19 Pandemic

(a) Early Warning

BlueDot, a Canada based AI infectious disease surveillance system, was the first to detect the spread of COVID-19. This platform sifts through data, for any possible large-scale disease spread and predicted the current outbreak at the end of 2019 issuing warnings to its clients even before the WHO (World Health Organisation) declared an emergency. BlueDot is also known to have made predictions about the Zika (2016) and Ebola (2014) in the past. Its systems merge varied AI tools with the knowledge of epidemiologists who identified where and how to look for evidence of emerging diseases. This information is based on over 40 pathogen-specific datasets reflecting disease mobility and outbreak potential.[13]

(b) Tracking and Prediction

The combination of advanced analytics and AI is being employed by various countries to check the spread of infection as well as to process high volumes of data that can offer insights and deeper knowledge about the disease and enable health and government officials to make informed decisions. For instance, in the 2015 Zika virus outbreak, a dynamic neural network was developed to predict its spread.[14]

These technologies can also be used to predict the hotspot where new diseases could emerge. It has been estimated by scientists that there are approximately 800,000 unknown animal viruses that could infect humans. AI and deep learning could be used to integrate various data about animal population, viruses, human demographics and cultural and social practices to predict future outbreaks. This would aid governments to be prepared beforehand. Considering "time" is a valuable asset during a pandemic outbreak, early detection could ramp up efforts to curb any outbreak.[15]

Due to the rapidly growing number of cases across the world, modelling the COVID-19's transmission dynamics and estimating its development were crucial for providing decision supports for public health departments and healthcare policy makers. Mathematical models are widely being used in evaluating epidemic transmissions, forecasting the trend of disease spread, and providing optimal intervention strategies and control measures. Many recent studies have contended to estimate COVID-19's scale and severity, several mathematical models and predicting approaches have also attempted to estimate the transmission of COVID-19.

A basic SEIR (susceptible-exposed-infected-removed) model and adjusted SEIR model is being used for prediction. Considering different model inputs may infer different model outputs different scenarios of epidemic development were undertaken especially focussing on short term predictions and peak predictions.

Figure 2: Basic SEIR-SEIRS Model

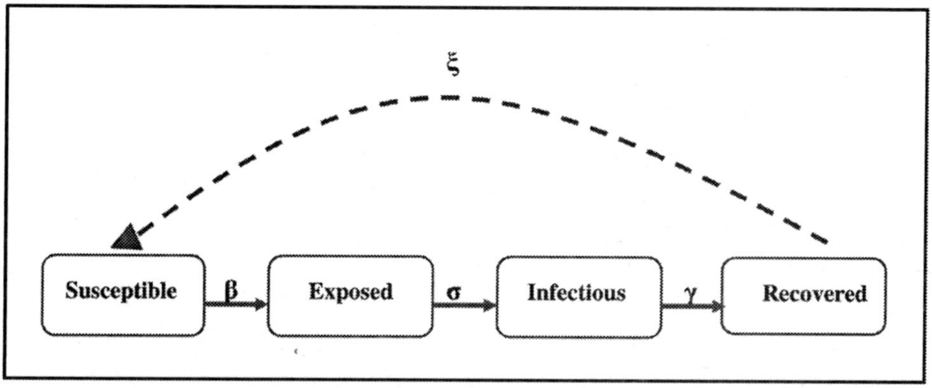

Source: https://www.idmod.org/docs/hiv/model-seir.html

β = The Infectious Rate (controls the rate of spread which represents the probability of transmitting disease between a susceptible and an infectious individual)

σ = The Incubation Rate (the rate of latent individuals becoming infectious (average duration of incubation is $1/\sigma$)

ξ = The rate which recovered individuals returns to the susceptible statue due to loss of immunity.

γ = Recovery Rate (calculated as $\gamma=1/D$)

D = The average duration of infection

A similar modified SEIR and AI prediction for noting the trend of COVID-19 is being used in China under public health interventions with the population migration data before and after 23 January. For implementing the AI approach, models were trained on the 2003 SARS data, to predict the epidemic.[16]

The majority of the published research tends to estimate the basic reproductive number R0, a key parameter to evaluate the potential of COVID-19 transmission. However, different models often yield different conclusions in terms of differences in model structure and input parameters. It is imperative and critical for improving early predictive and warning capability for the pandemic.[17]

AI is also being used to integrate travel and population data to predict where and how quickly a particular disease would spread.[18] After the Ebola outbreak, scientists created a travel census model that was able to correctly predict the exact county and even the likely hospital where an Ebola case could be found.[19]

(c) Diagnosis and Prognosis

Fast and accurate diagnosis of COVID-19 can save lives, limit the spread of the disease, and generate data on which AI models can be trained. The accuracy of AI could be as good as humans while making the process faster and cheaper as noted by researchers.[20]

An AI called COVID-Net is being used to detect COVID-19 in chest X-rays using data from patients with various lung conditions, including COVID-19.[21] Chinese e-commerce giant, Alibaba, has developed an AI-powered diagnosis system that can detect the coronavirus in Computed Tomography (CT) scans of a patient's chest with 96% accuracy against viral pneumonia cases.[22] And it merely takes 20 seconds for the AI to detect a case while a human takes about 15 minutes to do the same. AI in diagnostics is not yet carried over into practice, except for a few Chinese hospitals that have deployed AI-assisted radiology technologies and many researchers have expressed concern regarding the lack of data to train AI models.

Additionally, not all COVID-19 cases require intensive care. Hence, it is important to effectively forecast the severity of a patient and allocate resources accordingly. Researchers at China's Huazhong University of Science and Technology are using ML (machine learning) to develop a prognostic prediction algorithm to estimate the probability of someone surviving the infection.[23] And a team of researchers from Wenzhou and New York prepared an AI that can predict with 80 percent accuracy which person affected with COVID-19 will develop acute respiratory distress syndrome (ARDS).

(d) Treatments and Cures

Treatments and cures, in cases of newly discovered diseases, is a time-consuming process that is laden with trial and errors. AI can be used to examine data from similar viral diseases and then that data could be used to predict which types of vaccines and medicines are most likely to be effective. This can potentially shorten the normal drug discovery and development process by decades and saves hundreds and millions of dollars. In Australia, last year, an AI system developed a vaccine for humans.[24]

In the case of COVID-19, several research labs and data centers have indicated that they are recruiting AI to search for treatments and vaccines. Benevolent AI is known for using AI systems to build drugs that can fight the world's toughest diseases and is now assisting in efforts to find treatment for COVID-19.[25] Within weeks of the Corona outbreak, it used its predictive capabilities to propose existing drugs that might be useful.[26] Researchers from South Korea and the USA have published results from using ML to identify an existing drug, atazanavir, which could potentially be repurposed to treat COVID-19.[27] Even Google's DeepMind division has used its state-of-the-art AI algorithms and its computing power to understand the structure of the proteins that are associated with the COVID-19, and published the findings to help others develop vaccines.[28]

Using AI in the initial level of infection detection would reduce the contamination risk especially for the first line of healthcare workers. However, the full implementation of AI is still a distant dream. This is due to the lack of effective data to train the AI models. Then there is a humongous outlier data that needs to be evaluated before being put through clinical trials.

COVID-19 and Supercomputing

With an increasing number of fatalities due to coronavirus and no cure in the hindsight, many researchers are employing supercomputers to find a medical solution to the crisis. Supercomputers could be a standalone system or system of systems with a high level of performance.

Supercomputers have a long history of being used for various research purposes. With rapid advances in computing technology, supercomputers have also undergone a tremendous change in terms of speed of computing ability and volume of data being handled. Today, these high-performance computing systems allow researchers to run very large numbers of calculations in epidemiology, bioinformatics, and molecular modeling. These experiments would take years to complete if done manually, or months if handled on slower, traditional computing platforms.[29] The novel coronavirus has spikes on its surface, which it uses to invade cells in the human body. Supercomputers are looking for antiviral drugs that could potentially bind with those spikes, thus inhibiting the virus from infecting humans. Supercomputers are also helping in studying the structure and origin of the novel coronavirus, analysing the spread of the virus in a population, as well as how it interacts with cells in the human body.

In 2004, IBM's Blue Gene supercomputer was utilised for Human Genome's Sequencing Project.[30] This breakthrough realised major developments in the drugs sector and treatment methodologies. Blue Gene has helped to simulate approximately one percent of the human cerebral cortex, containing 1.6 billion neurons with approximately 9 trillion connections, leading to a greater understanding of the human brain.[31]

Going forward, the Blue Waters supercomputer of the National Centre for Supercomputing Applications (NCSA) at the University of Illinois at Urbana-Champaign was used in the analysis of the 2009 H1N1 flu pandemic (pH1N1). A very significant mathematical modelling effort was undertaken to understand the entire viral envelope of pH1N1. This was a major mesoscale simulation of pH1N1 and one of the largest biological systems ever to be simulated on that level. This powerful system has facilitated the understanding of researchers on how flu proteins interacted with one another on the surface of the virus and also for undertaking statistical analysis of viral protein movement. Supercomputers have also been used during past outbreaks, including the 2015 Zika epidemic and the 2014-16 Ebola epidemic.[32]

Currently, various supercomputing agencies are undertaking significant efforts. Summit (OLCF-4), the fastest supercomputer developed by IBM, commissioned in 2014 by the US Department of Energy commissioned the 'Summit' for solving some of the world's biggest problems using artificial intelligence (AI) and deep learning, is being used by scientists for drug analysis of COVID-19.[33] Simulations have been carried out on more than 8,000 compounds and some 77 compounds have been shortlisted for a possible vaccine. The research is still ongoing.

The US has also facilitated the creation of COVID-19 High-Performance Computing Consortium that has MIT, the University of California, San Diego, and Rensselaer Polytechnic Institute, New York along with other agencies to allow the research community involved in vaccine development access to supercomputer facilities. Currently, there are 16 supercomputers available in this network.

Another supercomputer cooperative network, C3.ai Digital Transformation Institute (DTI), established by Microsoft Corporation and various other US-based universities to take forward the new Science of Digital Transformation of Societal Systems. This has been made available for the use of scientists for research on COVID-19.

Even the Texas Advanced Computing Centre (TACC), developed during 2012 in response to the H1N1 swine flu crisis, working on issues connected with various disease outbreaks started dedicating its resources to predict the speed of the coronavirus outbreak when it was first labelled as an epidemic. The process involves simulating the spread of pandemic flu over an area of interest. This helps in forecasting the possible number of hospitalizations and determines where and when to place healthcare resources to maximize saving lives. Now, an updated model is available to predict the outcome of COVID-19. In fact, TACC has an existing tool called the Texas Pandemic Flu Toolkit, which uses supercomputers to optimize emergency healthcare response, and is most likely being used to handle the COVID-19 crisis.

Another project, Folding@home is spurring a global movement to commit powerful home computers and game consoles to the cause of mitigating COVID-19. Created by a lab at Stanford University, requests a piece of software that runs in the background on personal computers, gaming consoles and even some phones. When researchers need distributed computing resources for protein folding, drug development or other types of molecular dynamics, the process spins up across Folding@home's network of volunteer machines.[34]

Similarly, in May 2020, the OpenPandemics-COVID-19 partnership between Scripps Research and IBM's World Community Grid was launched. The partnership is a distributed computing project that allows anyone with a computer and an internet connection to donate their device's computing power to help scientists study the world's biggest problems in health and sustainability. By using this donated computing power, the scientists aim to identify promising chemical compounds for further laboratory testing. Additionally, scientists want to fight not only the current emergency but also prepare for the ones that will likely follow. Future pandemics could stem from a progressive accumulation of mutations, which can eventually lead to a new virus variant.[35]

In China, the supercomputer Tianhe-1 is being used to predict the trend of the infection and also to evaluate the effect of prevention and control. More importantly, an AI-based interface is allowing the Tianhe-1 supercomputer to go through hundreds of images (chest scans of the people with the suspected infection) generated by computed tomography (CT) and produce diagnosis within 10 seconds. This has proved to be of great assistance to the medical professionals both in cities and also in areas where limited medical facilities are available. Interestingly, the researchers are also known to be conducting a large sample calculation experiment to provide accurate data support for decision-making on the resumption of public and private activities and other works in the country.

Japan would be using the "Fugaku" supercomputer, government and the country's top research laboratory, which in the past was known to have the highest calculation speed in the world.[36] The Fugaku machine is noteworthy as it is the last big machine based on an all-CPU architecture, and it is also important to point out that despite all of the impressive features that come with the A64FX processor that is based on a modified ARM architecture tricked out with 512-bit vector engines, and despite the efficiencies that we expect in performance per watt from Fugaku running real-world applications, there is no way to scale any machine up to a real exascale of double-precision floating-point processing without being in the range of 60 megawatts to 80 megawatts of power consumption and perhaps costing close to 1.5 billion USD to 2 billion USD.[37] As of the end of April, five projects are running simulations on Fugaku relating to research on the coronavirus pandemic, including looking for drug candidates for treatments for COVID-19, indoor droplet infection simulations, a few different protein analyses of the SARS-CoV-2 virus that causes COVID-19, and statistical analysis of the spread of the disease in Japan and the economic damage of the lockdown.[38]

In India, the government owned Centre for Development of Advanced Computing (C-DAC) has announced that it would collaborate with laboratories of National Institute of Virology (NIV), IITs, Indian Institutes of Science Education and Research (IISER), labs operating under Council of Scientific and Industrial Research (CSIR), Department of Biotechnology (DBT), as well industries and start-ups for performing drug repurposing simulations required towards the discovery of a new drug for COVID-19 under the initiative called 'SAMHAR-COVID-19'. This can also help in finding solutions for identifying, tracking and forecasting outbreaks of COVID-19.[39] C-DAC with its proven record of Designing, Developing and Deploying Supercomputers under the National Supercomputing Mission (NSM) and record of many projects delivered in the area of AI, is in a unique position to exploit the benefits of this confluence and develop products for the societal benefits of our country.

COVID-19 and Space Technologies

Be it wartime, peacetime, humanitarian aid or relief work, space technology has always offered myriad solutions in terms of connectivity, resilience, and logistics. NASA (National Aeronautics and Space Administration) first started experimenting with satellite provision of healthcare as early as 1966 when the ATS-1 spacecraft was used to provide patient care to rural neighbourhoods in Alaska.[40] The major incentive for undertaking such a project was the need to demonstrate the value of satellite applications to state and federal agencies. Moreover, the lack of local medicine infrastructure and high rates of tuberculosis within the indigenous American-Indian community made it more pressing. Since this endeavour, satellite-based telemedicine was successfully used in India, Italy, Romania, Canada, Scotland, Australia, Russia and Albania.[41]

European Space Agency (ESA), in 1996, provided a satellite communication system to link Italian doctors with a field hospital to enable teleconsultations for both civilian and military patients Sarajevo and Bosnia. Indian Space Research Organisation (ISRO), in 2001, had set up a dedicated satellite-telemedicine network throughout India offering various medical facilities like mammography, X-ray, ophthalmology, radiology, cardiology, etc. using its GSAT-3, GSAT-12 and INSAT-3C spacecraft. Following the 2004 Tsunami, post relief mobile satellite-telemedicine stations were also setup on the Andaman and Nicobar Islands.

Understandably, the most important thing in a pandemic is access to healthcare services. Unfortunately for many deployed soldiers, access to healthcare services or specialized care could be limited. And that's not just the case overseas. Some soldiers and veterans in rural and geographically isolated locations within the country could also find themselves without access to specialized, quality healthcare services. Therefore, Telemedicine is also being used by the military to deliver quality care and specialized healthcare services to deployed soldiers, personnel on ships at sea, and veterans at home.[42] Unfortunately, in many of these geographically isolated places, the high bandwidth connectivity and terrestrial networks needed to carry the real-time, HD video necessary for effective telemedicine implementations are either unavailable or untrusted. In those places, SATCOM is helping to fill the connectivity vacuum and deliver essential telemedicine services. With today's advanced high-throughput satellites operating at orbits closer to Earth, the military can effectively deliver fiber-like connectivity to virtually anywhere on the planet. This connectivity could be used to deliver the real-time, high definition video teleconferencing that is needed for the delivery of telemedicine services.

Today, there are more than 2,200 active satellites support earthly infrastructure, economies, and national security systems, enabling hundreds of billions of dollars' worth of benefits over lifetimes.[43] Indeed, space technology has so deeply integrated into many facets of daily life that it is often invisible to the casual user. Therefore, many countries are turning towards space enabled solutions in the fight against COVID-19 as they can improve healthcare by providing high-bandwidth, multi-media patient information. These solutions may include remote visual and telephone consultation, use of satellite communications, navigation and positioning technologies, Earth observation satellites or technology derived from human spaceflight.

Combined with analytic tools and AI algorithms satellite data is helping the scientific community and public authorities to better understand the consequences of the crisis, formulate measures to mitigate its potential impacts and anticipate new models for the recovery period. The satellite data plays an instrumental role both at the macro as well as micro level by providing information about the success of the global response to the stay at home and policies of social distancing. Images from satellites are being used to keep a track of activities in crowded spaces like tourist destinations, highways, industrial sites, etc. Additionally, it is also being used to create population density maps which can be combined with census data to identify demographics of vulnerable population groups such as the young or elderly. Some countries are using geo-location to inform people if they have been in close contact with a carrier and to quarantine themselves.

Satellite navigation and positioning technologies are aiding the government agencies and first responders by pinpointing the high-risk zones, as well as geo-referencing patient data to be shared between doctors and patients. Even earth observation satellites are being used to provide contextual situational awareness data for epidemiological mapping. In an unprecedented collaboration ESA, NASA and JAXA (Japan Aerospace Exploration Agency) have created a 'COVID-19 Earth Observation Dashboard' that combines a wealth of information from earth observing satellites to monitor the worldwide impact of COVID-19.[44] The tri-agency platform gives the general public and policy makers a unique platform to explore the short and long term impacts of the coronavirus lockdown. The tool also allows users to explore and investigate how regional lockdowns and social distancing measures have affected Earth's air, land and water.[45]

Furthermore, monitoring of different services carried out at hospitals, ration-supply shops, sanitisation units to policing pickets is very much essential for timely decision making. Agencies are required to organise various types of activities from imposing quarantine measures to check the movement of migrant labours to ensure the continuing of food, water, electricity and other essential supplies. In case of a sudden jump in infections and deterioration in the health of many people, there would be a need to construct various makeshift facilities including temporary hospitals on open grounds/stadiums and even cremation facilities. Various satellite technologies are providing valuable assistance on such occasions. From communications to monitoring to providing geographical details of the locations and other relevant data inputs, various space-based platforms are proving to be much of use.

In China, BeiDou is helping to track patients and affected places, for containing the virus.[46] It is also helping in analyzing the pattern of the outbreak. With the help of reliable data and precise mapping and imagery, China has built thousands of new makeshift hospitals across the country. The European Union's flagship Earth Observation Programme – Copernicus – is offering over 16TB of free, full and open data through more than 30 owned satellites together with in situ (non-space) data. These vast amounts of data are being used to provide critical information to help service providers, public authorities and other international organisations to combat COVID-19. ESA has announced funding for companies to deploy space-based services to respond to the current global pandemic.[47] UK (United Kingdom) Space Agency in collaboration with ESA is investing some £2.6 million to develop space-enabled technology and services that can strengthen the National Health Service's response to coronavirus.[48]

COVID-19 and Cyberspace

In the backdrop of the COVID-19, the Internet has literally saved thousands of lives in the last few months. If it did not exist, sheltering in place would be nearly impossible. The idea of telecommuting or remotely working would be unimaginable. People would be forced by sheer economic necessity to go to work, grocery store, doctor or just go out, in general, to get work done which can now be done with a single click. Many would find it difficult, in some cases impossible, to check in on friends and loved ones around the world. Schools and colleges would simply collapse, or the administration would have no choice but to open schools and hope for the best.[49] The telephone was, in a sense, the Internet before it existed, but it had severe limitations for the exchange of ideas, and no capacity to transmit images or texts. Without the internet, the phone lines to state agencies and doctors, clinics and hospitals, would simply be overwhelmed.[50] It would have been nearly impossible for small businesses and individuals to survive the current economic shutdown. If only we had a metric to determine what supplies are now being supplied to the people through online shopping, and then contemplate the level of public mingling that would be required were such delivery systems not in place, and obviously the unimaginable death toll and infection rate due to these intermingling.

This sudden surge in 'digital usage and proximity' highlights how this necessity is affecting people's overall views about the role of the internet in their lives and society. It is important to note that the Internet and provision of Internet services is a business and like any other business it runs on money and trained manpower. Apart from medicine and food, the Internet will be the only other 'business' that would remain in demand as the world increasingly gets engulfed under the coronavirus cover. It has been estimated that the current pandemic may spike digital dependency in various sectors.

Unfortunately, this unexpected spike is also leading to the overcrowding of digital networks due to rapid traffic growth. There is an increasing fear that possibly the Internet may not be able to handle this additional strain. In some places, people are facing frequent Internet breakdowns and weak network connections. However, all this could be viewed more as tactical challenges. But it is also important to check if the 'arrangement of Internet' itself could survive the biggest threat ever posed to the entire humanity by the coronavirus.[51] The sheer growth in Internet-based applications including e-commerce, e-governance, e-learning, and videoconferencing tools, may to some extent, hinder the performance of broadband networks. More than a fixed broadband network, the traffic could be more on cellular networks. Broadly, it is expected that the entire system may not crash but witness some diminution in performance.

Although, it is difficult to gauge as to what would be the exact impact if there is a sudden surge. However, it is important to understand the possible impact on the existing Internet Ecosystem and analyse what may happen to this ecosystem if the COVID-19 threat picks up in a big way globally. Interests of almost 60 percent of the global population could be at stake if the global Internet architecture gets disturbed. The following table provides information about the increase in the global reach of the Internet in the recent past:

Figure 3: Internet Usage Stats

Date	Number of Users	% World Population
June 2017	3,885 million	51.7%
Dec 2017	4,156 million	54.4%
Jun 2018	4,208 million	55.1%
Dec 2018	4,313 million	55.6%
Mar 2019	4,383 million	56.8%
Jun 2019	4,536 million	58.8%
Jan 2020	4,574 million	58.7%

Source: Internet World Stats, available at https://www.internetworldstats.com/emarketing.htm#links, accessed on 24 June 2020.

It has been reported that the world's internet users will spend a cumulative 1.25 billion years online in 2020, with more than one-third of that time spent using social media.[52] According to the latest stats provided by Hootsuite, internet users saw a whopping surge of +7.1% (an approx. increase of 301 million) in April 2020 as compared to last year April 2019.[53]

Figure 4: Internet Usage in April 2020

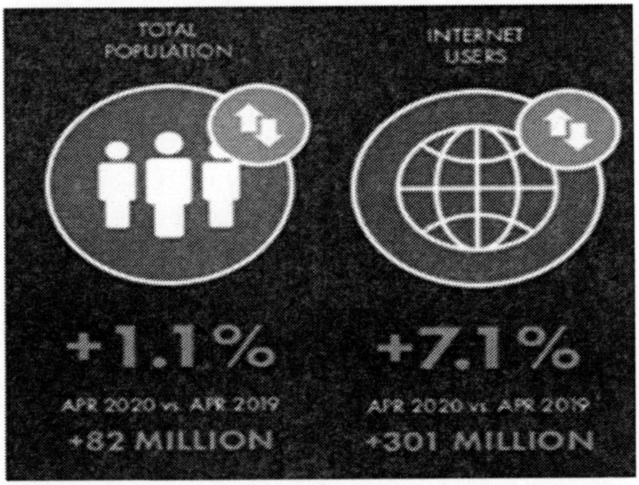

Source: Simon Kemp, 'Digital 2020: April Global Statshot,' available at https://datareportal.com/reports/digital-2020-april-global-statshot, accessed on 25 June 2020.

Internet is a mix of fixed-line and mobile networks run by governments, telcos, ISPs, cloud providers and academic institutions, supported by a constellation of internet exchange points or IXPs. It is a dynamic system consisting mainly of huge Data Centres. These are called the brains of the Internet. The present-day Data Centres are industry type facilities and houses many thousands of interconnected computers, servers, and other related technical systems. A single centre is known to consume electricity equivalent to the electricity required for the sustenance of a small town. The heart of the Internet system is data that exists in an Ocean. It is the underwater cables that are the invisible force driving the modern-day Internet. It is a network of around 380 underwater cables in operation around the world, spanning a length of over 1.2 million km. At present, this entire architecture is funded by Internet giants such as Facebook, Google, Microsoft, and Amazon. Cable failures happen each year and they happen both owing to human mistakes like ship movements or because of natural disasters like hurricanes or underwater earthquakes.

The distributed architecture means there is no imminent danger of a global or even regional internet blackout. There could be delays, lags, and congestion which could lead to temporary downtime or reduced download speeds.

With various sectors including healthcare ramping up its efforts towards adopting full digital mode thereby facilitating improved communication and different facilities. Especially in the healthcare sector, adapting potpourri of different technologies like AI, supercomputing, Big Data has been known to increase the overall efficiency of the healthcare services. The future health services could be exemplary hybrid models of digital and human efforts that would not only reduce contamination chances of the first line of healthcare providers but also render the requisite care to the patients. However, a major catch in such scenarios is the growing level of vulnerabilities across the sectors. Since February 2020, IBM X-Force has observed a 4,300 percent indicating that cybersecurity focus is being overshadowed and risks are rising in the corona era.[54]

Thousands of COVID-19 scams and malware sites have been created.[55] Many of these sites are being used to disseminate malware files, host phishing attacks, or commit financial fraud, including tricking individuals into paying for forged COVID-19 cures, kits, vaccines or supplements.[56] And the health sector will be most vulnerable because it holds a plethora of valuable and sensitive data. On 13 March, one of the Czech Republic's biggest testing laboratories, Brno University Hospital, was hit by a cyberattack.[57] As a result, the hospital had to postpone urgent surgical interventions and transfer patients with acute conditions to a different hospital while having to shut down their entire IT network. This attack also impacted other branches of the hospital, including the maternity and the children's wings.

Furthermore, many of the research institutes have been facing cyber espionage threats. Hackers have recently targeted California University leading COVID Research.[58] UCSF (University of California, San Francisco) has engaged in extensive sampling and antibody testing, including on the experimental antiviral drug remdesivir, which has shown signs of being effective early in the COVID-19 life cycle. Hackers are increasingly targeting institutions like UCSF not only for ransomware payments but also for possibly lucrative intellectual property, like research on a cure for COVID-19. Many reports have stated that Chinese hackers, possibly more at the individual level, are found to be targeting some universities, pharmaceutical and other healthcare businesses in the US.[59] Even Canada has warned that COVID-19 research is facing elevated "foreign" threats of hacking and spying without specifying any agencies or states.[60] Afterall, becoming the first country to develop a vaccine for COVID-19 would make a lot amount of economic sense besides, the significant geopolitical advantages. The state will get recognition as a global technology leader if the Chinese COVID-19 vaccine hits the market first.

As the COVID-19, has pushed businesses to operate remotely, video conferencing apps have seen a considerable uptick in its usage as well as breaching attempts. Even government meetings, online classes and family gatherings have shifted to video conferences. While some depend on commercial apps like Cisco WebEx, Classroom, Slack, Zoom, etc., many countries have also started launching their indigenous apps because of security, privacy and data protection concerns, for instance, India has recently launched a Say Namaste Video Conferencing App.[61]

Many of the freely available apps have a massive privacy and security threat as often the platform's default settings are not secure enough. Especially Zoom which has faced flak because of different issues including security flaws in the Windows 10 build of the platform's software, iPhone user data being sent to Facebook whether or not they had an account with the social media network, and a bug in URL (Universal Resource Locator) generation that permitted attackers to eavesdrop on private conferences have been uncovered.[62] Zoom has also acknowledged that the company's "end to end encryption" marketing practices masked the truth. AES-256 encryption was meant to be implemented to keep video calls secure, but instead, a substandard AES-128 key in ECB mode was actually in use. Encryption remains a sticking point that the company insists it is working on.[63] Additionally, the Zoom bombing activities, that is, disrupting online meetings and bombarding the attendees with disturbing pornographic and violent imagery was another prominent issue.[64]

Another downside of a digital world facing pandemic against which caution enabled by public information disseminated through digital platforms is the only safeguard, the disconnected have-nots are most at risk, both of suffering themselves and of amplifying the footprint of the infection. The Internet enables us to receive and share vital information about the pandemic and the measures being put in place to tackle it. It helps us to understand and scrutinise governments' actions. This is critical especially in light of the growing misinformation and fake news about COVID-19.

Many of the contact tracing apps designed to shield individuals and check the spread of COVID-19. Be it India's "Aarogya Setu," Singapore's "Trace together," Hong Kong's "StayHomeSafe" the whole idea has been to determine if users and their families were infected by the coronavirus, to chart out containment zones by tracing confirmed cases and alerting users if they come in contact with an infected person. However, many of these apps depend on smartphones and the internet, locking out a potentially vulnerable section of the society, putting significant constraints on their ability to access work and safeguard their health. Furthermore, many of the individuals likely from the older generation or low-income backgrounds may lack even basic technology skills, like not knowing how to download or open an app. Those people risk being shut out of attempts to build a smartphone-based contact-tracing, thereby, excluding the most vulnerable of society from any benefits these apps may bring. A central question in the digital divide debate is what role if any, should government play in helping those without access. Should states subsidize broadband access for those who currently lack access or should they urgently fund ways to bridge the gap with digital training and support. This indicates that a lack of proportionate response from the government towards the have-nots while providing the pandemic related information, those who have no access to digital technologies find themselves unable to respond to the ongoing crisis with the right information and in the right manner.

Limitations of Technology

Owing to space technology and global connectivity individuals can closely follow the course of the pandemic day by day, to analyse what works and does not work in other countries (and even states). In virtually all previous pandemics, people found it nearly impossible to know what was happening beyond their region. Fear, based on lack of reliable information, caused unnecessary panic. Computers are accelerating the development of antibodies, vaccines, and other ameliorative drugs. Various operations from businesses to entertainment are running with ease despite strict lockdown across the world. Satellites are not only allowing for safe monitoring and navigation but are also underpinning financial transactions and the protocols that keep data parcels in-sync across the internet and other networks. Without these space technologies, Internet speeds could slow, access to the cloud could deteriorate, and control systems for energy grids, water and transportation could begin to fail. However, this sudden shift to distance learning, working from home, staying in touch with loved ones, and accessing essential facilities have placed additional load on Internet applications.

With the sudden spike in internet usage, there have been debates and deliberations on the collapse of the internet which could mean reviving the old habits and infrastructure, payment, reachability. However, these doubts are misguided. Though there can be temporary lags and slowdowns, but the possibility of total blackout is impossible. The Internet has become an escape route in this pandemic and separating the Internet from everyday life is futile.

Another imminent issue that came to the forefront due to the COVID-19 situation is the changing needs of reliable energy and thus placing new importance on residential microgrids.[65] Energy use during the pandemic provides a glimpse into the challenges expected in the next five to ten years, with higher penetrations of renewable energy, a bigger duck curve and voltage issues. A study conducted by Global Workplace Analytics' Analysis noted that before the pandemic about 5 million people (approx. 3.6% of the workforce) worked from home. Currently, around 56% of workers are operating remotely which could add 3000 kWh per year to household electricity use in the US.[66] Due to the large influx of home workers, there could be a significant reconfiguration of electric demand patterns.

This pandemic has also exposed the limitations of advanced technologies made by the global powers, which otherwise the entire world is so proud about. Despite these rapid advances in Information and Communication Technologies, humans have continued to be on the frontline of the crisis. Though the technology has effectively assisted in each phase of dealing with the virus – be it treatment, diagnosis or just keeping a check on the rapid spread of the outbreak. Human input from various disciplines has been indispensable for the optimal utilisation of any technology application.

Various challenges bedevil the full implementation of technologies to control the rapid spread. The spectre of decision making is at all times in the hands of a human. Why so? This is because many of the technologies work by identifying patterns in data and require large amounts of unbiased data to find these patterns and train the models. The outputs are only as good as the training data, and in some cases, diagnostic claims have been called into question and some chatbots have given different responses to questions on symptoms. The fact that the characteristics of COVID-19 infections differ from those of previous pandemics adds to the challenges of data shortage. Then there is the challenge of too much noise and outlier data, and algorithmic dynamics which makes these technologies not very accurate and unreliable. To some extent tapping disruptive innovation or just employing these technologies have aided in building a coordinated response for this pandemic. Overcoming many of the prevalent constraints will require a more rigorous human-technology interaction.

Useful as these are, the same technologies are also putting individuals in an 'ethical quandary.' The fear is that once the outbreak is over, the erosion of data privacy would not be rolled back and that governments would continue to use the improved ability to survey their populations and use the data obtained for other purposes. Hence, there is a need for a careful balance between data privacy and public health concerns. The use of emergency measures should be carried out in full consultation with data protection authorities and respect the dignity and the private life of the users. The different biases of the various types of surveillance operations should be considered, as these may cause significant discrimination. In particular, the temporary measures of control and mass monitoring of the population by this technology should not be trivialized nor become permanent.

Mathematical Modelling and simulation exercises often carried out as tabletop exercises or integrated with advanced AI and supercomputers computing power aid in projecting the future number of infections, death and recovery. Additionally, these tabletop exercises illustrate the high-level strategic decisions and policies stakeholders would need to pursue to diminish the consequences of a severe pandemic. From Dark Winter in 2001 through Clade X in 2018 and Event 201 in 2019, these exercises have demonstrated the confusion, exodus of misinformation and disinformation, poor decision-making, and lack of coordination of resources and messaging that can undermine a response in the absence of crisis contingency planning and preparation.[67] Even simulations and mathematical modelling have their own limitations and may often vary in accordance with space, time and situations. Nonetheless, these exercises continue to be a vital point for future assessments more now with a real-life experience of a pandemic making governments as well as public more prepared. After all, the greatest message from these exercises may not be just to shock us into action now but to heed the warnings seriously in the future.

Conclusion

COVID-19 crisis should be regarded in a literal sense – 'A Global Reset Button.' This pandemic has not only been about healthcare but also businesses, livelihoods, wellbeing, innovation and resilience. The 21st century advances in technology came to the rescue as the much-needed hero in cape. Although, it is, very difcult to gauge the exact impact of ongoing technological integration for combating COVID-19. Nonetheless, the availability and use of sophisticated technologies under the close supervision of humans are in a lot of ways, proving to be helpful to constraint the spread of the pandemic, limit the economic damage from lockdowns, and avoid a re-occurrence of the virus once restrictions are relaxed.

There are significant lessons to be learnt from the ongoing crisis. As experts have predicted, this is just one of the many pandemics' humans are currently facing. Going forward these advances in technology are expected to revolutionize the entire experience of living through pandemics, wherein it would become extremely important that advanced computational and technological tools are being utilized regularly. Artificial intelligence, machine learning, supercomputing and other digital health approaches could be continuously employed for modelling potential outbreaks, and preparing for simultaneous identification, design and development of testing and therapeutic, if not preventative interventions. Such preparedness would be "ahead of the curve" if and when the pandemic began rather than having to "jump-start" such efforts in pandemic response amidst a rapidly evolving crisis. Thereby assuring that a sudden emergence of a virus may not push people to alter their regular lifestyle.

NOTES

1. Aditya Chaturvedi, 'The China Way: Use of Technology to Combat COVID-19,' *Geospatial World*, 11 May 2020, available at https://www.geospatialworld.net/article/the-sino-approach-use-of-technology-to-combat-covid-19/, accessed on 24 May 2020.
2. Shlomo Maital and D.V.R. Seshadri, 'Innovation Management: Strategies, Concepts and Tools for Growth and Profit,' 2007, v. 29.
3. K. Ganapathy, 'COVID-19 Innovations - Silver Lining in a Black Cloud,' *The Economic Times*, 8 May 2020, available at https://health.economictimes.indiatimes.com/news/industry/covid-19-innovations-silver-lining-in-a-black-cloud/75625835 accessed on 24 May 2020.
4. Sreevas Sahasranamam, 'How Coronavirus Sparked a Wave of Innovation in India,' *World Economic Forum*, 11 May 2020, available at https://www.weforum.org/agenda/2020/05/coronavirus-covid19-innovation-technology-india/, accessed on 25 May 2020.
5. Hong Luo and Alberto Galasso, 'The One Good Thing Caused by COVID-19: Innovation,' *Harvard*, 7 May 2020, available at https://hbswk.hbs.edu/item/the-one-good-thing-caused-by-covid-19-innovation, accessed on 24 May 2020.
6. Vangie Beal, 'The Birth of Internet,' *Webopedia*, available at https://www.webopedia.com/DidYouKnow/Internet/BirthoftheInternet.aspsw, accessed on 24 May 2020.
7. Brian Heater, 'Twitter says Staff can Continue Working from Home Permanently,' *Tech Crunch*, 12 May 2020, available at https://techcrunch.com/2020/05/12/twitter-says-staff-can-continue-working-from-home-permanently/, accessed on 24 May 2020.
8. See note 3.
9. 'Low Cost Test Kits to Sanitising Drones: IIT Innovations take Commercial Route to aid COVID-19 Fight,' *The Economic Times*, 14 June 2020, available at https://economictimes.indiatimes.com/news/science/low-cost-test-kits-to-santising-drones-iit-innovations-take-commercial-route-to-aid-covid-19-fight/articleshow/76368503.cms, accessed on 19 June2020.
10. Margaret Rouse, 'Artificial Intelligence,' *Tech Target*, available at https://searchenterpriseai.techtarget.com/definition/AI-Artificial-Intelligence, accessed on 25 May 2020.
11. Bernard Marr, 'Coronavirus: How Artificial Intelligence, Data Science And Technology Is Used To Fight The Pandemic,' *Forbes*, 13 March 2020, available at https://www.forbes.com/sites/bernardmarr/2020/03/13/coronavirus-how-artificial-intelligence-data-science-and-technology-is-used-to-fight-the-pandemic/#761cc4295f5f, accessed on 25 May 2020.
12. Call to Action to the Tech Community on New Machine Readable COVID-19 Dataset, *Office of Science and Technology Policy*, 16 March 2020, available at https://www.whitehouse.gov/briefings-statements/call-action-tech-community-new-machine-readable-covid-19-dataset/, accessed on 25 May 2020.
13. BlueDot, available at https://bluedot.global/, accessed on 25 May 2020.

14. Wim Naude, 'Artificial Intelligence Against COVID-19: An Early Review,' *Medium*, 01 April 2020, available at https://towardsdatascience.com/artificial-intelligence-against-covid-19-an-early-review-92a8360edaba accessed on 25 May 2020.
15. Steve Bennett, '4 ways Government can use AI to Track Coronavirus,' *GCN*, 10 March 2020, available at https://gcn.com/articles/2020/03/10/ai-coronavirus-tracking.aspx, accessed on 25 May 2020.
16. Zifeng Yang, Zhiqi Zeng, Ke Wang and et al., 'Modified SEIR and AI Prediction of the Epidemics Trend of COVID-19 in China under Public Health Interventions,' *Journal of Thoracic Disease*, vol. 12, no. 3, March 2020, available at https://www.ncbi.nlm.nih.gov/pmc/articles/PMC7139011/, accessed on 27 May 2020, pp. 165-174.
17. Xiang Zhou, Na Hong, Yingying Ma and et al., 'Forecasting the Worldwide Spread of COVID-19 based on Logistic Model and SEIR Model,' *medRxiv*, March 2020, available at https://doi.org/10.1101/2020.03.26.20044289, accessed on 28 May 2020.
18. Kritika Roy, 'Leveraging Technology to Fight Future Disease Outbreaks,' *CLAWS*, 02 April 2020, available at https://www.claws.in/leveraging-technology-to-fight-future-disease-outbreaks/#_edn12, accessed on 25 May 2020.
19. Ibid.
20. Joseph Bullock, Alexandra Luccioni and et. al., 'Fast and Accurate Diagnosis of COVID-19 can Save Lives, Limit the Spread of the Disease, and Generate Data on which to Train AI Models,' 24 April 2020, available at https://arxiv.org/pdf/2003.11336.pdf, accessed on 26 May 2020.
21. Linda Wang and Alexander Wong, 'COVID-Net: A Tailored Deep Convolutional Neural Network Design for Detection of COVID-19 Cases from Chest X-Ray Images,' available at https://arxiv.org/abs/2003.09871, accessed on 26 May 2020.
22. Tristan Greene, 'Alibaba's New AI System can Detect Coronavirus in Seconds with 96% Accuracy,' *The New Web*, available at https://thenextweb.com/neural/2020/03/02/alibabas-new-ai-system-can-detect-coronavirus-in-seconds-with-96-accuracy/, accessed on 26 May 2020.
23. See note 13.
24. Haron Masige, 'Australian Researchers Have Just Released the World's First AI-Developed Vaccine,' *Science Alert*, 13 July 2019, available at https://www.sciencealert.com/the-world-s-first-ai-developed-vaccine-could-prevent-another-horror-flu-season, accessed on 26 May 2020.
25. Justin Stebbing, Anne Phelan and et al., 'COVID-19: Combining Antiviral and Anti-Inflammatory Treatments,' *The Lancet*, vol. 20, no. 4, February 2020, available at https://www.thelancet.com/journals/laninf/article/PIIS1473-3099(20)30132-8/fulltext, accessed on 26 May 2020.
26. Peter Richardson, Ivan Griffin and et al., 'Baricitinib as Potential Treatment for 2019-nCoV Acute Respiratory Disease,' *The Lancet*, vol. 395, no. 10223, 04 February 2020, available at https://www.thelancet.com/journals/lancet/article/PIIS0140-6736(20)30304-4/fulltext, accessed on 26 May 2020.
27. Bo Ram Beck, Bonggun Shin and et. al., 'Predicting Commercially Available Antiviral Drugs that may Act on the Novel Coronavirus (2019-nCoV), Wuhan, China through a Drug-target Interaction Deep Learning Model,' *Cold Spring Harbour Laboratory*, available at https://www.biorxiv.org/content/10.1101/2020.01.31.929547v1.full, accessed on 26 May 2020.
28. Tiernan Ray, 'Google DeepMind's effort on COVID-19 Coronavirus Rests on the Shoulders of Giants,' *ZDNet*, 06 March 2020, available at https://www.zdnet.com/article/google-deepminds-effort-on-covid-19-coronavirus-rests-on-the-shoulders-of-giants/, accessed on 26 May 2020.

29. Dario Gil, 'Confronting the Coronavirus,' *IBM*, available at https://newsroom.ibm.com/IBM-helps-bring-supercomputers-into-the-global-fight-against-COVID-19, accessed on 27 May 2020.
30. Dave Turek, 'US Dept of Energy Brings the World's Most Powerful Supercomputer, the IBM POWER9-based Summit, Into the Fight Against COVID-19,' *IBM*, available at https://newsroom.ibm.com/US-Dept-of-Energy-Brings-the-Worlds-Most-Powerful-Supercomputer-the-IBM-POWER9-based-Summit-Into-the-Fight-Against-COVID-19, accessed on 27 May 2020.
31. Ajey Lele, 'Supercomputing Power Towards Resolving COVID-19 Crisis,' *SSPC*, 08 April 2002, available at https://www.sspconline.org/index.php/opinion-analysis/supercomputing-power-towards-resolving-covid-19-crisis-wed-04082020, accessed on 25 May 2020.
32. Explained: How Supercomputers are Being used to Understand and Prevent COVID-19, *The Indian Express*, 15 April 2020, available at https://indianexpress.com/article/explained/explained-supercomputers-used-prevent-covid-19-coronavirus-6360728/ accessed on 27 May 2020.
33. See note 27.
34. Oliver Peckham, 'Folding@Home Turns its Massive Crowdsourced Computer Network Against COVID-19,' *HPC Wire*, 16 March 2020, available at https://www.hpcwire.com/2020/03/16/foldinghome-turns-its-massive-crowdsourced-computer-network-against-covid-19/, accessed on 15 June 2020.
35. 'Open Pandemics-COVID-19,' *World Community Grid*, available at https://www.world communitygrid.org/research/opn1/overview.do, accessed on 15 June 2020.
36. See note 29.
37. Timothy Prickett Morgan, 'With Fugaku Supercomputer Installed, RIKEN Takes On Coronavirus,' *The Next Platform*, 18 May 2020, available at https://www.nextplatform.com/2020/05/18/with-fugaku-supercomputer-installed-riken-takes-on-coronavirus/, accessed on 23 June 2020.
38. Ibid.
39. 'Pune-based C-DAC Launches Supercomputing Based Research for Combating COVID-19,' *Punekar News*, 25 March 2020, available at https://www.punekarnews.in/pune-based-c-dac-launches-supercomputing-based-research-for-combating-covid19/, accessed on 30 May 2020.
40. Rajan Bedi, 'How Satellite Technology is Fighting COVID-19,' *EDN*, available at https://www.edn.com/how-satellite-technology-is-fighting-covid-19/#comments, accessed on 24 May 2020.
41. Ibid.
42. Ryan Schradin, 'Fighting COVID-19 From Space,'*MilSatMagazine*, June 2020, available at http://www.milsatmagazine.com/story.php?number=1848451628, accessed on 25 June 2020.
43. El Segundo, 'Study Explores Space's Impact on our Daily Lives,' *Space Daily*, 22 May 2020, available at https://www.spacedaily.com/reports/Study_explores_spaces_impact_on_our_daily_lives_999.html?mc_cid=7bf3b08297&mc_eid=8dbfe9f2ee, accessed on 28 may 2020.
44. 'Space Agencies Join Forces to Produce Global View of COVID-19 Impacts,' *Terra Daily*,26 June 2020, available at https://www.terradaily.com/reports/Space_agencies_join_forces_ to_produce_global_view_of_COVID_19_impacts_999.html, accessed on 29 June 2020.
45. Ibid.
46. Aditya Chaturvedi, 'The China Way: Use of Technology to Combat COVID-19,' *Geospatial World*, 11 May 2020, available at https://www.geospatialworld.net/article/the-sino-approach-use-of-technology-to-combat-covid-19/, accessed on 24 May 2020.

47. Space in Response to COVID-19 Outbreak, *The European Space Agency*, 01 April 2020, available at https://www.esa.int/Applications/Telecommunications_Integrated_Applications/Space_in_response_to_COVID-19_outbreak, accessed on 24 May 2020.
48. 'UK Launches Space-based Response to COVID-19,' *The European Space Agency*, April 14, 2020, available at http://www.esa.int/Enabling_Support/Preparing_for_the_Future/Space_for_Earth/Space_for_health/UK_launches_space-based_response_to_COVID-19, accessed on 24 May 2020.
49. Clay Jenkinson, "As the Pandemic Closes the World, the Internet Keeps It Open," *Governing*, 24 April 2020, available at https://www.governing.com/context/As-the-Pandemic-Closes-the-World-the-Internet-Keeps-It-Open.html accessed on 28 May 2020.
50. Ibid.
51. Ajey Lele, 'Could COVID- 19 Pandemic Lead to Long Term Disruption in Internet Services?' *SSPC Online*, 25 March 2020, available at https://sspconline.org/index.php/opinion-analysis/could-covid-19-pandemic-lead-long-term-disruption-internet-services-wed-03252020 accessed on 30 May 2020.
52. Simon Kemp, 'Digital trends 2020: Every Single Stat you Need to know about the Internet,' *The Next Web*, available at https://thenextweb.com/growth-quarters/2020/01/30/digital-trends-2020-every-single-stat-you-need-to-know-about-the-internet/ accessed on 30 May 2020.
53. Simon Kemp, Digital 2020: Global Digital Yearbook, *DataReportal*, 30 January 2020, available at https://datareportal.com/reports/digital-2020-april-global-statshot accessed on 30 May 2020.
54. Top 5 CyberTech Trends in India in Times of COVID-19, *CISOMag*, 14 May 2020, available at https://www.cisomag.com/cybertech-trends-in-india/, accessed on 28 May 2020.
55. Catalin Cimpanu, 'Thousands of COVID-19 Scam and Malware Sites are being created on a Daily Basis,' *ZDNet, 18* March 2020, available at https://www.zdnet.com/article/thousands-of-covid-19-scam-and-malware-sites-are-being-created-on-a-daily-basis/, accessed on 28 May 2020.
56. Catalin Cimpanu, 'Czech Hospital hit by Cyberattack While in the Midst of a COVID-19 Outbreak,' *ZDNet*, 13 March 2020, available at https://www.zdnet.com/article/czech-hospital-hit-by-cyber-attack-while-in-the-midst-of-a-covid-19-outbreak/, accessed on 28 May 2020.
57. Debra Pressey, 'C-U Public Health District's Website held Hostage by Ransomware Attack,' *The News Gazette, 11* March 2020, available at https://www.news-gazette.com/news/local/health-care/c-u-public-health-district-s-website-held-hostage-by/article_2dadedcd-aadb-5cb1-8740-8bd9e8800e27.htm, accessed on 28 May 2020.
58. Kartikay Mehrotra, 'Hackers Target California University Leading COVID Research,' *Bloomberg*, 4 June 2020, available at https://www.bloomberg.com/news/articles/2020-06-04/hackers-target-california-university-leading-covid-19-research accessed on 15 June 2020.
59. Dave Makichuk, 'China Trying to Steal Vaccine Research: Trump adviser," *Asia Times*, 26 May 2020, available at https://asiatimes.com/2020/05/trump-advisor-accuses-china-of-trying-to-steal-vaccine-research/, accessed on 28 May 2020.
60. Andrew Russell, 'Canadian COVID-19 Research Faces 'Elevated' Foreign Threat of Hacking, Spy Agencies Warn,' *Global News*, available at https://globalnews.ca/news/6947990/canadian-covid-19-research-foreign-spy-threats/, accessed on 28 May 2020.
61. Vanshika Malhotra, 'Say Namaste: Indian Video Calling App to Take on Zoom, Google Meet now on Android, iOS,' *India TV*, 11 June 2020, available at https://www.indiatvnews.com/technology/apps-say-namaste-indian-zoom-rival-video-calling-app-how-to-use-how-to-download-on-android-ios-625352, accessed on 22 June 2020.

62. Charlie Osborne, 'Zoom security: Your Meetings will be Safe and Secure if you do these 10 Things,' *ZDNet*, 22 April 2020, available at https://www.zdnet.com/article/make-sure-your-zoom-meetings-are-safe-by-doing-these-10-things/, accessed on 1 June 2020.
63. Ibid.
64. Adrian Kingsley-Hughes, 'How to Prevent your Zoom Meetings being Zoom-bombed (gate-crashed) by Trolls,' *ZDNet*, 23 March 2020, available at https://www.zdnet.com/article/how-to-prevent-your-zoom-meetings-being-zoom-bombed-gate-crashed-by-trolls/, accessed on 1 June 2020.
65. Microgrids is a group of interconnected loads and distributed energy resources within clearly defined electrical boundaries that acts as a single controllable entity with respect to the grid.
66. Elisa Wood, 'Could COVID-19 Give Rise to the Home Microgrid?' *Microgrid Knowledge*, 24 March 2020, available at https://microgridknowledge.com/residential-microgrids-covid19/ accessed on 15 June 2020.
67. Johns Hopkins Bloomberg School of Public Health, Centre for Health Security, available at https://www.centerforhealthsecurity.org/our-work/exercises/ accessed on 15 June 2020.

18

The Role of Biotechnology During Pandemics: The Case of COVID-19

Ronnie Ninan

The 21st century has recorded two highly pathogenic human coronaviruses (HCoVs), the severe acute respiratory syndrome coronavirus (SARS-CoV) in 2003, and the Middle East respiratory syndrome coronavirus (MERS-CoV) in 2012. These HCoVs, emerging from animal reservoirs, has infected people worldwide, reaching epidemic status. However, a novel HCoV was identified at the end of 2019, originating from Wuhan in China. The new HCoV is the third documented instance of an animal coronavirus spreading to humans in the last two decades and has been named coronavirus disease 19 (COVID-19) by the Coronaviridae Study Group (CSG) of the International Committee on Taxonomy of Viruses (ICTV).[1] Identifying the close similarities with the SARS-CoV, the new virus was named severe acute respiratory syndrome coronavirus 2 (SARS-CoV-2). The Director-General of the World Health Organization (WHO), Dr Tedros Adhanom Ghebreyesus, on 11 March 2020, characterized COVID-19 as a global pandemic, citing the spread of the novel virus enveloping more than 114 countries, with 18,000 confirmed cases, and more than 4000 deaths.[2] Although HCoV causing pandemics are not comparable to the death toll of other viral diseases such as the human immunodeficiency virus (HIV), which claimed close to 770,000 people in 2018,[3] or the influenza virus that kills close to 389,000 people each year,[4] the HCoV diseases such as the SARS outbreak of 2003 and MERS epidemic of 2012, and the ongoing COVID-19 pandemic has uncorked the demand for efficient medical products, faster detection techniques, and rigorous standards for the global health community.

Ever since a vaccine was developed to treat smallpox by Edward Jenner in 1796,[5] humanity has witnessed various advancements and additions in biotechnology. However, it is not restricted to vaccines or drugs in treating diseases but spreads across multiple domains including agriculture, marine life, chemical production, and healthcare. This chapter examines the threat posed by pandemics, especially viral outbreaks caused by coronaviruses, and focusses on the role played by biotechnology, specifically, medical biotechnology.

Biotechnology: An Overview

Biotechnology refers to the utilization of biological processes by the engineering of biological systems to augment human lives. The Organisation for Economic Co-operation and Development (OECD) defines biotechnology[6] as:

> "the application of science and technology to living organisms, as well as parts, products, and models thereof, to alter living or non-living materials for the production of knowledge, goods, and services."

It has matured into a profoundly essential aspect of human lives, in more ways than we realize. The field of biotechnology unites biochemistry, microbiology, and engineering[7] for the development and application with the goal of improving agriculture, food processing, waste treatment, and most importantly, medical technology.

Biotechnology: History and Evolution

The history of biotechnology begins with the Hungarian agricultural economist and engineer, Karl Erkey, who coined the term biotechnology in 1919.[8] However, the applications of biotechnology were recognized and practiced long before it got its title. During the initial years, biotechnology referred to the use of living organisms in producing new products from the raw materials of biological origins. The metamorphosis of biotechnology can be divided into three stages, which are ancient biotechnology, classical biotechnology, and modern biotechnology. [9]

Since prehistoric times, the ancient civilizations of Indus Valley and Egypt engaged in the domestication of animals along with the selection of plants to assure better yielding of crops and enhanced disease resistance.[10] Ancient biotechnology dating back between 5000 B.C. and 10,000 B.C., employed various methods of vegetation and breeding to produce specific plants.[11] The use of microorganisms to produce wine, cheese, and bread was a prevailing practice during this period.[12] Through the process of trial and error, this period fostered the future evolution of biotechnology.

The following period referred to as classical biotechnology, was characterized by various augmentations to the progress observed during ancient biotechnology.[13] Among these was the technology of fermentation, which played a significant part in stimulating industrial production of antibiotics, enzymes, and other organic acids such as citric acids, amino acids, vinegar, among others.[14] Moreover, this period witnessed the production of synthetic vitamins.[15] The French chemist Louis Pasteur studied the effect of yeast in the process of fermentation, during this period, investigating the ability of microorganisms to convert sugars, such as glucose, into alcohol like ethanol.[16] This period has marked the works of geneticists such as Gregor Johann Mendel, whose work on the basic principles of heredity revolutionized the field and prefaced controlled experiments on plant-breeding.[17]

Modern biotechnology arose with the discovery of DNA. The technique of recombinant DNA (rDNA) transformed the face of biotechnology, guiding it into the new era. [18] rDNA are DNA molecules created with two or more sources through genetic recombination methods like cloning, to form novel synthetic molecules. Another technique developed in this period is hybridoma technology,[19] which are hybrid cells with cells producing antibodies aimed against antigens. These innovative advancements in biotechnology generated a fresh wave in numerous sectors with industrial applications, such as biopharmaceuticals, virology, cancer, and parasitology. The period also marked the first cloned animal, a sheep named Dolly, in 1996;[20] the successful sequencing of the human genome in 2003;[21] and the rise of new techniques in vaccine and drug development. The principal driver of this evolution in biotechnology was the scientific progress witnessed during these periods.

Types of Biotechnology

The numerous fields of biotechnology can be broadly categorized into four domains namely green biotechnology, white biotechnology, blue biotechnology, and red biotechnology.[22]

Green biotechnology: Green biotechnology applies to the utilization of biotechnology in agriculture and is viewed as the next phase of the green revolution.[23] It focuses on diverse applications of genetic engineering, through the selection of designed traits, in plants and animals. This domain examines the evolution of disease resistance in animals and pest resistance in grains. Therefore, it incorporates plant biotechnology and animal biotechnology, under a unified umbrella.[24]

White biotechnology: White biotechnology, also termed as grey biotechnology, applies to the uses of biotechnology in industries associated with the processing and production of intermediate and final products from renewable materials, such as yeast, bacteria, and plants. These living cells would aid in synthesizing degradable products.[25] It also involves the creation and development of safer and renewable fuels for vehicles, assisting in the advancement of cleaner forms of energy, thereby reducing the strain on the environment. [26]

Blue biotechnology: Blue biotechnology, also referred to as marine biotechnology, applies to the application of technology in harnessing fresh and marine water resources.[27] The field of marine biotechnology has applications in the field of medicine, healthcare, cosmetics, and food supplements, among others.[28]

Red biotechnology: Red biotechnology, or medical biotechnology, refers to the appropriation of microorganisms in combating, diagnosing, and producing novel drugs to battle diseases. [29] The field also employs stem cells in the regeneration and replacement of injured tissues.[30] A celebrated footprint in the evolutionary chronicle of medical biotechnology is the Human Genome Project, launched in 1990, to sequence human DNA and witnessed its fruition in 2003.[31] The field of red biotechnology remains crucial, particularly in developing and producing drugs and vaccines to fight pandemics such as SARS, MERS, and the COVID-19. However, we need to take a closer look at pandemics, to understand the importance of medical biotechnology, in curtailing the consequences of diseases.

Origin and Threat of Pandemics

Pandemics are outbreaks of infectious diseases on large-scale, crossing international borders, with heightened mortality rates, leading to widespread disruptions in the social, economic, and political spheres.[32] Commonly, pandemics originate through zoonotic transmissions, where a pathogen transmission occurs from an animal reservoir to humans.[33] Zoonoses find their way from domestic, as well as wildlife animals, to humans.[34,35] These reservoirs, for the pathogen to skip into the human population, may arise due to hunting of wild species, its consumption, trade of wild animals, among other forms of contact with the wildlife.[36,37] Bats act as natural reservoir hosts of numerous zoonotic viruses such as the Nipah virus. Furthermore, several pieces of research have recognized bats to be the origin and reservoir host of the SARS-CoV.[38,39] Dromedary camels have been identified to be the animal host liable for the MERS-CoV, although its association to bats or other natural reservoirs remain contested.[40] In the case of the SARS-CoV-2, although the intermediate host remains unknown, it displays similarities to the SARS-CoV.[41]

Pandemics and its threats based on pathogens are broadly classified into three groups. The first group includes pathogens such as the influenza virus that may lead to the global transmission of the virus, with a prolonged asymptomatic period for further transmission, without detection. The second group consists of pathogens with a moderate transmission threat, such as the H5N1, H7N9 influenzas, and the Nipah virus. These pathogens do not show sustenance in human-to-human transmission, however, it can transmit efficiently, eyeing the pathogen's mutational and adaptation capacity. The third group of pathogens can cause regional epidemics, however, the chances of spreading to a global pandemic are restricted due to the slow rate of transmission. These pathogens include Ebola, Lassa, and Marburg, among others.[42] Moreover, the likelihood of pandemics will increase manifold in the future, due to the impact of globalization, societal mixtures, and ill-effects of human actions on the environment.[43,44] Humanity has experienced multiple pandemics over the years. These involve the bubonic plague or the black death pandemic of the 1300s, that enveloped Eurasia, with a high mortality rate of 30-50 percent;[45] the Spanish flu influenza pandemic during the early 1900s, that took the lives of 20 million to 100 million;[46] the Hong Kong flu influenza pandemic in 1968, which witnessed the deaths of about 1 million people;[47] the HIV/AIDS pandemic which continues to plague human lives;[48] and the swine flu influenza pandemic originating in the early 2000s, that claimed the lives of around 150,000 to 575,000 people worldwide.[49] The chapter will examine viral outbreaks caused by coronaviruses such as the SARS pandemic, MERS epidemic, and the ongoing COVID-19 pandemic, in the following sections.

A Brief Look at Coronavirus

Coronaviruses are the largest group of viruses that belong to the order of *Nidovirales* comprising of *Coronaviridae*, *Roniviridae*, *Arteriviridae*, and *Mesoniviridae* families.[50] The *Coronavirinae* are divided into four genera, which include α-coronavirus (alphaCoV), β-coronavirus (betaCoV), γ-coronavirus (gammaCoV), and δ-coronavirus (deltaCoV).[51,52]

Coronaviruses are enveloped pleomorphic viruses without significant symmetry, during the formation of the infectious particle. These viruses assume a broad spectrum of shapes, sizes, and compositions, varying from particle to particle, making each virion unique. The viral membrane of the coronavirus consists of the transmembrane glycoprotein (M), spike glycoprotein (S), and the envelope protein

(E). These viruses are RNA viruses, with a crown-like appearance because of glycoprotein spikes on its envelope.[53] Other examples of pleomorphic viruses include retroviruses such as HIV, paramyxoviruses such as measles, and orthomyxoviruses such as influenza.[54] Coronaviruses have been identified in several mammals including camels, mice, dogs, cats, and some avian hosts.[55] Previously, six HCoVs were recognized,[56] which are HCoV-NL63[57] and HCoV-229E,[58] belonging to the alphaCoV genus, and HCoV-HKU1,[59] HCoV-OC43 (OC43, known to cause the common cold[60]), SARS-CoV, and MERS-CoV, belonging to the betaCoV genus. The four HCoVs (229E, NL63, HKU1, and OC43) are endemic (restricted geographically and found regularly). They account for 10 percent to 30 percent of infections in the upper respiratory tract among adults.[61] Identifying the similarities of COVID-19 causing SARS-CoV-2 and SARS-CoV, the SARS-CoV-2 is classified as betaCoV.[62,63] The SARS-CoV and MERS-CoV were the two leading causes of severe cases of pneumonia in humans, and the SARS-CoV-2 has joined the list, accompanying its forerunners.

Fighting Pandemics using Medical (Red) Biotechnology: Drug and Vaccine Development

Within the realm of healthcare, the advancements in biotechnology have assisted in the development of vaccines and drug delivery. In the last few decades, we have seen many examples of pandemics enveloping the globe, followed by the race to produce vaccines and drugs, that may help in restricting the ill-effects of the outbreak across international boundaries. In this section, we will examine the stages of drug and vaccine development and production.

Drug Discovery and Development

The drug discovery stage covers three well-defined phases: target discovery, lead discovery and lead optimization.[64] These phases intend to discover a scientific link between the biological target, which can be proteins or nucleic acids, and the disease state model mimicking the pathological process in humans.[65] The target progression and validation process are required to select the drug target using known compounds. However, in the lead discovery and lead optimization phases, new compounds are identified. The lead optimization phase identifies a single compound for the drug development stage. Clinical trials have distinct phases to develop the final product. Phase I centres around the safety of the potential drug on selected healthy individuals.[66] The pharmacokinetics (movement of drugs in the body) and pharmacodynamics (response of the body to the drug) are observed in this phase. Phase II looks for the desired impact of the drug on a broader set of individuals. Phase II is further subdivided into Phase IIA, determining the dosage required for the desired therapeutic impact, and Phase IIB examines the potential drug based on its efficacy on the target population. Phase III is a randomized test on a larger group of individuals to ascertain the efficacy of the drug after Phase II. After the progress observed in Phase III, the drug is reviewed by the appropriate regulatory authority. Phase IV is the post-marketing surveillance of the drug[67], approved by the regulatory authority for production and marketing in case of rare adverse effects detected in larger populations during Phase III of clinical trials.[68,69] The discovery and development of drugs from the stage of target identification to its approval from regulatory authorities and marketing require approximately twelve years to complete,[70] with an estimated cost of 2.6 billion USD.[71]

Vaccines Simplified

The innate immunity acts as the first line of defence against unknown pathogens entering a living body. Vaccines function as an initiator of the innate immunity, replicating the form of natural infections, against the immune system.[72] This adaptive immunity, the second line of defence against pathogens,[73] is activated by an antigen in the vaccine stimulating subsets of the T lymphocytes and B lymphocytes, to produce specific antibodies killing the target cells. Thus, cell-mediated immunity aids in stopping attacks of an unknown pathogen entering the body, thereby commanding the immune system.[74]

Stages of Vaccine Development: There are five stages in the developmental cycle of a vaccine.[75,76,77,78] They are exploratory stage, pre-clinical stage, clinical development stage, regulatory review and approval stage, manufacturing stage, and quality control stage. Following the multiple steps can take approximately ten years, in developing a vaccine.[79]

The exploratory stage (discovery) is the research-intensive phase in vaccine development. It involves the target selection of natural or synthetic antigens, its findings, optimization of the data gathered on the antigen, and profiling of the antigen which include weakened strains of the virus.[80] The exploratory or discovery stage takes between two to five years, with upwards of a hundred candidate vaccines.[81,82] The second stage is the pre-clinical stage. This stage conducts research using cell-culture or tissue-culture, accompanied by trials on animals, to ascertain the immunity and safety offered by the candidate vaccine, known as immunogenicity. Along with immunogenicity, the toxicology of the candidate vaccine is tested to avoid harm on test subjects.[83] The pre-clinical stage generally needs at least two years for completion.[84] The following stage begins the clinical development of the vaccine. Being the most crucial stage in vaccine development is divided into different phases during the clinical trial of the vaccine. The clinical development stage comprising of three phases needs five to nine years, to finalize one potential vaccine candidate.[85,86] Phase I evaluates the reactogenicity and safety of human trials.[87] These trials are designed to be placebo-controlled, double-blind, and arbitrary. The safety and dosage range is ascertained in this phase, providing an optimal immune response. This phase intends to assess the safety of the candidate vaccine and the effects of the vaccine, identifying the immune responses.[88] Phase II centres around the immunogenicity of the components in the candidate vaccine.[89] This step ensures the vaccine's safety, the optimal dosage, and the schedule of the vaccine.[90] Therefore, the phase is divided into two, Phase IIA and Phase IIB. The efficacy of the vaccine, along with the number of doses, the interval between each dose, and the mode of delivery is examined.[91] Phase III is the final step in the clinical trial of the vaccine, before entering the regulatory review and approval stage.[92] This phase concentrates on the safety of the vaccine and its efficacy on a larger group of individuals.[93] During the regulatory review and approval stage, the vaccine is reviewed by a regulating authority for further approval. The regulatory review and approval stage requires two years, before entering the manufacturing and quality control stage.[94] The last stage before mass usage is the manufacturing and quality control stage. The drug manufacturers support in rendering necessary infrastructure, equipment, and personnel for mass production of the vaccine. It is necessary for the stakeholders involved in the cycle of vaccine development to adhere to adequate quality measures and reviewed for the performance, safety, and effectiveness of the vaccine.[95]

Drug Repurposing

To tackle the hurdles of high development costs and the lengthy-time required to develop novel drugs, the process of drug repurposing (also known as drug repositioning) is executed, especially when the demand for a drug is immediate.[96] There are numerous cases of drugs that were repurposed to serve the treatment requirements to suffice an immediate threat.[97] The Ebola epidemic witnessed the drug, sofosbuvir, which is commonly used in treating hepatitis C infection, being repurposed as a potential drug to fight the Ebola virus.[98] Favipiravir, an antiviral drug developed to treat the influenza virus, was a potential choice in treating the Zika virus.[99] Drug repurposing recognizes supplementary applications, outside the scope of licensed drugs or that are in the developmental stage. Amid a pandemic, when the demand for a drug is immediate, the application of drug repurposing serves as an assuring alternative to developing a wholly novel drug to fight the disease.

Other Applications of Medical Biotechnology

Reverse Transcription-polymerase Chain Reaction

Polymerase chain reaction (PCR) which is regarded as the gold standard[100] in the detection and diagnostics of diseases, was invented by Kary Mullis, an American biochemist in 1984.[101] Considered to be a revolutionary technology, the advancements in PCR led to the introduction of reverse transcription-polymerase chain reaction (RT-PCR). RT-PCR is an addition to the tool kit afforded by PCR, with reverse transcription of RNA to DNA in RT-PCT. This step provides for the amplification of DNA that is transcribed from RNA, especially in the case of pathogen strains that only contains RNA, but not DNA.[102] Since the early days of PCR, it has helped detect tuberculosis,[103] and chlamydia.[104] PCR has been upheld by infectious disease experts, due to the sensitivity of the technology, its specificity, and the speed with which it can amplify the nucleic acid, detecting the presence of a pathogen.[105,106] RT-PCR has been beneficial in the quick testing capability during outbreaks, such as Zika,[107] Ebola,[108] African swine fever,[109] MERS,[110] and several other diseases.[111]

Gene Editing using CRISPR

CRISPR-Cas (Clustered Regularly Interspaced Short Palindromic Repeats-CRISPR associated) is the tool to edit genomes, allowing researchers to modify the DNA sequences and alter the function of genes.[112] The CRISPR-Cas system is broadly categorized into two classes, Class 1 and Class 2. They are further subdivided, depending on the protein (e.g.: Cas9, Cas12, etc.) attached to it that would cut foreign DNA, into six variants (Type I, II, III, IV, V, and VI).[113] The most comprehensively developed and studied gene-editing tools within these variants are the CRISPR-Cas9 (Type II) and CRISPR-Cas12 (Type V) systems.[114,115] The applications of gene-editing range from reducing genetic problems like deafness in mice,[116] the treatment of sickle-cell anaemia,[117] and gene drives that could assist in managing the large-scale transmission of diseases, such as malaria.[118] Several researchers are applying gene editing applications using CRISPR-Cas to limit the spread of pandemics such as COVID-19.

Convalescent Plasma Therapy

Convalescent plasma therapy is a method of passive immunization antibody therapy.[119] Passive immunization is used to prevent and control the spread of a disease applying the concept of artificially acquired passive immunity. The treatment method dates back to the 20th century, for which the German physiologist, Emil von Behring, received the Nobel Prize in 1901 for physiology and medicine, acknowledging his work on the plasma in treating diphtheria.[120] The fundamental component of plasma in treatment are the antibodies produced by the immune system to fight the invading pathogen. The plasma of a recovered patient can be administered to other recipients and stimulate antibody production in their body to fight the specific pathogen.[121] Over the years, and witnessing a handful of outbreaks, such as SARS in 2003,[122] and Ebola in 2013,[123] convalescent plasma therapy has been used in trials, to encouraging results. The development of convalescent plasma therapy remains a viable option for treatment until vaccines of specific pathogens are developed.

Role Played by Biotechnology during SARS and MERS

The SARS outbreak of 2002 was the first recorded instance of a coronavirus reaching epidemic status, threatening the global health landscape, compelling researchers across the world, to work on vaccines and drugs to limit the spread of the disease. Most of the vaccines developed during the SARS epidemic were sub-unit vaccines (contains select antigen fragments of a pathogen)[124] targeting the S glycoprotein, recognizing the SARS-CoV uses this glycoprotein to bind and access the host cell. The pre-clinical stage, studies were conducted to develop live-attenuated vaccines (contains selectively weakened less virulent pathogens, mimicking the disease mildly),[125] inactivated vaccines (contains inactivated pathogens with retained immunogenicity), recombinant viral vector vaccines (includes live replicating viruses carrying extra genes from a specific pathogen),[126] and DNA vaccines.[127] The S protein of SARS-CoV binds with angiotensin-converting enzyme 2 (ACE2) receptor, a protein that facilitates the virus to bind with human cells.[128] Therefore, the candidate vaccines were based on the S glycoprotein, binding to the ACE2 receptor. Within the landscape of developing vaccines, inactivated, and DNA vaccines reached Phase I of the clinical trials. However, there are no commercially available vaccines for the SARS-CoV. The use of Ribavirin, an antiviral drug used in the treatment of Hepatitis C, was repurposed during the SARS outbreak,[129,130] demonstrating the role played by drugs in treating the disease.

Researchers around the world actively strived to develop a vaccine for the MERS-CoV, since its emergence in 2012. The vaccines that were in development to tackle the MERS epidemic were sub-unit vaccines based on the S glycoprotein of the virus, that binds on the Dipeptidyl-Peptidase 4 (DPP4) (protein) receptor present on macrophages (part of the white blood cells).[131] Alternatively, there were attempts to develop vaccines based on live attenuated viruses, recombinant viral vectors, and inactivated viruses.[132] However, the vaccines that entered Phase I of clinical trials were DNA-based vaccines.[133] Despite the concerted efforts to develop a vaccine to tackle the MERS-CoV, there are no commercial vaccines accessible for the MERS-CoV. There were attempts to repurpose drugs, such as Lopinavir,[134] an antiretroviral used in HIV treatment, that showed promising results against the MERS-CoV.[135] Another proposed treatment method to tackle the MERS outbreak was convalescent plasma therapy, revealed to be a likely therapeutic method to neutralize the MERS-CoV.[136] The research and advancements made in medical biotechnology during the SARS and MERS outbreaks have contributed a great deal in easing and advancing treatment methods, dissipating the effects of COVID-19.

COVID-19 and the Treatment Landscape Afforded by Biotechnology

During the tail-end of 2019, the world witnessed a highly pathogenic HCoV, emerging from Wuhan in China. The virus named SARS-CoV-2, brought with it COVID-19, sweeping the globe. Diverse strategies are in place, around the world, to develop a vaccine and drug to tackle COVID-19, which targets the S glycoprotein of the virus, as the SARS-CoV-2 shares genetic similarity to SARS-CoV, which binds to ACE2 receptor. Therefore, vaccines are being developed that would exhibit cross-reactivity.[137] Countries around the world have stepped up their efforts to develop vaccines, drugs, and additional treatment techniques to tackle COVID-19.

The US initiatives in the field of biotechnology have earned them a prominent position in the biotechnology industry. COVID-19, like other countries, has swept the US, and in search of a cure, the National Institutes of Health (NIH) entered clinical trials by developing an experimental vaccine. The vaccine called mRNA-1273 is being developed by the National Institute of Allergy and Infectious Diseases (NIAID) in collaboration with the biotechnology company, Moderna Inc.[138] Another candidate vaccine being developed by the NIAID is a sub-unit vaccine, in collaboration with Medigen Vaccine Biologics Corporation and Dynavax, which is in the pre-clinical stage.[139] A DNA-based vaccine, developed by an American biotechnology company, Inovio Pharmaceuticals, called INO-4800, has reached the clinical trial stage.[140] DNA vaccines help in producing therapeutic antibodies, thereby activating immune cells of the patient.[141] In terms of drug development, the U.S. Food and Drug Administration (FDA) has approved the use of the antiviral drug Remdesivir, previously explored to treat Ebola, MERS, and SARS patients,[142] as a potential treatment for COVID-19 patients.[143]

The National Health Commission of the People's Republic of China has devised a few strategies to tackle and curb the spread of COVID-19. These include the repurposing of anti-viral drugs citing the encouraging result in the early stages of animal testing. These anti-viral drugs include lopinavir/ritonavir, a combination of fixed-doses used as a medication to treat and prevent HIV/AIDS.[144] Ribavirin is another antiviral medication, that has been repurposed, generally used in the treatment of RSV (Respiratory Syncytial Virus) infection and hepatitis C, currently tested to treat COVID-19 patients.[145] Early testing of hydroxychloroquine and chloroquine, an anti-malarial medication, by the NHC, saw positive responses.[146,147] The draft landscape of vaccine development by the WHO, as of 18 June 2020, recognizes a few vaccines developed by China, which includes inactivated vaccines and viral vector vaccines.[148]

The European Commission, the executive arm of the European Union (EU), has been at the forefront of developing a vaccine for COVID-19. The Commission also called on global cooperation in the endeavour of finding a potential vaccine to avoid harmful competition in the global race trying to reach the finish line.[149] The EU has also earmarked 2.3 billion USD to fight the common cause.[150] The European Commission has offered financial support to CureVac, a biopharmaceutical company based in Germany, which is developing an mRNA vaccine, that has shown positive results in the pre-clinical trials.[151] Many EU countries (France, Germany, Italy, and the Netherlands) have also collaborated with AstraZeneca (developed by the University of Oxford), in the development of a vaccine that has entered Phase II of clinical trials.[152] To ensure quicker detection of the virus, BforCure, a biotechnology company based in France, has received a financial grant of close to 2 million USD, to develop swifter detection using RT-PCR technology.[153] Another addition to the rapid detection realm is the RT-LAMP technology, which is a variation of the RT-PCR, called CORONADX, and funded by the EU.[154]

India, known as the "world's pharmacy",[155] has created a stronghold in the field of biotechnology. As the threat posed by COVID-19 keeps intensifying around the world, researchers in India have initiated several steps to tackle the viral disease. These include efficient detection methods, development of vaccines, and drug development. The Regional Centre for Biotechnology (RCB) has collaborated with biotechnology companies, such as Bioheaven and InnoDx, to develop efficient and quicker COVID-19 detection kits based on the RT-PCR technique.[156] The vaccine development landscape in India looks promising. Zydus Cadila, an Indian pharmaceutical company, has been developing a DNA-based and viral vector vaccine, both of which are currently, in the pre-clinical stage.[157] A fully indigenous vaccine is in development, by Indian Council for Medical Research (ICMR) in collaboration with Bharat Biotech International Ltd (BBIL).[158] An international collaboration between the University of Wisconsin–Madison, FluGen, and BBIL, to develop a nasal vaccine called CoroFlu, which will be built on the backbone of a candidate flu vaccine called M2SR, with immunity against the influenza virus as well.[159] Drug development in India has also seen an impressive push, after the COVID-19 outbreak. Through drug repurposing, Favipiravir, an antiviral drug used in treating influenza, has been launched by Glenmark Pharmaceuticals under the name FabiFlu, after it received approval from the Drug Controller General of India (DCGI).[160]

Considering the global race to find a vaccine or drug that could be a potential treatment method for COVID-19, various advancements in medical biotechnology has been put to use to find other treatment methods. These methods include convalescent plasma therapy, which has shown effective results, especially in many severe cases.[161] The plasma therapy treatment would be advantageous in creating adequate buffer time until a commercial vaccine or drug is developed. The gene-editing tool, CRISPR-Cas12, has proven helpful in identifying the SARS-CoV-2 from extracted RNA samples. A novel advancement in CRISPR technology termed as SARS-CoV-2 DETECTR (DNA Endonuclease-Targeted CRISPR Trans Reporter), is regarded to be a quicker alternative to the RT-PCR, which is the most widely adopted technique to detect viruses.[162] The myriad of advancements in medical biotechnology, through the years, has proven to have a positive impact on global health security, especially in developing vaccines, designing new drugs, and the early detection of viruses, that remains helpful in tackling pandemics.

We have examined the advantages of applying medical biotechnology in addressing the issues posed by pandemics. However, the biotechnology industry faces a few challenges, which have been discussed further in this chapter.

Challenges Facing Biotechnology

Dual-use Dilemma

Biotechnology can be a double-edged sword when we parse the 'dual-use' dilemma. There is a need to evaluate the purpose of advancing biotechnology for the benefit of humanity, while promptly preventing the development of biological weapons used in bioterrorism, biowarfare, and bio-crimes. The Convention on the

Prohibition of the Development, Production and Stockpiling of Bacteriological and Toxin Weapons and their Destruction (BTWC) necessitates the ban on the development of biological weapons, though, permitting States to continue their activities on prophylactic biodefense, which remains questionable.[163] There have been several instances when States used bioweapons, threatening the positive development in biotechnology, such as South Africa,[164] Iraq,[165] and Syria.[166] Moreover, even terrorist organizations such as the Islamic State appropriated the possibilities of biotechnology to wage bioterrorism, exposing the capability of non-state actors to manipulate the technology.[167] Acknowledging advancements of biotechnology such as the CRISPR gene-editing tools enables the creation of designer bioweapons, which are much deadlier, using modified novel pathogens with higher pathogenicity and severity.[168] The potential of dual-use in biotechnology remains a challenge that needs to be addressed by the global community.

Lack of Time for Development Coupled with Rush for Monetization

Almost always, a pandemic that sweeps across national boundaries, force researchers to scramble for a vaccine or drug to curb the virus from spreading, although, the virus becomes the cash cow during this period. Assuming short term profits, a myriad of biotechnology firms would jump the gun, introducing or repurposing drugs, with inadequate clinical data on the virus.[169] The time required, from the development stage to the marketing stage of a vaccine, would on average demand ten years,[170] though the frenzy to develop a vaccine aggrandizes during a pandemic.[171] The race to develop the vaccine can be credited to the ever-rising cost (estimates between 200-million USD to 900-million USD) in research and development of the vaccine,[172] numerous technical hurdles, and biological challenges of obtaining a potential vaccine. Added to the fight against complex diseases, is the requirement of safety and efficacy through larger-scale clinical studies and the stringent regulatory environment.[173,174] It leads to the challenge of developing a quicker or precise vaccine.

Patent Regimes and Export Control

Researchers in the field of biotechnology face numerous challenges when they attempt to commercialize their research and patented products. Moreover, the lack of relevant amendments in the Patent Cooperation Treaty (PCT) International Application, researchers are required to tie-up with third-party firms, transferring their patented invention. Besides, when researchers conduct supplementary research on the same topic they are compelled to share intellectual property rights of their findings, attaching it to the original invention. These difficulties restrict the likelihood of prospective research on the topic.[175] Even the stakeholders encounter compliance-related challenges due to differing export control norms, globally. The dual-use dilemma misconstrues technologies as either being legitimate or prohibited, like the DNA synthesizers (used to assemble DNA) or equipment to store or grow pathogens, which can also be considered as a threat to the national security of a country.[176] Depending on the usage, which can vary, the control regimes remain ineffective in differentiating technologies. The dearth of awareness and diverging interpretations of norms in each regime add to the challenges facing advancements in biotechnology.[177]

The Way Forward

Since the beginning of the century, the world has witnessed three viral outbreaks caused by coronaviruses, the SARS-CoV in 2002, MERS-CoV in 2012, and the most recent, SARS-CoV-2 in 2019. At every instance, the global health community has joined arms in finding a cure for these outbreaks. Biotechnology, a term coined in the early 20th century, has become an indispensable part of human lives, covering fields such as food processing, agriculture, industrial chemicals, marine life, and medical technology. It is playing a critical role in advancing the frontiers of science, especially in the field of medicine and healthcare. The widespread panic caused by COVID-19 has driven many countries and international organizations to come forward with techniques of modern biotechnology to curb the spread of the SARS-CoV-2. Medical biotechnology has advanced through the years, most importantly, during a time of crisis such as pandemics. Ranging from advancements in vaccine and drug development, detection mechanisms afforded by RT-PCR, disease immunity using convalescent plasma therapies, to novel technologies like CRISPR-Cas for gene editing and quicker detection of pathogens, the world has seen the strides achieved in the field of medical biotechnology.

On 29 May 2020, the President of the United States, Donald John Trump, in the Rose Garden of the White House, announced the termination of ties between the United States and the WHO, during a press briefing.[178] The decision to discontinue relations would halt the US funds supporting WHO, the specialized agency of the United Nations, playing a crucial role during the COVID-19 pandemic. However, the chief scientist, and the Deputy Director-General for Programmes at WHO, Dr Soumya Swaminathan, addressed a press briefing from Geneva, discussing the possibilities of developing a vaccine against COVID-19 by the end of 2020.[179] The same optimism was echoed by Dr Anthony Fauci, an esteemed member of the US coronavirus taskforce and the Director of the National

Institute of Allergy and Infectious Diseases, expecting a commercial vaccine against the disease within 12 to 18 months.[180,181] Researchers in the field are striving to crunch the long and arduous process of vaccine and drug development, ordinarily demanding years, to a matter of months.

While countries around the world are following strict lockdown measures to control the spread of the virus, the global health community is striving around the clock to find vaccines, drugs, and alternative treatment mechanisms, to fight COVID-19. The future threat posed by pandemics is not far-fetched and can be a matter of global concern. Nevertheless, with the advancements witnessed in medical biotechnology through the years, there is hope for effective and quicker ways to approach the threat of diseases today, and pandemics of tomorrow.

NOTES

1. Coronaviridae Study Group of the International Committee on Taxonomy of Viruses, 'The species Severe acute respiratory syndrome-related coronavirus: classifying 2019-nCoV and naming it SARS-CoV-2', *Nature microbiology*, Vol. 5, No. 4, 2020, pp. 536–544.
2. World Health Organization, 'WHO Director-General's Opening Remarks at the Media Briefing on COVID-19', 11 March 2020, available at https://www.who.int/dg/speeches/detail/who-director-general-s-opening-remarks-at-the-media-briefing-on-covid-19--11-march-2020, accessed on 6 June 2020.
3. World Health Organization, 'Number of deaths due to HIV/AIDS', 2020, available at https://www.who.int/gho/hiv/epidemic_status/deaths_text/en/, accessed on 3 June 2020.
4. John Paget, Peter Spreeuwenberg, Vivek Charu and et al., 'Global Mortality Associated with Seasonal Influenza Epidemics: New Burden Estimates and Predictors from the GLaMOR Project', *Journal of Global Health*, vol. 9, no. 2, 2019.
5. Alexandra Minna Stern and Howard Markel, 'The History of Vaccines and Immunization: Familiar Patterns, New Challenges', *Health Affairs (Project Hope)*, vol. 24, no. 3, 2005, pp. 611–621.
6. OECD, 'Biotechnology', OECD Factbook 2013: Economic, Environmental and Social Statistics, 2013, available at https://doi.org/10.1787/factbook-2013-63-en, accessed on 3 June 2020.
7. John Desmond Bu'Lock and Bjorn Kristiansen (eds.), *Basic biotechnology*, Academic press, 1987.
8. Robert Bud, 'History of Biotechnology', *Nature*, vol. 337, no. 10, 1989.
9. Ashish Swarup Verma, Shishir Agrahari, Shruti Rastogi et al., 'Biotechnology in the Realm of History,' *Journal of Pharmacy & Bioallied Sciences*, vol. 3, no. 3, 2011, pp. 321–323.
10. Jared Diamond, 'Evolution, Consequences and Future of Plant and Animal Domestication', *Nature*, vol. 418, 2002, pp.700-707.
11. Klaus Buchholz and John Collins, 'The Roots: A Short History of Industrial Microbiology and Biotechnology', *Applied Microbiology and Biotechnology*, vol. 97, no. 9, 2013, pp. 3747–3762.
12. Edwin George, Michael Hall, and Geert-Jan De Klerk (eds.), *Plant Propagation by Tissue Culture*, United Kingdom: Springer, 2008.
13. Icolyn I. Amarakoon, Cindy Leigh C. Hamilton, Sylvia Mitchell et al., 'Technological Applications Using Biological Systems,' *Pharmacognosy: Fundamentals, Applications and Strategies*, 2017, pp. 549-563.

14. B.A. Law, 'Biotechnology in Food Manufacture', *Chem Ind.*, 1994, pp. 502-505.
15. Raymond Zilinskas and Carl Lundin, 'Marine Biotechnology and Developing Countries', *World Bank Discussion Papers*, 1993, p. 6, available at http://documents.worldbank.org/curated/en/737571468740402364/Marine-biotechnology-and-developing-countries, accessed on 10 June 2020.
16. Luisa Alba-Lois and Claudia Segal-Kischinevzky, 'Yeast Fermentation and the Making of Beer and Wine', *Nature Education*, vol.3, no. 9, 2010.
17. Margaret W. Rossiter and Robert Bud, 'The Uses of Life: A History of Biotechnology', *The American Historical Review*, vol. 99, 1994, pp. 1642-1643.
18. See note 13.
19. N.R. Ling, 'Properties of the Monoclonal Antibodies Produced by Hybridoma Technology and their Application to the Study of Diseases', *Immunology*, vol. 49, no. 1, 1983, pp. 202–203.
20. Karen Weintraub, '20 Years after Dolly the Sheep Led the Way-Where Is Cloning Now?', *Scientific American*, 5 July 2016, available at https://www.scientificamerican.com/article/20-years-after-dolly-the-sheep-led-the-way-where-is-cloning-now/, accessed on 6 June 2020.
21. Heidi Chial, 'DNA sequencing technologies key to the Human Genome Project' *Nature Education*, vol. 1, no.1, 2008, pp. 219.
22. Saurabh Bhatia, 'History, Scope and Development of Biotechnology', *Introduction to Pharmaceutical Biotechnology*, vol. 1. 2018, pp 1-5.
23. Kevan M.A. Gartland and Jill S. Gartland, 'Contributions of Biotechnology to Meeting Future Food and Environmental Security Needs', *The EuroBiotech Journal*, vol. 2, no. 1, 2018, pp. 2-9.
24. See note 13.
25. Giovanni Frazzetto, 'White biotechnology', *EMBO reports*, vol. 4, no. 9, 2003, pp. 835–837.
26. See note 13.
27. Foresight Marine Panel, 'A Study into the Prospects for Marine Biotechnology Development in the United Kingdom', vol. 2, 2005, available at https://www.biobridge.co.uk/ClientArea/files/Publications/MARINE%20BIOTECHNOLOGY%20DEVELOPMENT%20in%20UK%20M%20Lloyd-Evans%20Jan%202005%20Vol%202.pdf,, accessed on 7 June 2020.
28. See note 13.
29. Edgar J. DaSilva, 'The Colours of Biotechnology: Science, Development and Humankind', *Electronic Journal of Biotechnology*, vol. 7, no. 3, 2004, pp. 1-2.
30. Ajit Kumar Saxena, Divya Singh, and Jyoti Gupta, 'Role of Stem Cell Research in Therapeutic Purpose: A Hope for New Horizon in Medical Biotechnology', *Journal of Experimental Therapeutics & Oncology*, vol. 8, no. 3, 2010, pp. 223–233.
31. Leroy Hood and Lee Rowen, 'The Human Genome Project: Big Science Transforms Biology and Medicine', *Genome Medicine*, vol. 5, no. 9, 2013.
32. Stephen S. Morse, 'Factors in the Emergence of Infectious Diseases', *Emerging Infectious Diseases*, vol. 1, no. 11, 1995, pp. 7-15.
33. F.A. Murphy, 'Emerging Zoonoses', *Emerging Infectious Diseases*, vol. 4, no.3, 1998, pp. 429–435.
34. Mark E.J. Woolhouse and Sonya Gowtage-Sequeria, 'Host Range and Emerging and Re-emerging Pathogens', *Emerging Infectious Diseases*, vol. 11, no. 12, 2005, pp. 1842–1847.
35. Nita Madhav, Ben Oppenheim, Mark Gallivan et al., 'Pandemics: Risks, Impacts, and Mitigation', in Dean T. Jamison, Hellen Gelband, Susan Horton, Prabhat Jha, Ramanan Laxminarayan, Charles N Mock, and Rachel Nugent (eds.), *Disease Control Priorities: Improving Health and*

Reducing Poverty, 3rd edition, 2017, Washington DC: The International Bank for Reconstruction and Development/The World Bank.

36. James M. Hughes, Mary E. Wilson, Brian L. Pike et al., 'The Origin and Prevention of Pandemics', *Clinical Infectious Diseases*, vol. 50, no. 12, 2010, pp. 1636–1640.
37. Nathan D. Wolfe, Claire Panosian Dunavan, and Jared Diamond, 'Origins of Major Human Infectious Diseases', *Nature*, vol. 447, 2007, pp. 279–283.
38. Li W, Shi Z, Yu M, et al., 'Bats are Natural Reservoirs of SARS-like Coronaviruses', *Science*, vol. 310, 2005, pp. 676-679.
39. Shu-ran Gong, and Lin-lin Bao, 'The Battle against SARS and MERS Coronaviruses: Reservoirs and Animal Models', *Animal models and Experimental Medicine*, vol. 1, no. 2, 2018, pp. 125–133.
40. Hamzah A. Mohd, Jaffar A. Al-Tawfiq and Ziad A. Memish, 'Middle East Respiratory Syndrome Coronavirus (MERS-CoV) Origin and Animal Reservoir', *Virology Journal*, vol. 13, no. 87, 2016.
41. Yan-Rong Guo, Qing-Dong Cao, Zhong-Si Hong et al., 'The Origin, Transmission and Clinical Therapies on Coronavirus Disease 2019 (COVID-19) Outbreak - an Update on the Status', *Military Medical Research*, vol. 7, no. 1, 2020.
42. See note 35.
43. Kate E. Jones, Nikkita G. Patel, Marc A. Levy et al., 'Global Trends in Emerging Infectious Diseases', *Nature*, Vol. 451, 2008, pp. 990–993.
44. See note 35.
45. Sharon N. DeWitte, 'Mortality Risk and Survival in the Aftermath of the Medieval Black Death', *PloS one*, vol. 9, no. 5, 2014.
46. Niall P.A. S. Johnson and Juergen Mueller, 'Updating the Accounts: Global Mortality of the 1918-1920 "Spanish" Influenza Pandemic', *Bulletin of the History of Medicine*, vol. 76, no. 1, 2002, pp. 105–115.
47. John D. Mathews, Joanne M. Chesson, James M. McCaw et al., 'Understanding Influenza Transmission, Immunity and Pandemic Threats', *Influenza and other Respiratory Viruses*, vol. 3, no. 4, 2009, pp. 143–149.
48. World Health Organization, 'Number of Deaths due to HIV/AIDS', available at https://www.who.int/gho/hiv/epidemic_status/deaths_text/en/, accessed on 4 June 2020.
49. Fatimah S. Dawood, A. Danielle Iuliano, Carrie Reed et al., 'Estimated Global Mortality Associated with the First 12 Months of 2009 Pandemic Influenza A H1N1 Virus Circulation: A Modelling Study', *The Lancet Infectious Diseases*, vol. 12, no. 9, 2012, pp. 687-695.
50. Anthony R. Fehr and Stanley Perlman, 'Coronaviruses: An Overview of their Replication and Pathogenesis', in Helena Jane Maier, Erica Bickerton and Paul Britton (eds.), *Methods in Molecular Biology*, New York: Springer, 2015, pp. 1–23.
51. Luis P. Villarreal, 'How Viruses Shape the Tree of Life', *Future Virology*, vol. 1, 2006, pp. 587–595.
52. Francesco Di Gennaro, Damiano Pizzol, Claudia Marotta et al., 'Coronavirus Diseases (COVID-19) Current Status and Future Perspectives: A Narrative Review', *International Journal of Environmental Research and Public Health*, vol. 17, no. 8, 2020.
53. Stanley Perlman and Jason Netland, 'Coronaviruses post-SARS: Update on Replication and Pathogenesis', *Nature reviews. Microbiology*, vol. 7, no. 6, 2009, pp. 439–450.
54. Carmen San Martín, 'Structure and Assembly of Complex Viruses', in Mauricio G. Mateu (ed.), *Structure and Physics of Viruses*, Dordrecht: Springer, 2013, pp. 329-360.

55. Roujian Lu, Xiang Zhao, Juan Li et al., 'Genomic Characterisation and Epidemiology of 2019 Novel Coronavirus: Implications for Virus Origins and Receptor Binding', *Lancet*, vol. 395, 2020, pp. 565–574.
56. Zhiqi Song, Yanfeng Xu, Linlinn Bao et al., 'From SARS to MERS, Thrusting Coronaviruses into the Spotlight', *Viruses*, vol. 11, no. 1, 2019, pp. 59.
57. Sahar Abdul-Rasool and Burtram C Fielding, 'Understanding Human Coronavirus HCoV-NL63', *The open Virology Journal*, vol. 4, 2010, pp. 76–84.
58. Sarah L. Warnes, Zoë R. Little and William Keevil, 'Human Coronavirus 229E Remains Infectious on Common Touch Surface Materials', *mBio*, vol. 6, no. 6, 2015.
59. Samuel R. Dominguez, Susmita Shrivastava, Andrew Berglund et al., 'Isolation, Propagation, Genome Analysis and Epidemiology of HKU1 betacoronaviruses', *The Journal of General Virology*, vol. 95, 2014, pp. 836–848.
60. Susanna K.P. Lau, Paul Lee, Alan K.L. Tsang et al., 'Molecular Epidemiology of Human Coronavirus OC43 Reveals Evolution of Different Genotypes Over Time and Recent Emergence of a Novel Genotype due to Natural Recombination', *Journal of Virology*, vol. 85, no. 21, 2011, pp. 11325–11337.
61. Catharine I. Paules, Hilary D. Marston, and Anthony S. Fauci, 'Coronavirus Infections-More Than Just the Common Cold', *JAMA*, vol. 323, no. 8, 2020, pp. 707-708.
62. Jun Zheng, 'SARS-CoV-2: An Emerging Coronavirus that Causes a Global Threat', *International Journal of Biological Sciences*, vol. 16, no. 10, 2020, pp. 1678–1685.
63. Xintian Xu, Ping Chen, Jingfang Wang et al., 'Evolution of the Novel Coronavirus from the Ongoing Wuhan Outbreak and Modelling of its Spike Protein for Risk of Human Transmission', *Science China. Life sciences*, vol. 63, no. 3, 2020, pp. 457–460.
64. Benjamin E. Blass, 'Drug Discovery and Development: An Overview of Modern Methods and Principles', in *Basic Principles of Drug Discovery and Development*, Academic Press, 2015, pp. 1-34.
65. P. Hughes, S. Rees, S.B. Kalindjian and K.L Philpott, 'Principles of Early Drug Discovery', *British Journal of Pharmacology*, vol. 162, no. 6, 2011, pp. 1239–1249.
66. See note 64.
67. See note 64.
68. Ingrid Torjesen, 'Drug Development: The Journey of a Medicine from Lab to Shelf', *The Pharmaceutical Journal*, 12 May 2015, available at https://www.pharmaceutical-journal.com/publications/tomorrows-pharmacist/drug-development-the-journey-of-a-medicine-from-lab-to-shelf/20068196.article, accessed on 4 June 2020.
69. R.G. Hill and H.P. Rang, 'Drug Development: Introduction', in *Drug Discovery and Development*, Churchill Livingstone, 2013, pp. 203-209.
70. J.A. DiMasi, L. Feldman, A. Seckler and A. Wilson, 'Trends in Risks Associated with New Drug Development: Success Rates for Investigational Drugs', *Clinical Pharmacology and Therapeutics*, vol. 87, no. 3, 2010, pp. 272–277.
71. Joseph A. DiMasi, Henry G. Grabowski and Ronald W. Hansen, 'Innovation in the Pharmaceutical Industry: New Estimates of R&D Costs', *Journal of Health Economics*, vol. 47, 2016, pp. 20–33.
72. C.A. Siegrist, 'Vaccine Immunology', *Vaccines*, vol. 5, no. 1, 2008, pp. 17-36.
73. Angela S. Clem, 'Fundamentals of Vaccine Immunology', *Journal of Global Infectious Diseases*, vol. 3, no. 1, 2011, pp. 73–78.
74. Volker Vetter, Gulhan Denizer, Leonard R. Friedland et al., 'Understanding Modern-day

Vaccines: What you Need to Know', *Annals of Medicine*, vol. 50, no. 2, 2018, pp. 110–120.
75. Stanley Plotkin, James M. Robinson, Gerard Cunningham et al., 'The Complexity and Cost of Vaccine Manufacturing - An overview', *Vaccine*, vol. 35, no. 33, 2017, pp. 4064–4071.
76. Centers for Disease Control and Prevention, 'Vaccine Testing and Approval Process', *CDC*, 2020, available from https://www.cdc.gov/vaccines/basics/test-approve.html, accessed on 4 June 2020.
77. International Federation of Pharmaceutical Manufacturers & Associations, 'The Complex Journey of a Vaccine: The Steps Behind Developing a New Vaccine', *IFPMA*, 2020, available at https://www.ifpma.org/wp-content/uploads/2019/07/IFPMA-ComplexJourney-2019_FINAL.pdf, accessed on 6 June 2020.
78. GW Staff, 'Producing Prevention: The Complex Development of Vaccines', *Milken Institute School of Public Health*, 2020, available at https://publichealthonline.gwu.edu/blog/producing-prevention-the-complex-development-of-vaccines/#:~:text=Exploratory%3A%20This%20research%2 Dintensive%20phase,strains%20of%20a%20particular%20virus., accessed on 7 June 2020.
79. Esther S. Pronker, Tamar C. Weenen, Harry Commandeur et al., 'Risk in Vaccine Research and Development Quantified', *PloS one*, vol. 8, no. 3, 2013.
80. See note 77.
81. Douglas Broom, '5 Charts that Tell the Story of Vaccines Today', *World Economic Forum*, 2 June 2020, available at https://www.weforum.org/agenda/2020/06/vaccine-development-barriers-coronavirus/, accessed on 5 June 2020.
82. Stuart A. Thompson, 'How Long will a Vaccine Really Take?', *The New York Times*, 30 April 2020, available at https://www.nytimes.com/interactive/2020/04/30/opinion/coronavirus-covid-vaccine.html, accessed on 2 June 2020.
83. See note 78.
84. See note 81.
85. See note 81.
86. See note 75.
87. Karen B. Goetz, Michael Pfleiderer, and Christian K. Schneider, 'First-in-human Clinical Trials with Vaccines: What Regulators Want', *Nature Biotechnology*, vol. 28, no. 9, 2010, pp. 910–916.
88. Seunghoon Han, 'Clinical Vaccine Development', *Clinical and Experimental Vaccine Research*, vol. 4, no. 1, 2015, pp. 46–53.
89. Ibid.
90. The College of Physicians of Philadelphia, 'Vaccine Development, Testing, and Regulation', 17 January 2018, available at http://www.historyofvaccines.org/content/articles/vaccine-development-testing-and-regulation, accessed on 12 June 2020.
91. Seunghoon Han, 'Clinical Vaccine Development', *Clinical and Experimental Vaccine Research*, vol. 4, no. 1, 2015, pp. 46–53.
92. World Health Organization, 'Guidelines on Clinical Evaluation of Vaccines: Regulatory Expectations', 2003, available at http://www.who.int/biologicals/publications/trs/areas/vaccines/clinical_evaluation/en/, accessed on 12 June 2020.
93. See note 87.
94. See note 81.
95. See note 78.
96. Sudeep Pushpakom, Francesco Iorio, Patrick A. Eyers et al., 'Drug Repurposing: Progress,

Challenges and Recommendations', *Nature Review Drug Discovery*, vol. 18, no. 1, 2019, pp. 41–58.

97. Tudor I. Oprea, Julie E. Bauman, Cristian G.Bologa et al., 'Drug Repurposing from an Academic Perspective', *Drug Discovery Today Therapeutic Strategies*, vol. 8, no. 3-4, 2011, pp. 61–69.
98. Sandra E. Reznik, Amit K. Tiwari and Charles R. Ashby Jr., 'Sofosbuvir: A Potential Treatment for Ebola', *Frontiers in Pharmacology*, vol. 9, 2018, pp. 1139.
99. Camilly P. Pires de Mello, Xun Tao, Tae Hwan Kim et al., 'Clinical Regimens of Favipiravir Inhibit Zika Virus Replication in the Hollow-Fiber Infection Model', *Antimicrobial Agents and Chemotherapy*, vol. 62, no. 9, 2018.
100. Ian M. Mackay, Katherine E. Arden, and Andreas Nitsche, 'Real-time PCR in Virology', *Nucleic Acids Research*, vol. 30, no. 6, 2000, pp. 1292–1305.
101. S.A. Deepak, K.R. Kottapalli, R. Rakwal et al., 'Real-Time PCR: Revolutionizing Detection and Expression Analysis of Genes', *Current Genomics*, vol. 8, no. 4, 2007, pp. 234–251.
102. Nicole Jawerth, 'How is the COVID-19 Virus Detected using Real Time RT-PCR?', *IAEA Office of Public Information and Communication*, 27 March 2020, available at https://www.iaea.org/newscenter/news/how-is-the-covid-19-virus-detected-using-real-time-rt-pcr, accessed on 9 June 2020.
103. R.F. D'Amato, A.A. Wallman, L.H. Hochstein et al., 'Rapid Diagnosis of Pulmonary Tuberculosis by Using Roche AMPLICOR Mycobacterium Tuberculosis PCR test', *Journal of Clinical Microbiology*, vol. 33, no. 7, 1995, pp. 1832–1834.
104. Samuel Yang and Richard E. Rothman, 'PCR-based Diagnostics for Infectious Diseases: Uses, Limitations, and Future Applications in Acute-care Settings', *The Lancet Infectious diseases*, vol. 4, no. 6, 2004, pp. 337–348.
105. M. Louie, L. Louie, and A. E. Simor, 'The Role of DNA Amplification Technology in the Diagnosis of Infectious Diseases', *CMAJ : Canadian Medical Association journal = journal de l'Association medicale canadienne*, vol. 163, no. 3, 2000, pp. 301–309.
106. J.C. Post and G.D. Ehrlich, 'The Impact of the Polymerase Chain Reaction in Clinical Medicine', *JAMA*, vol. 283, no. 12, 2000, pp. 1544–1546.
107. Oumar Faye, Ousmane Faye, Anne Dupressoir et al., 'One-step RT-PCR for Detection of Zika virus', *Journal of Clinical Virology: The Official Publication of the Pan American Society for Clinical Virology*, vol. 43, no. 1, 2008, pp. 96–101.
108. E.M. Leroy, S. Baize, C.Y. Lu et al., 'Diagnosis of Ebola Haemorrhagic Fever by RT-PCR in an Epidemic Setting', *Journal of medical virology*, vol. 60, no. 4, 2000, pp. 463–467.
109. Montserrat Agüero, Jovita Fernández, Luis José Romero et al., 'A Highly Sensitive and Specific Gel-Based Multiplex RT-PCR Assay for the Simultaneous and Differential Diagnosis of African Swine Fever and Classical Swine Fever in Clinical Samples', *Veterinary research*, vol. 35, no. 5, 2004, pp. 551–563.
110. Shirato Kazuya, Naganori Nao, Shutoku Matsuyama et al., 'Ultra-Rapid Real-Time RT-PCR Method for Detecting Middle East Respiratory Syndrome Coronavirus Using a Mobile PCR Device', *Japanese Journal of Infectious Diseases*, vol. 73, no. 3, 2020, pp. 181-186.
111. Christoph Steininger, Michael Kundi, Stephan W. Aberle et al., 'Effectiveness of Reverse Transcription-PCR, Virus Isolation, and Enzyme-linked Immunosorbent Assay for Diagnosis of Influenza A virus Infection in Different Age Groups', *Journal of Clinical Microbiology*, vol 40, no. 6, 2002, pp. 2051–2056.
112. Aparna Vidyasagar, 'What is CRISPR?', *Live Science*, 2018, available at https://www.livescience.com/58790-crispr-explained.html, accessed on 5 June 2020.

113. Ruilian Yaoa, Di Liub, Xiao Jiaa et al., 'CRISPR-Cas9/Cas12a Biotechnology and Application in Bacteria', *Synthetic and Systems Biotechnology*, vol. 3, no. 3, 2018, pp. 135–149.
114. Fancheng Yan, William Wang, and Jiaqiang Zhang, 'CRISPR-Cas12 and Cas13: The Lesser known Siblings of CRISPR-Cas9', *Cell Biology and Toxicology*, vol. 35, no. 6, 2019, pp. 489–492.
115. Jeffrey R. Strich and Daniel S. Chertow, 'CRISPR-Cas Biology and Its Application to Infectious Diseases', *Journal of Clinical Microbiology*, vol. 57, no. 4, 2019.
116. Xue Gao, Yong Tao, Veronica Lamas et al., 'Treatment of Autosomal Dominant Hearing Loss by in-Vivo Delivery of Genome Editing Agents', *Nature*, vol. 553, 2018, pp. 217–221.
117. Nikhil Swaminathan, 'Blood Diseases Could Show Crispr's Potential as Therapy', *Wired*, 20 November 2016, available at https://www.wired.com/2016/11/blood-diseases-show-crisprs-potential-therapy/, accessed on 8 June 2020.
118. Stephanie James, Frank H. Collins, Philip A. Welkhoff et al., 'Pathway to Deployment of Gene Drive Mosquitoes as a Potential Biocontrol Tool for Elimination of Malaria in Sub-Saharan Africa: Recommendations of a Scientific Working Group†', *The American journal of tropical medicine and hygiene*, vol. 98, no. 6, 2018, pp. 1–49.
119. The Lancet Haematology, 'The Resurgence of Convalescent Plasma Therapy', *The Lancet: Haematology*, vol. 7, no. 5, 2020.
120. Claudio Nunes-Alves, 'Blood is a Very Unusual Fluid', *Nature Immunology*, vol. 17, no. 1, 2016.
121. Giuseppe Marano, Stefania Vaglio, Simonetta Pupella et al., 'Convalescent Plasma: New Evidence for an Old Therapeutic Tool? *Blood transfusion*, vol. 14, no. 2, 2016, pp.152–157.
122. Y. Cheng, R. Wong, Y.O.Y. Soo et al., 'Use of Convalescent Plasma Therapy in SARS Patients in Hong Kong', *European Journal of Clinical Microbiology & Infectious*, vol, 24, no. 1, 2005, pp. 44–46.
123. World Health Organization, 'Use of convalescent whole blood or plasma collected from patients recovered from Ebola virus disease for transfusion, as an empirical treatment during outbreaks: interim guidance for national health authorities and blood transfusion services' (No. WHO/HIS/SDS/2014.8), *World Health Organization*, 2014, available at https://www.who.int/csr/resources/publications/ebola/convalescent-treatment/en/, accessed on 4 June 2020.
124. Volker Vetter, Gülhan Denizer, Leonard R. Friedland et al., 'Understanding Modern-day Vaccines: What you need to know' *Annals of Medicine*, vol. 50, no. 2, 2018, pp. 110–120.
125. Philip D. Minor, 'Live Attenuated Vaccines: Historical Successes and Current Challenges', *Virology*, vol. 479-480, 2015, pp. 379–392.
126. James J. Bull, Scott L. Nuismer, and Rustom Antia, 'Recombinant Vector Vaccine Evolution', *PLoS computational biology*, vol. 15, no. 7, 2019.
127. Eriko Padron-Regalado, 'Vaccines for SARS-CoV-2: Lessons from Other Coronavirus Strains', *Infectious Diseases and Therapy*, vol. 9, no. 2, 2020, pp. 1–20.
128. Hong Peng Jia, Dwight C. Look, Lei Shi, Melissa Hickey et al., 'ACE2 Receptor Expression and Severe Acute Respiratory Syndrome Coronavirus Infection Depend on Differentiation of Human Airway Epithelia', *Journal of Virology*, vol. 79, no. 23, 2005, pp. 14614–14621.
129. Christopher M. Booth, Larissa M. Matukas, George A. Tomlinson et al., 'Clinical Features and Short-term Outcomes of 144 patients with SARS in the Greater Toronto area', *JAMA*, vol. 289, no. 21, 2003, pp. 2801–2809.
130. Susan M. Poutanen, Donald E. Low, Bonnie Henry et al., 'Identification of Severe Acute Respiratory Syndrome in Canada', *The New England Journal of Medicine*, vol. 348, no. 20, 2003, pp. 1995–2005.

131. Ahmed A. Al-Qahtani, Konstantina Lyroni, Marina Aznaourova et al., 'Middle East Respiratory Syndrome Corona Virus Spike Glycoprotein Suppresses Macrophage Responses via DPP4-mediated Induction of IRAK-M and PPARγ', *Oncotarget*, vol. 8, no. 6, 2017, pp. 9053–9066.
132. Eriko Padron-Regalado, 'Vaccines for SARS-CoV-2: Lessons from Other Coronavirus Strains', *Infectious Diseases and Therapy*, vol. 9, no. 2, 2020, pp. 1–20.
133. Kayvon Modjarrad, Christine C. Roberts, Kristin T. Mills et al., 'Safety and Immunogenicity of an anti-Middle East Respiratory Syndrome Coronavirus DNA Vaccine: A Phase 1, Open-label, Single-arm, Dose-escalation Trial', *The Lancet. Infectious Diseases*, vol. 19, no. 9, 2019, pp. 1013–1022.
134. Ashish Chandwani and Jonathan Shuter, 'Lopinavir/ritonavir in the Treatment of HIV-1 Infection: A Review', *Therapeutics and Clinical Risk Management*, vol. 4, no. 5, 2008, pp. 1023–1033.
135. TianTian Yao, JianDan Qian, WenYan Zhu et al., 'A Systematic Review of Lopinavir Therapy for SARS Coronavirus and MERS Coronavirus-A possible Reference for Coronavirus Disease-19 Treatment Option', *Journal of Medical Virology*, vol. 92, no. 6, 2020, pp. 556–563.
136. International Severe Acute Respiratory & Emerging Infection Consortium, 'Treatment for MERS-CoV: Decision support tool', 2013, available at https://media.tghn.org/articles/Decision_Support_Document_v1_1_20130729.pdf, accessed on 5 June 2020.
137. Kuldeep Dhama, Khan Sharun, Ruchi Tiwari et al., 'COVID-19, An Emerging Coronavirus Infection: Advances and Prospects in Designing and Developing Vaccines, Immunotherapeutics, and Therapeutics', *Human Vaccines & Immunotherapeutics*, 2020, pp. 1–7.
138. National Institutes of Health, 'NIH clinical trial of Investigational Vaccine for COVID-19 Begins', *NIH*, 16 March 2020, available at https://www.nih.gov/news-events/news-releases/nih-clinical-trial-investigational-vaccine-covid-19-begins, accessed on 8 June 2020.
139. World Health Organization, 'Draft Landscape of COVID-19 Candidate Vaccines', *WHO*, 18 June 2020, available at https://www.who.int/publications/m/item/draft-landscape-of-covid-19-candidate-vaccines, accessed on 19 June 2020.
140. 'Inovio Accelerates Timeline for COVID-19 DNA Vaccine INO-4800', *Inovio*, 2020, available at http://ir.inovio.com/news-releases/news-releases-details/2020/INOVIOs-COVID-19-DNA-Vaccine-INO-4800-Demonstrates-Robust-Neutralizing-Antibody-and-T-Cell-Immune-Responses-in-Preclinical-Models/default.aspx, accessed on 6 June 2020.
141. Dominika Hobernik and Matthias Bros, 'DNA Vaccines: How Far from Clinical Use?', *International Journal of Molecular Sciences*, vol. 19, no. 11, 2018.
142. Yeming Wang, Dingyu Zhang, Guanhua Du et al., 'Remdesivir in Adults with Severe COVID-19: A Randomised, Double-blind, Placebo-controlled, Multicentre trial', *The Lancet*, vol. 395, no. 10236, 2020, pp. 1569-1578.
143. Food and Drug Administration, 'Coronavirus (COVID-19) Update: FDA Issues Emergency Use Authorization for Potential COVID-19 Treatment', *FDA*, 1 May 2020, available at https://www.fda.gov/news-events/press-announcements/coronavirus-covid-19-update-fda-issues-emergency-use-authorization-potential-covid-19-treatment, accessed on 9 June 2020.
144. Nanshan Chen, Min Zhou, Xuan Dong et al., 'Epidemiological and Clinical Characteristics of 99 Cases of 2019 Novel Coronavirus Pneumonia in Wuhan, China: A Descriptive Study', *Lancet (London, England)*, vol. 395, no. 10223, 2020, pp. 507–513.
145. Fujun Peng, Lei Tu, Yongshi Yang et al., 'Management and Treatment of COVID-19: The Chinese Experience', *The Canadian Journal of Cardiology*, vol. 36, no. 6, 2020, pp. 915–930.
146. Jia Liu, Ruiyuan Cao, Mingyue Xu et al., 'Hydroxychloroquine, A Less Toxic Derivative of

Chloroquine, is Effective in Inhibiting SARS-CoV-2 Infection in Vitro', *Cell discovery*, vol. 6, 2020, pp. 16.

147. Manli Wang, Ruiyuan Cao, Leike Zhang et al., 'Remdesivir and Chloroquine Effectively Inhibit the Recently Emerged Novel Coronavirus (2019-nCoV) in Vitro', *Cell Research*, vol. 30, no. 3, 2020, pp. 269–271.
148. See note 139.
149. European Union, 'Von der Leyen on European Vaccine Strategy: Making the World safe from the Coronavirus', *European Commission*, 17 June 2020, available at https://ec.europa.eu/commission/presscorner/detail/en/ac_20_1120, accessed on 18 June 2020.
150. Francesco Guarascio, 'EU Calls for Global Alliance to Buy COVID-19 Vaccines up front', *Reuters*, 17 June 2020, available at https://in.reuters.com/article/health-coronavirus-eu-vaccine-von-der-le/eu-calls-for-global-alliance-to-buy-covid-19-vaccines-up-front-idINKBN23O309, accessed on 18 June 2020.
151. European Union, 'Coronavirus: Commission offers Financing to Innovative Vaccines Company CureVac', *European Commission*, 16 March 2020, available at https://ec.europa.eu/commission/presscorner/detail/en/IP_20_474, accessed on 9 June 2020.
152. Reuters, 'AstraZeneca Agrees to Supply Europe With 400 Million Doses of COVID-19 Vaccine', *The New York Times*, 13 June 2020, available at https://www.nytimes.com/reuters/2020/06/13/world/europe/13reuters-health-coronavirus-vaccines.html, accessed on 15 June 2020.
153. Office of the Minister of the Armed Forces, 'Communiqué_Lutte contre le COVID-19 : Le ministère des Armées soutient une nouvelle technologie de détection rapide du virus, développée par BforCure', *Ministry of the Armed Forces*, 7 April 2020, available at https://www.defense.gouv.fr/salle-de-presse/communiques/communique_lutte-contre-le-covid-19-le-ministere-des-armees-soutient-une-nouvelle-technologie-de-detection-rapide-dú-virus-developpee-par-bforcure, accessed on 9 June 2020.
154. CORDIS, 'Three Rapid Diagnostic tests (Point-of-Care) for COVID-19 Coronavirus, Improving Epidemic Preparedness, Public Health and Socio-economic Benefits', *EU*, 10 April 2020, available at https://cordis.europa.eu/project/id/101003562, accessed 10 June 2020.
155. Edmond Differding, 'The Drug Discovery and Development Industry in India-Two Decades of Proprietary Small-Molecule R&D", *ChemMedChem*, vol. 12, no. 11, 2017, pp. 786–818.
156. Regional Centre for Biotechnology, 'COVID-19 Related Research Activities at Rcb', *RCB*, 12 April 2020, available at https://rcb.res.in/upload/RCB%20Media%20Report% 2012%20April%202020.pdf, accessed on 7 June 2020.
157. See note 139.
158. The Hindu, 'Coronavirus | ICMR, Bharat Biotech Tie up for Indian COVID-19 Vaccine', *The Hindu*, 10 May 2020, available at https://www.thehindu.com/sci-tech/health/coronavirus-icmr-bharat-biotech-tie-up-for-indian-covid-19-vaccine/article31547614.ece, accessed on 8 June 2020.
159. Eric Hamilton, 'UW–Madison, FluGen, Bharat Biotech to Develop CoroFlu, A Coronavirus Vaccine', *University of Wisconsin–Madison*, 2 April 2020, available at https://news.wisc.edu/uw-madison-flugen-bharat-biotech-to-develop-coroflu-a-coronavirus-vaccine/, accessed on 4 June 2020.
160. Lalatendu Mishra, 'Coronavirus | Glenmark's Antiviral Drug Fabiflu to be Used for Patients with Mild and Moderate Symptoms', *The Hindu*, 20 June 2020, available at https://www.https//www.thehindu.com/business/Industry/coronavirus-glenmarks-antiviral-drug-fabiflu-to-be-used-for-patients-with-mild-and-medium-symptoms/article31876147.ece, accessed on 20 June 2020.

161. Kai Duan, Bende Liu, Cesheng Li et al., 'Effectiveness of Convalescent Plasma Therapy in Severe COVID-19 Patients', *Proceedings of the National Academy of Sciences*, vol. 117, no. 17, 2020.
162. James P. Broughton, Xianding Deng, Guixia Yu et al., 'CRISPR-Cas12-based detection of SARS-CoV-2', *Nature Biotechnology*, 2020.
163. Ronald M. Atlas and Malcolm Dando, 'The Dual-use Dilemma for the Life Sciences: Perspectives, Conundrums, and Global Solutions', *Biosecurity and Bioterrorism: Biodefense Strategy, Practice, and Science*, vol. 4, no. 3, 2006, pp. 276–286.
164. C. Gould and A. Hay, 'The South African Biological Weapons Program'. in Mark Wheelis, Lajos Rozsa, Malcolm Dando (eds.) *Deadly Cultures: Biological Weapons Since 1945*, Cambridge Mass: Harvard University Press, 2006, pp. 191–212.
165. G.S. Pearson, 'The Iraqi Biological Weapons Program', in Mark Wheelis, Lajos Rozsa, Malcolm Dando (eds.) *Deadly Cultures: Biological Weapons Since 1945*, Cambridge Mass: Harvard University Press, 2006, pp. 169–190.
166. Annie Sparrow, 'Bashar al-Assad Is Waging Biological War – By Neglect', *Foreign Policy*, 24 October 2018, available at https://foreignpolicy.com/2018/10/24/bashar-al-assad-is-waging-biological-war-by-neglect/, accessed on 4 June 2020.
167. Aimee Amiga and Ruth Schuster, 'EU Report: ISIS Could Commit Chemical or Biological Terror Attack in West', *Haaretz*, 2018, available at https://www.haaretz.com/middle-east-news/isis/eu-isis-could-commit-chemical-biological-attack-in-west-1.5436111, accessed on 7 June 2020.
168. Kate Charlet, 'The New Killer Pathogens: Countering the Coming Bioweapons Threat', *Foreign Affairs*, 2018, available at https://www.foreignaffairs.com/articles/2018-04-16/new-killer-pathogens, accessed on 7 June 2020.
169. Peg Brickley, 'The SARS Cash Cow: How Four Letters Bettered Some Biotechnology Companies' Stock Values', *The Scientist*, vol. 17, no. 15, 2003, pp. 48-50, available at https://www.the-scientist.com/profession/the-sars-cash-cow-51275, accessed on 20 June 2020.
170. See note 79.
171. Shaun Tan Yi Jie, 'Fastest or Most Precise?', *Asia-Pacific Biotech News*, vol. 24, no. 3, 2020, available at https://www.asiabiotech.com/24/2403/24030022x.html#gsc.tab=0, accessed on 5 June 2020.
172. F.E. André, 'How the Research-based Industry Approaches Vaccine Development and Establishes Priorities', *Developments in Biologicals*, vol. 110, pp. 25–29.
173. Ismail Kola and John Landis, 'Can the Pharmaceutical Industry Reduce Attrition Rates?', *Nature reviews Drug Discovery*, vol. 3, no. 8, 2004, pp. 711–715.
174. Joseph A. DiMasi and Henry G. Grabowski, 'The Cost of Biopharmaceutical R&D: Is Biotech Different?', *Managerial and Decision Economics*, vol. 28, no. 45, 2007, pp. 469-479.
175. Avinash Arivazhahan and Gerard M. Raj, Intellectual Property Rights in Drug Development and Biotechnology', in Harikesh Bahadur Singh, Alok Jha, and Chetan Keswani (eds.) *Intellectual Property Issues in Biotechnology*, United Kingdom: CABI, pp. 239-244.
176. Belay Seyoum, 'Export Controls and International Business: A Study with Special Emphasis on Dual-Use Export Controls and Their Impact on Firms in the US', *Journal of Economic Issues*, vol. 51, no. 1, 2017, pp. 45-72.
177. Sibylle Bauer, Kolja Brockmann, Mark Bromley, and Giovanna Maletta, 'Challenges and Good Practices in the Implementation of the EU's Arms and Dual-use Export Controls: A Cross-sector Analysis, *SIPRI*, 2017, pp. 21-23, available at https://www.sipri.org/publications/2017/

challenges-and-good-practices-implementation-eus-arms-and-dual-use-export-controls-cross-sector, accessed on 8 June 2020.

178. Steve Holland and Michelle Nichols, 'Trump Cutting U.S. Ties with the World Health Organization over Virus', *Reuters*, 30 May 2020, available at https://in.reuters.com/article/health-coronavirus-trump-who/trump-cutting-u-s-ties-with-world-health-organization-over-virus-idINKBN23602N, accessed on 8 June 2020.
179. Press Trust of India, 'WHO Hopeful Coronavirus Vaccines could be Available Before end of 2020', *LiveMint*, 18 June 2020, available at https://www.livemint.com/science/health/who-hopeful-coronavirus-vaccines-could-be-available-before-end-of-2020-11592500002892.html, accessed on 19 June 2020.
180. Brakkton Booker, 'Fauci Says It's 'Doable' To Have Millions Of Doses Of COVID-19 Vaccine By January', *NPR*, 30 April 2020, available at https://www.npr.org/sections/coronavirus-live-updates/2020/04/30/848478507/fauci-says-its-doable-to-have-millions-of-doses-of-covid-19-vaccine-by-january, accessed on 8 June 2020.
181. Marcos E. García-Ojeda, 'What Needs to go Right to get a Coronavirus Vaccine in 12-18 months', *The Conversation*, 8 May 2020, available at https://theconversation.com/what-needs-to-go-right-to-get-a-coronavirus-vaccine-in-12-18-months-136816, accessed on 9 June 2020.

19

Decoding the Effectiveness of Contact Tracing Apps

Kritika Roy

With the sudden outbreak of COVID-19 governments across the world have put in place stringent measures to control the transmission. From closing the international borders to facilitating strict lockdowns, the major idea has been to flatten the curve such that it does not put unnecessary pressure on the healthcare facilities. Epidemiologists have established that the spread of highly contagious COVID-19 virus has to be controlled by bringing down the elusive number R0, or simply the number of new infections an affected person will cause by contagion. Often these means to achieve the objective requires innovative methods that can be implemented quickly, dynamically, and often remotely. Several strategies like testing, social distancing, screening, restricting movement, tracing and lockdown have been employed to restrict the transmission. Among these strategies, digital applications (apps) based tracing for infected persons have gained ground with every major country launching an app to digitally trace the infected individual as well as those with whom the infected individual would have come in contact. These apps and technological measures have been envisaged to limit the transmission rate, yet such data-intensive technology is positing a dilemma of privacy and public health among citizens.

With governments and societies taking extraordinary measures, aided by technology, to limit the spread of the virus, this chapter tries to examine the precedents being set for the foreseeable future. The chapter dwells into the technological know-how of contact tracing apps, the effectiveness of these technological solutions and the prevalent concerns of using the same. Additionally, the chapter also throws light on the issue of securitization of health and how such a framing typically precedes "extraordinary" invasive measures that could slowly become ordinary.

Understanding the Technology behind Contact Tracing Apps

Tracing is a technique that has been used to identify carriers of infectious disease and then further aid in uncovering who else they may have exposed, in an effort to "break the chain" of transmission. This tracing can be done either manually or technologically. Human contact tracers have been effective since the bubonic plague.[1] Tracing is a time-tested investigation method used to successfully fight outbreaks of diseases like Ebola, measles and HIV.[2] A similar model was created using the digital platform in an attempt to help stem the pandemic in its earliest days. With the announcement of the outbreak, groups of academic researchers and corporate software engineers popped up worldwide to figure out the technology behind digital contact tracing.[3] The basic need of a contact tracing app is to try and track down people and alert them if they have been in close contact with a COVID-19 positive person and if they need to self-quarantine. Digital tracing also helps to identify anonymous contacts, such as encounters on public transport and public places. Often digital means of tracing are employed to enhance the efficiency of human tracers by accentuating the speed, accuracy and scale of the endeavour.

Following are the popular means that have been employed using technology[4]

Bluetooth Based Proximity Beacons: Bluetooth could help to notify individuals who have been in close contact with the infected through Bluetooth signals that transmit an anonymous ID. These low energy Bluetooth signals perform a "digital handshake" when two users come into close contact. The focus of this approach is not on locating; rather, it is to compile a list of who all a person was in proximity with (infected individual), at varied times of the day.[5]

Telecom Data of Subscribers Geolocation: The mobile phone works by connecting to the closest cell tower. Therefore, the mobile service provider always has a record of user movements as logged by the sequence of cell towers that the mobile is connected to. This data collection cannot be turned off and hence it is required that the phones continue to work. Mobile service providers (or carriers) store this data for periods ranging from a few months to a couple of years. This kind of location data is accurate to the order of a few hundred meters. This data, normally, cannot be shared with anyone except law enforcement, under specific laws or court orders.

App-Based Geolocation Data: Location can be tracked best by using satellite-based systems. Here, a special radio in the smartphone communicates directly with a network of satellites, and the technique is commonly known as 'Global Positioning System' or GPS. Basically, location is determined using triangulation which uses the distance of a mobile phone from multiple cell phone towers or public WiFi hotspots. Overall, the accuracy of the location ranges from a few to tens of meters.

In terms of data collection, COVID-19 apps tend to fall into three categories.[6]

Firstly, those that are not doing digital contact tracing but rather allow users to voluntarily record and check their symptoms.

Secondly, apps which use a much less invasive decentralized models of Bluetooth contact tracing like that developed by Google and Apple. Under this model, data is stored on people's phones, rather than on a centralized database.

The third, and most serious for human rights are contact tracing apps, which are centralized, meaning they log data captured via the phone's Bluetooth sensor or GPS (or both) and upload this data to a centralized government database, and in some cases are mandatory.

Other than apps, location data can be accessed from advertisement servers, hardware beacons that detect the proximity of a mobile (typically installed in shops and malls), license plate readers, and points of sale (example: credit card use at a store).[7]

Are these Apps Effective Enough?

How well such apps will work, and whether people will install them in sufficient numbers to be useful, remains an open question. Despite some surveys indicating people are skeptical of the technology itself, yet more than 45 countries have (few of them listed in table 1), or plan to, rollout COVID-19 contact tracing apps.

For the apps to work effectively it must be adopted by a majority in a given area. The experience with contact tracing apps across the countries has been mixed. Wherein many countries saw an uneven adoption of the apps. This could be attributed to, first the prevalent digital divide among societies, the obvious lack of technology literacy and the privacy and data protection concerns. Additionally, there are concerns about the accuracy of the technology itself – if it could provide the level of precision necessary to calculate people's risk of exposure.

Table 1: List of Apps Deployed Across the Countries

Country	*Apps*
Austria	Stopp Corona
Australia	Covidsafe
Bahrain	BeAware
China	Close Contact Detector
Denmark	Smittestop
France	StopCovid
Germany	CoronaWarnApp
Hong Kong	StayHomeSafe
India	Aarogya Setu
Iran	AC19
Japan	COCOA (COVID-19 Contact App)
Kuwait	Shlonik
Qatar	EHTERAZ
Russia	Social Monitoring (name as translated to English)
Singapore	Trace Together
South Korea	Corona 100m (Co100)
Taiwan	Electronic Fence
Tunisia	E7mi
North and South Dakota (US)	Care19
Utah (US)	Healthy Together

Source: Compiled by the Author.

Note: Individual states in the US have adopted individual apps/ methods rather than a single national contact tracing technology. Additionally, more than 45 countries are in the process of adopting and rolling out apps but have not announced a name yet like the UK.

Following is a detailed assessment of all the mentioned factors:

(a) Socio-Economic Factor

As states pour their resources into contact tracing tools, they are missing half of one of the most vulnerable populations, that is, old, migrant workers, technologically deprived sections. There is a real disparity here. Any kind of contact tracing that relies heavily on smartphones may just exacerbate inequalities, discriminating against people who do not either have sophisticated phones or lack even basic skills like not even knowing how to download or open an app. Industry analysts estimate that up to 2 billion mobile phone users worldwide do not own devices that are configured to support Bluetooth-based tracing, a popular version of the technology. Disparities in access could further undermine uptake, for instance, only a limited population in Latin America, sub-Saharan Africa and Asia use mobile internet regularly.[8] Some of those at high risk of COVID-19 exposure live in conditions that are thoroughly incompatible with digital contact tracing. Aid workers and community leaders rely on internet-based communication tools to coordinate emergency services and share important information in the camps. A central question in the digital divide debate is what role if any, should government play in helping those without access. Should states subsidize broadband access for those who currently lack access or should they urgently fund ways to bridge the gap with digital training and support. In this regard, Indian Health Ministry has launched 'Aarogya Setu Interactive Voice Response System (IVRS)' to include citizens with feature phones and landline connections. The Aarogya Setu Interactive Voice Response System (IVRS)' is a toll-free service, available across the country, wherein citizens can give a missed call to a given number.[9] They will get a call back requesting for inputs regarding their health. However, this only solves a part of the problem. A more holistic and inclusive means would be needed to address the issue at the grassroot level.

Additionally, internet shutdown in places prevents effective dissemination of pandemic related instructions and impedes aid workers' ability to conduct "contact tracing" to contain transmission of the virus.[10] For instance, Rohingya refugees in Bangladesh are facing an internet blackout and the country has confiscated camp residents' SIM cards, ostensibly for security reasons. Refugees living in camps elsewhere are known to switch between multiple SIM cards to cope with unreliable connections, which would thwart the purpose of contact-tracing apps.[11] Often a large number of migrant workers do not have a phone or not enough credit balance to use the devices. Sometimes a single device is shared among many.

Further compounding the problem is the lack of sufficiently developed digital infrastructure leaving a major chunk of populace unconnected or unable to use services that require an internet connection especially, in the case of developing countries.

If the app becomes a one-stop solution for accessing services or freedoms, such as permission to return to work, to use public transport, or to enjoy other freedoms, this would drastically alter the value proposition of the app and potentially introduce new levels of inequity which would need to be identified and addressed by respective countries.[12]

(b) Technology Factor

Although there have not been any nationwide surveys to convey the effectiveness of the apps, however, people have been awry of the technical inconsistencies the app might have. The app could be very well susceptible to generate erroneous results like false positives and negatives. For instance, Russia's 'Social Distancing' app was noted to be deeply flawed on many levels and results in many fines automatically issued to people who are in fact fully complying with self-quarantine regulations. The app randomly sends push notifications to users instructing them to immediately take and send a selfie as proof of being at home. If users miss a notification, they are automatically fined 4,000 rubles (approximately 56 USD). Some users said that the notification would arrive in the middle of the night while they were sleeping and they would have been fined by the time they woke up. Another problem is that the screen tends to freeze while taking a selfie or the selfie would not send triggering an automatic fine. As of 20 May, there had been 60,000 installations of the app and 53,000 fines have been issued. Thirty percent of the fined users have also received multiple fines.[13]

Then there can be instances where people did not encounter someone with the virus but received a notification anyway, and instances where people were actually exposed but were not notified. By definition, a contact tracing app would also fail to detect where COVID-19 was transmitted by other means, such as through delivered food or contaminated surfaces.

Scientists have also found that when people sat across a table from each other, signal strength was much lower if their phones were in their pockets than if they put the phones on the table. Sometimes, the strength of the signal increased as people moved farther apart – potentially because of reflection off the metal surfaces such as supermarket shelves. Additionally, momentary instances of crossing paths at the signal or in the grocery store will be substantially more common and substantially less likely to cause transmission. However, certain tracing apps tend to leave out these encounters, which could mean not warning people about their possible exposure to the virus. Then there were obvious worries about Bluetooth-based apps either failing to alert people of risky encounters or flooding them with false alarms.[14] As such a situation could lead to panic or frustration if people are asked to repeatedly quarantine themselves.

(c) Security and Privacy Factor

The name 'contact tracing' itself has been a topic of debate owing to the negative connotation of tracking population while also possibly lowering expectations of what the apps were actually going to do. Efforts to rename the apps as "exposure notification" have been made, in effect, removing the stigma that it is more about controlling/tracking population, not about coronavirus. Privacy and data protection have been a major concern over a worldwide adoption of such measures.

In South Korea, the government uses several sources, such as location data, CCTV, and credit-card records, to broadly monitor citizens' activity. When somebody tests positive, local governments send out an alert, that reportedly includes the individual's last name, sex, age, district of residence, and credit-card history, with a minute-to-minute record of their comings and goings from various local businesses.[15] There have been reports of socially inappropriate targeting of individuals when South Korea released anonymised but detailed location trails about COVID-19 patients into the public sphere. This led to a series of online harassments of patients, who could now be easily figured out due to the detailed location trails.[16] In China, citizens have been required to download the software that broadcasts their location to several authorities, including the local police. The app interlinks geo-tracking with other data, such as travel bookings, to designate citizens with color codes ranging from green (low risk) to red (high risk). High-risk individuals can be banned from apartment complexes, offices, and even grocery stores.[17] In a recent incident, personal information of more than 7000 people who returned home from Wuhan, for the holidays, was leaked.[18] In India, a Karnataka government app for contact tracing – using location data – revealed the names and addresses of all patients on a map showing location trails, leading to harassment by neighbours.[19]

Amnesty international, conducted a study, on the contact tracing apps of 11 countries (Algeria, Bahrain, France, Iceland, Israel, Kuwait, Lebanon, Norway, Qatar, Tunisia, and United Arab Emirates).[20] It was found that three of these apps (Bahrain, Kuwait and Norway) collected satellite location data from users, instead of simply relying on Bluetooth signals, and matched accounts with real identities. These apps were following an invasive centralized approach, by capturing location data through GPS and uploading this to a central database, tracking the movements of users in real-time.[21] Bahrain's app was even linked to a national television show called "Are You at Home?", wherein prizes were offered to individuals who stayed at home during Ramadan. Ten phone numbers were randomly selected every day using a computer programme using contact details gathered from the app, and those numbers were called live on air to check if the app users were at home. Inclusion in the television programme draw was initially mandatory until Bahrain's Information and eGovernment Authority added an option to its BeAware Bahrain app allowing users to 'opt out' of participating in the show.[22]

Furthermore, surveillance and cyber-intelligence firms like Cellebrite have tried to sell repurposed spy and law enforcement tools to track the virus and enforce quarantines.[23] The concerned officials declined to specify which countries have purchased their surveillance products, citing confidentiality agreements with governments. However, executives at four of the companies said they are piloting or in the process of installing products to counter coronavirus in more than a dozen countries in Latin America, Europe and Asia.[24] As per the BBC Russian Service, Russia's app has been developed by the Gaskar Integration company. This company has contracts with the department of information technology, including an agreement for 180 million Rubles, concluded in January with GKU "Information City."[25] This app during installation asks for geolocation, camera, memory, calls and indicators of phone sensors. Also, the application gets the opportunity to view any data and has access to any settings. To register in it, you must specify the phone number to which SMS will come, as well as take a picture. The application transmits all received information in open form to the servers of the Moscow City Hall. For face recognition, servers in Estonia and Germany are used.[26]

Additionally, the desperation to quickly launch an app, often undermines the core cyber security measures that are vital. For instance, a critical weakness that was noticed in Qatar's contact tracing app, as discovered by Amnesty's Security Lab, would have allowed cyber attackers to access highly sensitive personal information, including the name, national ID, health status and location data of more than one million users.[27]

Location data collected via these apps are gold trove and can reach the data markets because it may not be shielded well, or the app design permits leakage, or the servers are hacked. From the data market, it can reach anyone – advertisers, stalkers, criminals or political opponents.

In North and South Dakota, United States authorities are promoting the use of an app called Care19, which can "anonymously cache the individual's locations throughout the day," storing information about where people spent at least 10 minutes at a time.[28] According to the Jumbo report, the app has been sharing this information with other parties including, Foursquare (a leading location-data provider), Bugfender (a Barcelona based service) and Google without disclosing the same in their privacy policy.[29] Many apps have vague or open ended privacy policy because of which data is often shared with third parties, law enforcement or tax authorities and can be used for coercive purposes that it was never intended for. Additionally, many countries do not even have an established national data privacy and protection law. For instance, in India, the personal data protection bill is yet to be passed in the parliament, which makes matters more complicated.

These challenges indicate that there is a need for a pragmatic and modest approach towards deployment of technology meant for contact tracing such that it facilitates data protection and privacy in a manner, that these tracing apps do not end up becoming Orwellian nightmare.

Securitisation of Health

Infectious diseases have been common phenomena in human history, yet it is only in the past twenty-five years that certain health issues have been propelled onto the security agenda through the process of 'securitization.'[30] By labelling something as a 'security' threat, it conveys a sense of urgency, giving an issue saliency and prioritization on the political agenda and therefore greater attention and resources from the international community.[31] Often the Western powers have elevated only the specific health concerns that they believe threaten their own security- often at the expense of the issues most pertinent to developing states like HIV/AIDS. Securitisation, therefore, enables those in power to "gain control" over an issue, its framing and its response.

Government administrations have already declared 'war' on the disease and such a framing generally precedes "extraordinary" invasive measures that slowly become ordinary.[32] The world would be well headed towards a 'new normal' characterised by more invasive health screenings, where people can check your entire health history through a digital certificate, where it is acceptable to expose the personal information of people online for a disease they may have no control over, where governments and citizens laud violent action against individuals with no power.[33] Such measures often stoke fear that governments are willing to create a Panopticon society for their personal gains. After all, history stands witness to the fact that once the government has surveillance tools, it will never maintain modesty and caution when using them.

The Way Forward

Pertinent questions about data protection and privacy like '*Who is acquiring this data? How will it be secured? Who all will have access to it? Can it be used for some other purpose? What can happen if this data were hacked or leaked? Most importantly, how will my identity and privacy be protected?*' highlights a visible scepticism regarding a full-fledged adoption of this technology.

Governments across the world rushing out to launch contact tracing apps that are too often poorly designed and lack privacy safeguards, making them susceptible to vulnerabilities. Often, many components of the tool go beyond the common requirements of contact tracing and could result in pervasive surveillance. A major question remains why the app needs to access all of this data – is it just to monitor compliance with self-isolation or keep a tab on citizens. Further compounding the issue is that many countries have made them mandatory. While there has been no public sunset clause when the app would cease to be mandatory. Thereby giving rise to deep concerns that often blur the line between voluntary and mandatory and between privacy-preserving and privacy-invading. These will surely have long term consequences.

In a rare joint move, the smartphone operating system rivals Google and Apple have released details on building a "privacy-preserving contact tracing," which is slated to be added to their phone software. These apps are built to track exposed users without compromising their privacy.[34] Although this is a notable move, however, it solves just a part of the problem.

The absence of a cohesive national plan for contact tracing, the lack of which has hobbled states as they have searched for money and resources to launch their own programs. Rather than focussing on building apps that would collect as little personal information as possible and keep any data that was collected secure, all while reassuring potential users that they were safe. There is a need to bring together the best minds in public health, academia and private industry to design a program that can help lower the risk for COVID-19. There has to be a credible institutional oversight and transparency while deploying such instruments. Many countries have been attempting to build an element of trust and transparency by making open source applications that are open for data protection audits or data protection impact assessment by academia, researchers, developers, non-profit organisations and anyone with genuine concern. Thus, making these apps 'data protection friendly' to a large extent rather than making the pandemic an excuse to introduce a blanket system of surveillance.

Going forward, these data-intensive apps should be consent-based and voluntary. For instance, tracing apps from countries such as France, Iceland and the United Arab Emirates (UAE) use a centralized model, but information on contact between devices is uploaded only when users voluntarily decide to report themselves as symptomatic or at the request of the health authorities. Such voluntary and consensual uploads at least reduce the risk of mass surveillance, as data is not automatically uploaded.

Another drawback of these applications is that these are state driven approaches and lack a single nation approach, considering many countries would soon start opening borders to accelerate economic recovery even without a vaccine in sight. In such a scenario technology should be made with some sort of cross border interoperability feature.

Furthermore, using a blanket approach rather than a multi-prong approach that does not account for different operating areas would not help in deterring the current situation. Afterall technology is no silver bullet. Experiments with unproven technology could displace funds for basic measures that are known to be effective in protecting those most vulnerable in the pandemic. Secondly, such tracking could open a dangerous new front in the surveillance and repression of marginalized groups. The idea that users are uniquely linked to their phones – an implicit assumption of contact-tracing apps – is frequently out of step with how they use technology. The internet shutdown often obstructs crucial information about symptoms and prevention, or end up risking the lives of refugees, host communities, and healthcare workers. Then there are still some phones in use that might not have the necessary Bluetooth or the latest operating system. The lack of appropriate digital readiness not only excludes individuals from opportunities to overcome the social and economic limitations of self-isolation but also limits the ability of governments to effectively manage the pandemic and its economic fallout. For economically weaker sections and low-income countries, digital readiness among populace continues to be a work in progress. Therefore, blindly, relying on technology to counter the pandemic may not have the desired effect. This showcases the importance of human tracers where digital platforms can only augment their capabilities not completely replace them.

Conclusion

There has been no doubt that in the Twenty-first century data is power and we go around carrying that power in our pockets. Are you willing to trade this power in the name of health and security? There is a plausible chance that these apps may come pre-installed in smartphones with a no-uninstall option. This pandemic is making acceptance of so many 'new normals' easy and swift with barely any questions asked. This is the starting point of building 'panopticon societies' where the question of privacy is also about creating power asymmetries.

These apps should be about healthcare and should be meant to complement the pandemic response. These apps should have built-in privacy and data protection by design, meaning any data collected must be the minimum amount necessary and securely stored. If contact tracing apps are to play an effective part in combating COVID-19 people need to have confidence that their privacy will be protected. Understandably, in a battle against the virus, an overemphasis on privacy could prove fatal for a large populace, however, even at this time of emergency, privacy has to be balanced in context with other human rights and due process and reasonability needs to be applied. Technology might be a small step but would surely become a giant step in combating current and future pandemics.

Will things return to 'old normal' when the pandemic subsides? Is a question that would continue to linger for long.

NOTES

1. David Ingram, 'Coronavirus Contact Tracing Apps were Tech's Chance to Step Up. They Haven't,' available at https://www.nbcnews.com/tech/tech-news/coronavirus-contact-tracing-apps-were-tech-s-chance-step-they-n1230211, accessed on 8 June 2020.
2. Patrick Howell O'Neill, "Five Things We Need to do to Make Contact Tracing Really Work" *MIT Review*, 28 April 2020, available at https://www.technologyreview.com/2020/04/28/1000714/five-things-to-make-contact-tracing-work-covid-pandemic-apple-google/, accessed on 5 June 2020.
3. See note 2.
4. Brijesh Singh and Khushboo Jain, 'COVID-19 Contact Tracing and Privacy Concerns: Here's What Experts Think,' *ET*, 13 April 2020, available at https://telecom.economictimes.indiatimes.com/news/covid-19-contact-tracing-technology-and-privacy-concerns/75119433, accessed on 10 June 2020.
5. Anurag Mehra, 'Contact Tracing, Location Data Markets and the Perils of Being Tracked,' *The Wire*, 14 May 2020, available at https://thewire.in/tech/contact-tracing-location-data-markets-and-the-perils-of-being-tracked, accessed on 10 June 2020.
6. 'Bahrain, Kuwait and Norway Contact Tracing Apps Among Most Dangerous for Privacy,' *Amnesty International*, 16 June 2020, available at https://www.amnesty.org/en/latest/news/2020/06/bahrain-kuwait-norway-contact-tracing-apps-danger-for-privacy/
7. Ibid.
8. Amos Toh and Deborah Brown, 'How Digital Contact Tracing for COVID-19 Could Worsen Inequality,' *Human Rights Watch*, 4 June 2020, available at https://www.hrw.org/news/2020/06/04/how-digital-contact-tracing-covid-19-could-worsen-inequality, accessed on 12 June 2020.
9. Aarogya Setu IVRS, Ministry of Health and Family Welfare, Government of India, available at https://www.mohfw.gov.in/pdf/AAROGYASETUIVRS1921.pdf accessed on28 June 2020.
10. 'Bangladesh: Internet Ban Risks Rohingya Lives,' 26 March 2020, *Human Rights Watch*, available at https://www.hrw.org/news/2020/03/26/bangladesh-internet-ban-risks-rohingya-lives, accessed on 12 June 2020.
11. Ibid.
12. Alex Hern, 'Millions Risk being Locked out of COVID-19 Contact Tracing App,' *The Guardian*, 15 May 2020, available at https://www.theguardian.com/technology/2020/may/15/millions-risk-locked-out-covid-19-contact-tracing-app, accessed on 12 June 2020.
13. 'Russia: Intrusive Tracking App Wrongly Fines Muscovites,' *Human Rights Watch*, 21 May 2020, available at https://www.hrw.org/news/2020/05/21/russia-intrusive-tracking-app-wrongly-fines-muscovites, accessed on 22 June 2020.
14. Kelly Servick, 'COVID-19 Contact Tracing Apps are Coming to a Phone Near You. How Will we Know Whether they Work?' *Science*, 21 May 2020, available at, https://www.sciencemag.org/news/2020/05/countries-around-world-are-rolling-out-contact-tracing-apps-contain-coronavirus-how, accessed on 12 June 2020.

15. Derek Thompson, 'The Technology that Could Free America from Quarantine,' *The Atlantic*, 7 April 2020, available at https://www.theatlantic.com/ideas/archive/2020/04/contact-tracing-could-free-america-from-its-quarantine-nightmare/609577/, accessed on 14 June 2020.
16. See note 5.
17. See note 13.
18. Jeffrey Ding, 'Privacy in the Time of Coronavirus,' *ChinAI Newsletter*, 9 March 2020,available at https://chinai.substack.com/p/chinai-85-privacy-in-the-time-of, accessed on 12 June 2020.
19. Alithea Stephanie Mounika and Sanyukta Dharmadhikari, 'Karnataka's App for Contact Tracing Reveals Home Addresses of COVID-19 Patients,' *The News Minute*, 27 March 2020, available at https://www.thenewsminute.com/article/karnataka-s-app-contact-tracing-reveals-home-addresses-covid-19-patients-121241, accessed on 12 June 2020.
20. 'Bahrain, Kuwait and Norway Contact Tracing Apps Among Most Dangerous for Privacy,' *Amnesty International*, 16 June 2020, available at https://www.amnesty.org/en/latest/news/2020/06/bahrain-kuwait-norway-contact-tracing-apps-danger-for-privacy/
21. Ibid.
22. See note 16.
23. Joel Schectman, Christopher Bing and Jack Stubbs, 'Special Report: Cyber-intel Firms Pitch Governments on Spy Tools to Trace Coronavirus,' *Reuters*, 28 April 2020, available at https://www.reuters.com/article/us-health-coronavirus-spy-specialreport/special-report-cyber-intel-firms-pitch-governments-on-spy-tools-to-trace-coronavirus-idUSKCN22A2G1, accessed on 12 June 2020.
24. Ibid.
25. 'The Application "Social Monitoring" from the Moscow City Hall has appeared on Google Play. It Requires Access to Geolocation and Phone Sensors,' *Meduza*, 1 April 2020, available at https://meduza.io/news/2020/03/31/v-google-play-poyavilos-prilozhenie-sotsialnyy-monitoring-ot-merii-moskvy-ono-trebuet-dostup-k-geolokatsii-i-pokazatelyam-datchikov-telefona, accessed on 26 June 2020.
26. Ibid.
27. 'Qatar: Contact Tracing App Security Flaw Exposed Sensitive Personal Details of more than one million,' *Amnesty International*, 26 May 2020, available at https://www.amnesty.org/en/latest/news/2020/05/qatar-covid19-contact-tracing-app-security-flaw/, accessed on 16 June 2020.
28. Steven Melendez, 'North Dakota's COVID-19 App has been sending Data to Foursquare and Google,' *Fast Company*, 21 May 2020, available at https://www.fastcompany.com/90508044/north-dakotas-covid-19-app-has-been-sending-data-to-foursquare-and-google, accessed on 12 June 2020.
29. Ibid.
30. Colin McInnes and Kelly Lee, 'Health, Security and Foreign Policy,' *Review of International Studies*, vol. 32, no. 1, February, 2006, pp. 5-6.
31. Debra L. DeLaet, 'Whose Interests is the Securitization of Health Serving?', *Routledge Handbook of Global Health Security ed. Simon Rushton and Jeremy Youde*, August 2014, p. 342.
32. 'What we Will Lose to COVID-19,' *ORF*, 25 March 2020, available at https://www.orfonline.org/expert-speak/what-we-will-lose-covid19-63685/, accessed on 25 June 2020.
33. Ibid.
34. Google, available at https://www.apple.com/covid19/contacttracing, accessed on 14 June 2020.

SECTION IV

POLITICS AND COVID-19

20

US-China Power Politics in a COVID-19 Context

Namrata Goswami

United States (US)-China relations have always been fraught because of their two very different political systems (democratic versus authoritarian), societal values, and political culture.[1] Across several presidential administrations, China has been perceived as a strategic adversary or competitor at best, with an aim to undo the US-led international order.[2] While President George H.W. Bush Senior is remembered as an 'old friend of China' having spent years cultivating personal diplomatic relations, since his time as US ambassador to China, even he started getting skeptical of China's intentions.[3] Bush Sr. played a critical role in the 1982 Taiwan Straits crisis, the 1989 Tiananmen square crisis, and visited China after becoming President.[4] His successor, President Bill Clinton forwarded his policy of comprehensive engagement with China and supported China's entry into the global economy with the hope that this would lead to China's political democratisation.[5] It never happened. George W. Bush Jr aspired to normalize trade relations with China especially after its entry into the World Trade Organization (WTO) in 2001, based on conditions that it would regulate the flow of Chinese exports. Some argue that China kept its currency exchange rate at artificially low levels thereby offering it competitive advantage known as the 'China Shock" theory.[6] Despite that, under Bush Jr, there was hope that China would become further integrated into the global economy and abide by the rules. Bush Jr was distracted by the 2001 War on Terror and the 2003 Iraq war. The 2008 financial crisis had a role to play in this regard as well.[7] When Barack Obama became President, he was optimistic about a good relationship with China to include mulling over the idea of a G2 during his first term,[8] subsequently going on to oversee a 'pivot to Asia' policy in his second term as a 'containment of China' strategy.[9] In 2010, as this concept of Asian pivot was introduced to the world by Secretary of State, Hilary Clinton at the ASEAN (Association of Southeast Asian Nations) Regional Forum held in Hanoi on 23 July 2010,[10] China surpassed the US to become the lead manufacturer of the world.

US-China Power Politics

Donald Trump's presidential campaign in 2016 emphasized the need to call out China as a currency manipulator and bring back manufacturing to the United States. He pledged to break up unfair trade deals with China, accused China of stealing American jobs, engaging in cyber espionage, as well as non-transparent trade practices. When Trump was elected President, President Xi Jinping visited him at Mar-a-Lago in April 2017 and Trump agreed at that time to resist from designating China a currency manipulator.[11] During that visit, the US, and China set up the United States-China Comprehensive Dialogue process based on four pillars: the Diplomatic and Security Dialogue; the Comprehensive Economic Dialogue; the Law Enforcement and Cybersecurity Dialogue; and the Social and Cultural Dialogue.[12] Trump visited China in November 2017 and was accorded a 'state plus' visit by China. During this visit, both countries recognized the critical importance of their economic relationship to each other's prosperity as well as the importance of the international trading system.[13] Companies from both sides signed deals worth 250 billion USD during the visit. Trump however cautioned that the US will be taking steps to balance the trade deficit and create a level playing field.[14] The cordial nature of those visits did not last for long. In June 2018, the Trump Administration imposed 25 percent tariffs on 50 billion USD of Chinese goods. China responded by imposing sanctions on 34 billion USD worth of US exports. China cleverly selected items that affected Trump's voter base, especially in the agriculture and automobile industry, with the calculated expectation that it would put pressure on Trump.[15]

The relationship has spiraled downhill since then with growing competition across politics, economic, US criticism of China's handling of the pro-democracy protests in Hong Kong, and rivalry in outer space. The US Treasury designated China a currency manipulator in August 2019,[16] though that decision was reversed in January 2020.[17] Then the COVID-19 pandemic hit, across the globe, with the US becoming the most affected country in the world by March 2020. Originating in Wuhan, China, COVID-19 at first affected China in December 2019 beginning

2020 but then gradually spread to Europe with Italy, Spain and the UK (United Kingdom) worse hit, further spreading to the US. As of 30 June 2020, the US deaths from COVID-19 reached 130,123 deaths with more than two million impacted.[18] The closures of town and cities from the virus have resulted in massive unemployment across the US, devastating economic loss and brought in an economic recession.[19] There were widespread suspicions in the US to include statements from US Secretary of State, Mike Pompeo[20] and Republican Senator from Arkansas Tom Cotton[21] that COVID-19 was manufactured in a Wuhan lab as part of China's bioweapon warfare program despite scientists remaining skeptical of such an origin theory.[22] This Wuhan lab origin theory took on such a hold in US policy and public discourses that the US Office of the Director of National Intelligence issued a rare public statement maintaining that COVID-19 was not manmade or genetically modified.[23]

It is in the context of the COVID-19 pandemic that this chapter offers a diagnosis of current US-China politics. The chapter argues that there have been four attendant consequences as a result of COVID-19 in regard to US posture vis-à-vis China. These include an elite consensus across bipartisan lines to hold China responsible; the impact of the virus on everyday Americans and they now have a stake in making China pay; the US has woken up to the reality of having to depend on China for critical virus related medical supplies to include ventilators; and finally, the US banning of travel between the US and China has not been as devastating as it was forecasted to be. For China, President Xi Jinping and the Communist Party of China (CPC) has run a highly effective propaganda campaign displaying how China has come to the rescue of the world during the virus by sending over doctors and equipment; that the country continues to have economic growth and good relationship with other countries, including US allies like Germany and the UK. China is also investing heavily in an alternate world order where strategic dips in its relationship with the US would not prove catastrophic for its existence. The chapter examines whether this Chinese strategy is working. Finally, the chapter ends with a diagnosis of how the pandemic has created a world order skeptical of the benign role of a CPC led China.

COVID-19 Pandemic and Impact on US-China Relationship

The COVID-19 pandemic has taken the US off guard. In the beginning, when there were numerous stories of the virus impacting Wuhan and other cities in China (end of 2019 early 2020), both the World Health Organisation (WHO) and Trump downplayed the global impact of the pandemic. WHO as late as 28

January 2020 praised China's response and hesitated to declare it a global pandemic for fear of economic repercussions.[24] This was despite delays by China in releasing the genetic map or genome of the virus and resisting in making COVID-19 patients data available for further diagnosis.[25] Trump on 24 January 2020 praised China tweeting, "China has been working very hard to contain the Coronavirus. The United States greatly appreciates their efforts and transparency. It will all work out well. In particular, on behalf of the American People, I want to thank President Xi!" He continued to assert that President Xi was handling the coronavirus situation well, and that it will be soon under control by April 2020. Things changed however when the US cases of coronavirus started rising fast, with the first death reported on 28 February 2020. On 13 March 2020, Trump declared a national emergency. This was followed by the closure of businesses across the US, to include limitations on public gatherings and 'stay at home' orders.

Elite Consensus across Bipartisan Lines to hold China Responsible

COVID-19 changed the way the US elite viewed China. Before the onslaught of the pandemic, there have been divergent perspectives on China and the CPC, with calls from US elites, ranging from policy, academia to mainstream media for more engagement with China to bring it into the international liberal order. Others have issued warnings about guarding against China's intellectual property theft and unfair trade practices. COVID-19 has created the structural conditions for the US to offer a more comprehensive national security engagement strategy with China. This was evident in the months following the rise of COVID-19 cases across Europe and the US Steve Bannon, Trump's former White House Chief Strategist, accused China of spreading the virus globally while containing it within their own provinces where the country did not suffer from much internal spread beyond Wuhan. Bannon asserted that "the Chinese Communist Party is going to have to pay…I think the world's going to hold them in judgement, and that judgement is not going to be very pretty. They owe trillions, if not tens of trillions of dollars."[26] The US intelligence community, in a report to the White House, asserted that China deliberately hid the actual number of infected patients and deaths, which is suspected to be far higher than the fake numbers provided by the Chinese state.[27] As per a Pew Research Survey that was conducted between 03 March and 29 March 2020, both Republicans and Democrats expressed a growing negative view of China. As per the survey, two-thirds of those surveyed had this negative view, the highest since the Pew Center starting asking this question in 2005.[28] In his book, *Trump Vs China*, Newt Gingrich identified China as the US's greatest threat, especially in its desire to become the world's preeminent superpower.[29] Gingrich, who routinely advises Trump, expressed concern that "in America, the news media, businesses, much of academia, and many of our political leaders (down to the state, county, and city levels) have fallen for a 'nice, new China' model and have ignored the fact that the country is ruled by a communist totalitarian dictatorship."[30] The Trump Administration released the 'United States Strategic Approach to the People's Republic of China' in May 2020. In this approach, it is made clear that the US engagement with China was made with the hope that China would become a free and democratic society as it integrated with the world. However, the CPC has utilized this access to acquire economic and military resources with an aim to reshape the international order in its own image and ideology. The approach identified is premised on a competitive approach where the US is primarily aimed at ensuring the resiliency of US institutions, alliances and partnerships, and compelling China to give up actions harmful to US vital interests. The strategy calls for cooperation with the US Congress, state and local actors, to include academia and the private sector to partner in this competitive endeavor vis-a-vis China. The document recognizes India's Security and Growth for All in the Region Policy as a common vision in the Indo-Pacific. The document calls out on China's predatory economic policies, its Belt and Road Initiative (BRI) at norm building, and specifies that "Beyond the media, the CCP uses a range of actors to advance its interests in the United States and other open democracies. CCP United Front organizations and agents target businesses, universities, think tanks, scholars, journalists, and local, state, and Federal officials in the United States and around the world, attempting to influence discourse and restrict external influence inside the PRC."[31] Such a document has support across several elite stakeholders especially, in the COVID-19 context. The US State Department echoed the White House's strategy regarding China. In a document titled "Competitive Strategy vis-à-vis China and Russia",[32] Christopher A. Ford, US Assistant Secretary of State, asserted that China and Russia presented systemic threats to the US and to the rules-based international order. Therefore, the US must ensure that the revisionist tendencies of these two states are countered by a whole of government US approach. Ford states:

> The PRC seeks to have a military more capable than any other in the world by 2049, hegemony in the Asia-Pacific region (and one that implicitly erodes US presence), leading positions within international organizations, and a dominant position in the advanced technologies essential to military power. With these achievements, the PRC hopes to claim what it sees as its natural hegemonic place at the center of the world system that generally defers to Beijing's interests.[33]

Given these efforts by China to seek comprehensive national power through a combination of political, economic, military and soft power, Ford recommends the US must build upon its allies and partnerships to meet the China challenge. The US has already banned the Chinese 5G company Huawei, and restrict the transfer of technology.[34] On 15 May 2020, Trump issued an executive order to secure the information and communications supply chain, stating that cyber and industrial espionage by foreign adversaries is weakening the US resilience. Trump identified that an unrestricted acquisition of information and communications technology developed by foreign adversaries constituting an "extraordinary threat to the national security, foreign policy, and economy of the United States."[35] Florida Representative W. Gregory Steube sponsored the Chinese Government COVID-19 Accountability Act in the US, House of Representative and US Senators Lindsey Graham (R-S.C.), Thom Tillis (R-N.C.), Cindy Hyde-Smith (R-Miss.), Mike Braun (R-Ind.) and Rick Scott (R-Fla.) introduced the COVID-19 Accountability Act to the Senate. The Proposed Act sought to "authorize the President to impose sanctions on the People's Republic of China if China fails to cooperate and provide a full accounting of the events leading up to the outbreak of COVID-19."[36] The recommendations of the Act are stringent, to include a ban on issuance of student visas to Chinese nationals, prohibit US financial institutions from making loans to Chinese controlled entities, unless they are involved in human right issues, and "oppose any loan from the international financial institution that would benefit any Chinese controlled or directed entity."[37] This split spread out to the WHO with Trump signaling that the US will exit the WHO due to its closeness to China and the mishandling of the pandemic.[38] We can analyze from the statements made by Trump, the several strategy documents signed by him, as well as overall hearings on China in the US Congress that in this context of the pandemic, the concerns about the threat China constitutes, not just politically and militarily but also at the societal level, has spiked in the US.[39] The official documents and policy statements are occurring in an American societal context where negative perceptions of China have increased.

Impact of the Virus on Americans' Perspective on China

The COVID-19 pandemic has drastically altered the opinion of Americans across demographics and their perspectives on China. Most now view China led by President Xi Jinping as not being able to do the right thing. This perspective is across different age groups.[40] Amid the COVID-19 crisis, two-thirds of Americans polled in a Pew Research Survey had negative views of China, the highest in such negative perceptions since the Pew Center started asking that question in 2005.

They believed that the CPC deliberately misled the world in this crisis and that the US is a much better option to be a world leader than China. They viewed China as a threat to the US especially when it came to cyber espionage and cyber-attacks, human rights, environment and space. Americans also viewed China's military and technological prowess as serious concerns. Especially due to the COVID spread and fiasco, Americans now firmly believe that the world is better off under US leadership. For the first time in 12 years, Americans believe the US is the world's economic powerhouse and militarily dominant with China, a distant second. While the Pew report specified that Republicans had a more negative opinion of China than Democrats, interestingly, because of the COVID-19 impact, Democrats have registered an increase in negative opinions of China.[41]

During the ongoing COVID-19 crisis, social media in the US has ignited with calls to hold China accountable for the COVID crisis. Anger was expressed against Chinese social media propaganda during the pandemic touting China's so-called impressive response to COVID-19.[42] Anger at the CPC was high when the death of Chinese whistleblower Wuhan doctor was made known.

Gauging the American public's overarching sentiment, American mainstream media ran several articles calling out for holding China accountable.[43] This is a new development and clearly indicates that Americans have been deeply affected by the COVID-19 on a personal basis, with loss of family, colleagues, friends, jobs, to the virus. They have lost their business and millions have filed for unemployment. Long term uncertainty continues with the pandemic still spreading and no vaccine in sight. Usually, the American's electorate and general public's perception of China has been limited to trade and cheap goods available in department stores. That perspective has changed with the onset of the pandemic.

Bring Back Manufacturing to the US

The US has woken up to the reality of having to depend on China for critical virus-related medical supplies to include ventilators. This stark reality was evident with hospitals and several US states running out of medical supplies and having to depend on Chinese manufacturers to respond to desperate orders for more ventilators. This extends to pharmaceutical drugs.[44] Peter Navarro, the Trump Administration's Trade Adviser is aiming to introduce and tighten 'buy American' laws so that US federal agencies have to buy American made medical products and pharmaceuticals. Navarro in an interview with *The New York Times* stated that "China has managed to dominate all aspects of the supply chain using the same unfair trade practices that it has used to dominate other sectors – cheap sweatshop labor, lax environmental regulations and massive government subsidies...as President Trump has said, what we need to do is bring those jobs home so that we can protect the public health and the economic and national security of the country."[45] Navarro is the brainchild behind Trump's trade war and trade sanctions with China.[46] His book *Death by China* has been pretty influential.[47] Chinese pharmaceutical companies supply more than 90 percent of US vitamin C, ibuprofen and hydrocortisone, antibiotics and more than 70 percent of acetaminophen, and 40 to 45 percent of heparin in recent years.[48] The fear from such dependence has escalated especially in a worst case scenario if China decides to ban the export of critical life-saving drugs and ventilators to the US. Decoupling with China would however mean rapture in a global supply chain of medical supplies and limited access to cheaper drugs. Manufacturing in the US implies much more expensive drugs creating a chokehold on people who do not have insurance or higher co-pays on insurance coverage. Despite that, there are calls for decoupling the US-China economy, because of the virus. When President Trump came to office, one of the campaign rallying points was 'America First' and bringing back manufacturing to the US to create jobs. The pandemic has instigated long term trends for such decoupling as suggested by Trump but the US dependence on China for crucial supplies remains for now. The White House airlifted crucial supplies like N-95 masks, thermometers, gloves from Shanghai in March 2020, and China has established several new factories that are manufacturing medical supplies to meet the rising global demand.[49] There are growing concerns within the US that China, whose COVID-19 cases have dropped, will selectively utilize its hold on critical medical supplies, to offer it to countries based on political calculations. Rosemary Gibson, in her testimony to the US-China Economic and Security Review Commission (USCC), specified how China could even weaponize the weapons stating that "medicines can be made with lethal contaminants or sold without any real medicine in them, rendering them ineffective. These products can be distributed to specific targets."[50] In this context, I argue that the US will have learnt lessons from the COVID-19 context and encourage the manufacturing of critical supplies in the US and/or diversify medical imports from other countries. Already such moves are on in several sectors across the country.

Impact of US Travel Bans between the US and China

On 2 February 2020, Trump issued a travel ban from China into the US. While there are criticisms that the ban was ineffective in limiting the spread of COVID-19, with nearly 430,000[51] people traveling to the US from China in January amid a virus spread in Wuhan, the travel ban has not been economically disastrous as some thought it to be. There were criticisms however that the ban should have been imposed much early especially given the Center for Disease Control and the US intelligence community warned Trump of an impending pandemic.[52] By the time Trump imposed the ban, another 40,000 people entered the US from China. Trump might have been delaying a ban as he wanted to get his trade deal with China inked at that time. However, as the pandemic peaked in the US around April 2020, Americans have come to the realization that a China travel ban has not been as devastating as made out to be for the US economy. Cargo traffic has continued between the US and China.[53] In a display of pressure tactics however, Trump issued notification of a travel ban for Chinese passenger airline carriers entering the US in response to China not responding to American airlines seeking approval to fly to China.[54] And that pressure tactic worked. 12 hours from the announcement of the ban on Chinse carriers, the Chinese Aviation Authority issued a notification that it will allow all foreign carriers to choose from a list of 37 approved airports to fly into China.[55]

China's Response to US-China Tensions during the Pandemic

China has been on the backfoot due to the origin and spread of the COVID-19 from Wuhan, China. The US Congressional moves against China's handling of Hong Kong has added to China's anxiety. However, the Chinese response to accusations of a manufactured virus has been strong and dismissive. In response to Mike Pompeo's accusations that COVID-19 originated in a Wuhan lab, the Chinese state funded *Global Times* ran an op-ed that stated that Pompeo's had no basis for such an accusation; neither did he have any evidence and was simply bluffing.[56] The op-ed asserted that:

> The Trump administration continues to engage in unprecedented propaganda warfare while trying to impede global efforts in fighting the COVID-19 pandemic. The most urgent tasks for international communities are to prevent the virus from spreading and to save lives while restarting the world economy. Ironically, Washington has put forth the weakest efforts in accomplishing the aforementioned tasks. As the US presidential election campaigns are underway, the Trump administration has implemented a strategy designed to divert attention from the incompetence it has displayed in fighting the pandemic. It is clear that their goal is to blame China for the pandemic by pinpointing the country as the source of the COVID-19.[57]

When Pompeo later retracted his statements on the Wuhan lab origins of the virus, Chinese news media specified that the U.S. strategy to create conspiracy theories had backfired. Hua Chunying, a spokesperson for China's Ministry of Foreign Affairs highlighted that the Wuhan lab was an experiment between China and France and that the US Secretary of State was full of lies.[58] Wang Yanyi, Wuhan Institute of Virology Director, asserted that the lab received its first sample of COVID-19 on 30 December 2019. There was no knowledge of the virus before that.[59]

The rhetoric on the origin of the virus got shriller when Zhao Lijian, a spokesperson of China's Ministry of Foreign Affairs (MOFA) tweeted in March 2020 that the US military had brought the virus to Wuhan during the Military World Games hosted in Wuhan in October 2019. This conspiracy theory had large takers in Chinese social media. When US national security adviser, Robert O'Brien blamed China for its initial coverup of COVID-19, another Chinese Foreign Minister spokesperson, Geng Shuang asserted that the US blame game was immoral and irresponsible.[60]

Diplomatic Offensive on Social Media

Chinese diplomats, including ambassadors, participated in a social media offensive with China's Consul General in Kolkata promoting a Russian media article blaming the US for COVID-19.[61] Chinese ambassadors in Europe blamed the US for spreading conspiracy theories against China on social media. Analyses of social media statements by *Politico* revealed that China's diplomats were actively creating a counter-narrative that showed China as responsible, and dismissing criticism of China's handling of the pandemic. Most diplomats took to twitter hailing China's response and help offered during the COVID-19. The usage of social media by Chinese diplomats between December 2019 and April 2020 increased ten folds. The social media strategy was a coordinated move by China to dismiss and spread counter-narratives by tweeting articles from foreign sources that help salvage China's COVID-19 reputation.[62]

China's Medical Diplomacy

China utilised its counter-narrative of being the COVID-19 savior of the world to downplay the COVID-19 originator theory. When Italy was reeling under COVID-19, China was the first country to send in doctors and supplies of ventilators and masks. A grateful Italy acknowledged China's help especially given Chinese doctors had experience dealing with the pandemic and could teach skills to Italian doctors.[63] Similar Chinese COVID-19 medical responses were witnessed in Spain,[64] and Brazil. More importantly, China ramped up COVID-19 related shipments to countries along its BRI.[65] Significantly, China became the world's supplier of ventilators, masks and other COVID-19 related medical supplies,[66] creating this situation where China's cooperation in fighting the virus became critical, so much so that many countries perceived China as taking leadership position where the Trump administration failed by putting 'America first'.[67] Chinese medial supply companies have also reaped enormous profits from the sale of medical supplies, especially in a context where the world is dependent on them.

President Xi Jinping stressed on building the Health Silk Road embedded into the BRI, envisioned since 2017. This health framework for Eurasia is built along with China's maritime and land silk routes. As part of this health framework, Xi offered medical help to 89 countries, spreading across Africa, Latin America, East Asia to Europe.[68] European countries like Italy, Greece, Austria, Bulgaria, Cyprus, Estonia, Hungary are part of the BRI.[69] Some view China's health silk road as an alternative to the WHO but led by China. Such interconnections are further buttressed by existing China-related connections including Chinese factories setting up shop in countries like Italy to ensure a 'made in Italy' tag.[70] Several are starting to perceive the Health Silk Road as a lifeline during the times of COVID-19. In June 2020, the State Council Information Office of the People's Republic of China (PRC) issued a White Paper titled *Fighting COVID-19 China in Action*. The document asserted that China's response to the virus was swift during the early stages (27 December 2019 to 19 January 2020), to the period (18 March- 28 April 2020) where the country registered an initial victory in Wuhan and Hubei province as a whole.[71] China credited this to an efficient command and control system and its ability to impose tight restrictions on societal movements. The report highlighted the unified effort of a billion Chinese people in fighting the virus, coupled with China's efforts in building that global health community through international partnerships. The report highlighted the resilience of the Chinese people and their role in establishing stringent mechanisms to contain the virus. The report states:

> Having forged the idea that the world is a global community of shared future and believing that it must act as a responsible member, China has fought shoulder to shoulder with the rest of the world. In an open, transparent, and responsible manner and in accordance with the law, China gave timely notification to the international community of the onset of a new coronavirus, and shared without reserve its experience in containing the spread of the virus and treating the infected...The Communist Party of China (CPC) and the Chinese government have addressed the epidemic as a top priority, and taken swift action. General Secretary Xi Jinping has taken personal command, planned the response, overseen the general situation and acted decisively, pointing the way forward in the fight against the epidemic. This has bolstered

> the Chinese people's confidence and rallied their strength. Under the leadership of the CPC, the whole nation has followed the general principle of "remaining confident, coming together in solidarity, adopting a science-based approach, and taking targeted measures", and waged an all-out peoples war on the virus...As of 24:00 of May 31, 2020, a cumulative total of 83,017 confirmed cases had been reported on the Chinese mainland, 78,307 infected had been cured and discharged from hospital, and 4,634 people had died. This demonstrates a cure rate of 94.3 percent and a fatality rate of 5.6 percent.[72]

The paper exonerates China of any responsibility stating:

> In a timely manner, China informed the WHO and other countries, including the US, of the developing situation, and released the genome sequence of the novel coronavirus. After community spread and clusters of cases emerged in Wuhan and confirmed cases were reported in other Chinese regions, which were due to virus carriers traveling from the city, a nationwide program of epidemic prevention and control was launched.[73]

The White Paper is clearly aimed at addressing criticism of China's reticence at releasing information about the virus's genome sequence during its early stages,[74] the arrest of a Wuhan doctor Li Wienliang who tried to warn his colleagues, and later died of the virus,[75] and China's clever strategic move to declare Wienliang a martyr.[76] The White paper offers a detailed timeline of how China responded to the virus, without any souring of course, and praises the CPC's astute handling of the unfolding crisis, specifically Xi Jinping's leadership in steering China through the crisis and establishing international partnerships. The document highlights China's Center for Disease Control (CDC) responding to the U.S. Center for Disease Control (CDC) request for sharing of information on prevention and control on 12 February 2020.[77] The document, in almost every second page, highlights Xi's leadership in setting up COVID-19 task forces, to issuing guidelines, to specifying how he personally offered mechanisms based on science to deal with this public health emergency. The White paper highlighted the WHO's praise of China's response.

> The WHO-China Joint Mission on COVID-19 released a report about its field study trip in China. The report described China's (sic) control efforts. It said, "In the face of a previously unknown virus, China has rolled out perhaps the most ambitious, agile and aggressive disease containment effort in history... As striking, has been the uncompromising rigor of strategy application that proved to be a hallmark in every setting and context where it was examined... Achieving China's (sic) exceptional coverage with and adherence to these containment measures has only been possible due to the deep commitment of the Chinese people to collective action in the face of

> this common threat. At a community level this is reflected in the remarkable solidarity of provinces and cities in support of the most vulnerable populations and communities."

We, of course, are aware of how much criticism the WHO faced for outward praise of China's COVID-19 response while internal documents have now surfaced that there was much skepticism within WHO internal structures on the efficacy of China's response.[78] Nowhere in the White Paper is there a discussion on the origins of COVID-19 or why there was so much criticism within China of Xi's lack of leadership.[79] Instead, the document forcefully asserts how Xi took command from the word go.[80] It also takes a swipe at Trump's advocacy of different medical responses, sometimes on his own,[81] by specifying China's trust in purely science-based responses to the virus. And that China has been transparent with regard to the virus, clearing responding to criticisms that China has hidden virus related figures and did not warn the world of the upending pandemic.

But any criticism or a case for compensation,[82] is now cleverly put into a context of dishonoring those who are battling, and those who died from the virus.[83]

> China has suffered tremendously but has contributed generously to the global efforts to combat the virus. Its efforts should be duly recognized, and it should not be criticized groundlessly. Since the early days of the outbreak, China has informed the rest of the world of every development in clear and unambiguous terms. *Certain countries ignored this information, and now blame China for their own failure to respond to the epidemic and protect their people's (sic) lives* [emphasis added] Those who are intent on maligning others will easily find a pretext. China has always acted with openness, transparency and responsibility, and informed the international community of developments of the epidemic in a timely manner. The baseless accusation that China concealed epidemic information and death figures is a calculated slur on the 1.4 billion Chinese people, including those killed by the virus, and on millions of Chinese medical workers. China categorically rejects any such accusation...It is both irresponsible and immoral to play the blame game in an attempt to cover up one's (sic) own shortcomings. China will never accept any frivolous lawsuits or compensation claims.[84]

In continuance of this counter-offensive and efforts to salvage China's reputation, Xi reinforced in May 2020 the need for 'the military to think about worst-case scenarios, scale up training and battle preparedness, promptly and effectively deal with all sorts of complex situations and resolutely safeguard national sovereignty, security and development interests."[85] What Xi is messaging here is that China will use military force if it faces a situation of an attack on its mainland, Hong Kong, or attendant disputed islands. This is a continuation of Xi's military thinking since

2017 when he made it clear to the Chinese military that it has to organize to win wars.[86]

Conclusion

It is clear that US-China relations were tensed when Trump became president with escalating trade tensions, South China Sea issues, accusations of Chinese cyber espionage, and subversion of American social systems to include US academic institutions through Chinese research funding under programs like the 'Thousands Talent Program'.[87] On 29 May 2020, the White House released a statement asserting that President Trump was protecting the US from Chinese intellectual property thefts by issuing a proclamation that would block Chinese nationals that work within China's civil-military fusion strategy from obtaining J or F visas.[88] The US has also designated Chinese media outlets as state entities and brought them under stricter rules.[89]

The COVID-19 context builds upon those US-China tensions. It is clear from policy statements across US bipartisan lines that there is a deep distrust of China. This elite perspective is supported by American public opinion whose perception of China and Xi has become more negative than when he first assumed power in 2013. As Trump enters his second presidential campaign phase, rhetoric on China can be expected to get stricter and more combative. Trump will portray himself as the strong president who stood up to China. China, on its part, will work behind the scenes taking advantage of the US open democratic system by routinely placing its own perspective on Trump and try to reach out especially to Democrats who are perceived as less hostile than Republicans. China's White paper on the COVID-19 crisis is clearly a response to the dominant narrative in the US and the rest of the world of China's culpability in regard to the virus spread. The intertwined nature of US-China businesses could see a decoupling. COVID-19 is a wakeup call to the US to bring back manufacturing, specifically of key medical supplies, to the US or locate them in countries other than China. We will see far more national security focused strategy vis-à-vis China with the US aimed at building alliances and partnerships with countries like Japan, Australia, and India in its efforts to contain China. In the long run, Americans will perceive US leadership as good for the world and will work towards limiting Chinese influence and the CPC led and dominated authoritarian international order that foretells.

NOTES

1. G. John Ikenberry, *Liberal Leviathan: The Origin, Crisis, and Transformation of the American World Order*, New Jersey: Princeton University Press, 2012, pp. 1-35; Michael Pilsbury, *The Hundred-Year Marathon: China's Secret Strategy to Replace America as a Global Superpower*, New York: Henry Holt and Co, 2015.
2. Terri Moon Cronk, 'China Poses Largest Long-Term Threat to U.S., DoD Policy Chief Says,' *U.S. Department of Defense*, 23 September 2019, available at https://www.defense.gov/Explore/News/Article/Article/1968704/china-poses-largest-long-term-threat-to-us-dod-policy-chief-says/; accessed on 10 June 2020; James Fallow, 'China's Great Leap Backward,' *The Atlantic*, December 2016, available at https://www.theatlantic.com/magazine/archive/2016/12/chinas-great-leap-backward/505817/ accessed on 10 June 2020.
3. Shi Jiangtao, 'George H.W. Bush-the Foreign Policy Realist and 'Old Friend' of China,' *South China Morning Post*, 01 December 2018, https://www.scmp.com/news/china/diplomacy/article/2175965/george-h-w-bush-foreign-policy-realist-and-old-friend-china, accessed 10 June 2020.
4. Ibid.
5. "Transcript: Clinton Outlines China Policy," *CNN*, 7 April 1999, available at http://edition.cnn.com/ALLPOLITICS/stories/1999/04/07/clinton.china/transcript.html, accessed on 09 June 2020.
6. Jeffrey Frankel, 'The Currency Manipulation Game,' *Project Syndicate*, 9 August 2019, available at https://www.project-syndicate.org/commentary/america-china-currency-manipulation-by-jeffrey-frankel-2019-08?barrier=accesspaylog accessed on 10 June 2020.
7. Paul Blusten, "The Untold Story of How George W. Bush Lost China," *Foreign Policy*, 02 October 2019, available at https://foreignpolicy.com/2019/10/04/the-untold-story-of-how-george-w-bush-lost-china/, accessed on 10 June 2020.
8. Cheng Li, 'Assessing U.S.-China Relations under the Obama Administration,' *Brookings*, 30 August 2016, https://www.brookings.edu/opinions/assessing-u-s-china-relations-under-the-obama-administration/ accessed 10 June 2020.
9. Ibid.
10. Catherine Puzz and Shannon Tiezzi, 'Did Hilary Clinton's Pivot to Asia Work?', *FiveThirtyEight*, 14 April 2016, available at https://fivethirtyeight.com/features/did-hillary-clintons-pivot-to-asia-work/, accessed on 10 June 2020.
11. David Nakamura, 'At Mar-e-Lago, Trump Welcomes China's Xi in First Summit," *The Washington Post*, 7 April 2017, https://www.washingtonpost.com/politics/at-mar-a-lago-trump-to-welcome-chinas-xi-for-high-stakes-inaugural-summit/2017/04/06/0235cdd0-1ac2-11e7-bcc2-7d1a0973e7b2_story.html, accessed on 10 June 2020.
12. The White House, 'President Donald J. Trump's Visit to China,' 10 November 2017, available at https://www.whitehouse.gov/briefings-statements/president-donald-j-trumps-state-visit-china/ accessed on 10 June 10, 2020.
13. Ibid.
14. Ibid.
15. Jacob Pramuk, 'Trump to Slap 25% Tariffs on up to $50 billion of Chinese goods; China Retaliates," *CNBC*, 15 June 2018, available at https://www.cnbc.com/2018/06/15/trump-administration-to-slap-a-25-percent-tariff-on-50-billion-of-chinese-goods-threatens-more.html, accessed on 10 June 2020.
16. U.S. Department of Treasury, 'Treasury Designates China as a Currency Manipulator,' 5 August 2019, available at https://home.treasury.gov/news/press-releases/sm751, accessed on 10 June 2020.

17. 'US Reverses China 'Currency Manipulator' Label,' *BBC*, 14 January 2020, available at https://www.bbc.com/news/business-51098294, accessed on 10 June 2020.
18. Worldometer, United States Coronavirus, available at https://www.worldometers.info/coronavirus/country/us/, accessed on 10 June 2020.
19. Scott Horsley, 'Its Official: The U.S. Economy is in a Recession,' *NPR*, 8 June 2020, available at https://www.npr.org/sections/coronavirus-live-updates/2020/06/08/872336272/its-official-scorekeepers-say-u-s-economy-is-in-a-recession, accessed on 10 June 2020.
20. Zachery Basu, 'Pompeo says there's "enormous evidence" Coronavirus Originated in Wuhan Lab," *Axois*, 3 May 2020, available at https://www.axios.com/pompeo-coronavirus-wuhan-lab-5f305526-9ceb-49af-943a-fd8291a6d5d9.html, accessed on 10 June 2020.
21. Tom Cotton, 'Coronavirus and Laboratories in Wuhan,' *The Wall Street Journal*, 21 April 2020, available at https://www.wsj.com/articles/coronavirus-and-the-laboratories-in-wuhan-11587486996, accessed on 10 June 2020.
22. Jack Brewster, ' A Timeline of the Covid-19 Wuhan lab Origin Theory,' *Forbes*, 24 May 2020, available at https://www.forbes.com/sites/jackbrewster/2020/05/10/a-timeline-of-the-covid-19-wuhan-lab-origin-theory/#2935de5c5aba, accessed on 10 June 2020; Eliza Barclay, ' Why these Scientists Still Doubt that Coronavirus Leaked from a Chinese Lab,' Vox, 29 April 2020, available a https://www.vox.com/2020/4/23/21226484/wuhan-lab-coronavirus-china, accessed on 10 June 2020.
23. Office of the Director of National Intelligence, 'Intelligence Community Statement on Origins of Covid 19,' 30 April 2020, available at https://www.dni.gov/index.php/newsroom/press-releases/item/2112-intelligence-community-statement-on-origins-of-covid-19, accessed on 10 June 2020.
24. 'WHO, China Leaders Discuss Next Step in Battle Against Coronavirus Outbreak,' *World Health Organization*, 28 January 2020, available at https://www.who.int/news-room/detail/28-01-2020-who-china-leaders-discuss-next-steps-in-battle-against-coronavirus-outbreak; accessed on 15 June 2020; Stuart Lau, ' Coronavirus: WHO Head Stands by his Praise for China and Xi Jinping on Response to Outbreak,' *South China Morning Post*, 13 February 2020, available at https://www.scmp.com/news/china/science/article/3050351/coronavirus-who-head-stands-his-praise-china-and-xi-jinping, accessed on 15 June 2020.
25. 'WHO, China Leaders Discuss Next Steps in Battle against Coronavirus Outbreak,' n.24.
26. Kevin Stankiewicz, 'They Owe Trillions' Steven Bannon says China must be Held Accountable for Coronavirus Spread,' *CNBC*, 30 April 2020, available at https://www.cnbc.com/2020/04/30/steve-bannon-china-must-be-held-accountable-for-coronavirus-spread.html, accessed on 10 June 2020.
27. Sonam Sheth and Isaac Scher, 'The US Intelligence Community has Reportedly Concluded that China Intentionally Misrepresented its Coronavirus Numbers,' *Business Insider*, 1 April 2020, available at https://www.businessinsider.com/us-intelligence-found-china-misrepresented-coronavirus-stats-report-2020-4
28. https://www.pewresearch.org/global/2020/04/21/u-s-views-of-china-increasingly-negative-amid-coronavirus-outbreak/ accessed on 10 June 2020.
29. Newt Gingrich with Claire Stevenson, *Facing America's Greatest Threat*, New York and Nashville: Center Street, 2019.
30. Gingrich, *Trump Vs. China*, p. 7.
31. The White House, 'The United States Approach to the People's Republic of China,' p.6. 2020, available at https://www.whitehouse.gov/wp-content/uploads/2020/05/U.S.-Strategic-Approach-to-The-Peoples-Republic-of-China-Report-5.20.20.pdf, accessed on 10 June 2020.

32. Christopher A. Ford, 'Competitive Strategy vis-à-vis China and Russia,' Arms Control and International Security Papers, Vol.1, No.2, 11 May 2020, available at https://www.state.gov/wp-content/uploads/2020/05/T-paper-series-6-Strategic-competition.pdf, accessed on 10 June 2020.
33. Ibid.
34. Christopher A. Ford, 'U.S. National Security Export Controls and Huawei: The Strategic Context in Three Findings', Arms Control and International Security Papers, Vol.1, No.8, 22 May 2020, available at https://www.state.gov/wp-content/uploads/2020/05/T-Paper-Series-U.S.-National-Security-Export-Controls-and-Huawei.pdf, accessed on 10 June 2020.
35. The White House, Executive Order on Securing the Information and Communications Technology and Services Supply Chain, 15 May 2020, available at https://www.whitehouse.gov/presidential-actions/executive-order-securing-information-communications-technology-services-supply-chain/, accessed on 10 June 2020.
36. H.R. 6405, Chinese Government COVID-19 Accountability Act 2019-2020, available at https://www.congress.gov/bill/116th-congress/house-bill/6405, accessed on 10 May 2020.
37. The COVID-19 Accountability Act in the Senate Summary, 2019-2020, available at https://www.hydesmith.senate.gov/sites/default/files/2020-05/COVID-19%20Accountability%20Act%20-%20Summary.pdf, accessed on 10 June 2020.
38. Trump: U.S. Ending Relationship with World Health Organization,' *CNN*, 29 May 2020, available at https://www.cnn.com/videos/politics/2020/05/29/donald-trump-us-world-health-organization-sot-vpx.cnn, accessed on 10 June 2020.
39. Jennifer Haberkorn and Tracy Wilkinson, 'Congress Looks at Options to Punish China over the Coronavirus Outbreak,' *Los Angeles Times*, 30 April 2020, available at https://www.latimes.com/politics/story/2020-04-30/congress-looks-at-options-to-punish-china-over-the-corornavirus-outbreak, accessed on 10 June 2020.
40. Kat Devlin, Laura Silver, and Christine Huang, ' U.S. Views of China Increasingly Negative Amid Coronavirus Outbreak,' *Pew Research Center*, 21 April 2020, available at https://www.pewresearch.org/global/2020/04/21/u-s-views-of-china-increasingly-negative-amid-coronavirus-outbreak/, accessed on 15 June 2020. https://link.springer.com/article/10.1007/BF00993437; Mathew S. Hirschberg, 'Consistency and Change in American Perceptions of China,' *Political Behavior*, No. 15 (1993), pp. 247-263.
41. Ibid.
42. Li Yuan, 'With Selective Coronavirus Coverage, China's Builds a Culture of Hate,' *The New York Times*, 22 April 2020, available at https://www.nytimes.com/2020/04/22/business/china-coronavirus-propaganda.html, accessed on 12 June 2020.
43. John Yoo, 'How to Make China pay for COVID-19,' American Enterprise Institute, 28 April 2020, available at https://www.aei.org/op-eds/how-to-make-china-pay-for-covid-19/, accessed on 12 June 2020. Marc A. Thiessen, 'China Should be legally Liable for the Pandemic Damage it has Done,' *The Washington Post*, 9 April 2020, available at https://www.washingtonpost.com/opinions/2020/04/09/china-should-be-legally-liable-pandemic-damage-it-has-done/, accessed on 12 June 2020; Riley Walters and Dean Cheng, 'How to Hold China Accountable for Covid-19,' The Heritage Foundation, 21 April 2020, available at https://www.heritage.org/asia/commentary/how-hold-china-accountable-covid-19, accessed on 12 June 2020.
44. Aime Williams, 'US Lawmakers Push to Reclaim Medical Supply Chains from China,' *The Financial Times*, 02 April 2020, available at https://www.ft.com/content/d71c01db-5333-470b-abcd-0df126864447, accessed on 12 June 2020.
45. Ana Swanson, 'Coronavirus Spurs US Efforts to End China's Chokehold on Drugs,' *The New*

York Times, 11 March 2020, available at https://www.nytimes.com/2020/03/11/business/economy/coronavirus-china-trump-drugs.html, accessed on 12 June 2020.

46. Bob Sellers, 'Tariff Man Behind Trump Economic Adviser Peter Navarro's Long Quest to Ratchet Up the Trade War with China,' *Fortune*, 27 August 2019, available at https://fortune.com/2019/08/27/tariff-man-behind-trump-economic-advisor-peter-navarros-long-quest-to-ratchet-up-the-trade-war-with-china/, accessed on 12 June 2020.
47. Peter Navarro and Greg Autry, *Death by China: Confronting the Dragon: A Global Call to Action*, New Jersey: Pearson FT Press, 2011.
48. Ana Swanson, 'Coronavirus Spurs US Efforts to End China's Chokehold on Drugs,' n.45.
49. Ana Swanson, 'White House Airlifts Medical Supplies from China in Coronavirus Fight,' *The New York Times*, 29 May 2020, available at https://www.nytimes.com/2020/03/29/business/economy/coronavirus-china-supplies.html, accessed on 12 June 12, 2020. Yasmeen Serhan and Kathy Gilsinan, 'Can the West Actually Ditch China,' *The Atlantic*, 24 April 2020, available at https://www.theatlantic.com/politics/archive/2020/04/us-britain-dependence-china-trade/610615/, accessed on 12 June 2020.
50. Testimony of Rosemary Gibson, Senior Advisor, The Hastings Center and Author, "China Rx: Exposing the Risks of America's Dependence on China for Medicine" Before the US-China Economic and Security Review Commission "Exploring the Growing U.S. Reliance on China's Biotech and Pharmaceutical Products," 31 July 2019, available at https://www.uscc.gov/sites/default/files/RosemaryGibsonTestimonyUSCCJuly152019.pdf, accessed on 12 June 2020.
51. Steve Eder, et.al, '430, 000 People have Travelled from China to US Since Coronavirus Surfaced,' *The New York Times*, 4 April 2020, available at https://www.nytimes.com/2020/04/04/us/coronavirus-china-travel-restrictions.html, accessed on 12 June 2020.
52. Will Ragland, "Trump's travel Restrictions on China Failed to Stop the Spread of Coronavirus,' *Center for American Progress*, 20 April 2020, https://www.americanprogressaction.org/issues/security/news/2020/04/20/177454/trumps-travel-restrictions-china-failed-stop-spread-coronavirus/
53. Morgan Krakow, 'International Air Cargo Traffic Continues through Anchorage amid new travel restrictions,' *Anchorage Daily News*, 8 February 2020, available at https://www.adn.com/alaska-news/aviation/2020/02/09/international-air-cargo-traffic-continues-through-anchorage-amid-new-travel-restrictions/, accessed on 12 June 2020.
54. United States of America Department of Transportation Office of the Secretary, Washington D.C. Issued by the Department of Transportation, 3 June 2020, available on https://www.transportation.gov/sites/dot.gov/files/2020-06/China%20Part%20213%20Phase%20Order%2020120-6-1%20Final.pdf accessed on 12 June 2020; Evelyn Cheng, 'China's Aviation Authority to allow more foreign flights after the U.S. bans Chinese Carriers,' CNBC, 4 June 2020, available at https://www.cnbc.com/2020/06/04/china-to-allow-more-foreign-flights-after-us-bans-chinese-carriers.html, accessed on 10 June 2020.
55. Ibid.
56. 'Pompeo's anti-China Bluff Strategy Reveals all-or-nothing Mentality to fool US Voters: Global Times Editorial,' *The Global Times*, 04 May 2020, available at https://www.globaltimes.cn/content/1187359.shtml, accessed on 10 June 2020.
57. Ibid.
58. Zhao Yusha, 'Washington's 'blame China Initiative' faces Setback', *The Global Times*, 07 May 2020, available at https://www.globaltimes.cn/content/1187705.shtml, accessed on 12 June 2020; 'Coronavirus : Chinese State media take aim at US 'lab theory', BBC, 05 May 2020, available at https://www.bbc.com/news/world-asia-52540737 accessed on 12 June 2020. Zhao

Yusha and Cao Siqi, 'More Virus Evidence Slaps Trump's China Theory,' *The Global Times*, 06 May 2020, available at https://www.globaltimes.cn/content/1187604.shtml, accessed on 12 June 2020.

59. 'CGTN Exclusive: Director of Wuhan Institute of Virology Says, 'Let Science Speak,' *CGTN*, 25 May 2020, available at https://news.cgtn.com/news/2020-05-23/Exclusive-with-head-of-Wuhan-Institute-of-Virology-Let-science-speak-QJeOjOZt4Y/index.html' accessed on 15 June 2020.
60. Joyce Huang, 'Chinese Diplomat Accuses US of Spreading Coronavirus,' *Voice of America*, 13 March 2020, available at https://www.voanews.com/science-health/coronavirus-outbreak/chinese-diplomat-accuses-us-spreading-coronavirus; accessed on 15 June 2020.
61. Russia Television, @RT_com, 9 April 2020, available at https://twitter.com/RT_com/status/1248434273587060738?s=20; accessed on 15 June 2020.
62. Mark Scott, 'Chinese Diplomacy Ramps up Social Media Offensive in COVID 19 Info War,' *Politico*, 29 April 2020, available at https://www.politico.eu/article/china-disinformation-covid19-coronavirus/; accessed on 15 June 2020.
63. Johnny Wood, ' China is Sending Medical Experts and Supplies to Help Italy Fight Coronavirus,' *World Economic Forum*, 16 March 2020, available at https://www.weforum.org/agenda/2020/03/coronavirus-covid-19-italy-china-supplies/, accessed on 15 June 2020.
64. 'China Sends Medical Aid to Spain,' *Reuters*, 12 Mach 2020, available at https://www.reuters.com/article/us-health-coronavirus-spain-aid/china-sends-medical-aid-to-spain-and-italy-idUSKBN20Z27G, accessed on 15 June 2020.
65. Tomas Navia, ' China is Sending Medical Supplies Around the World so You'll Forget They Kept Coronavirus a Secret,' *Vice*, 17 April 2020, available at https://www.vice.com/en_us/article/y3m8qj/china-is-sending-medical-supplies-around-the-world-so-youll-forget-they-kept-coronavirus-a-secret, accessed on 15 June 2020.
66. John Edwards, 'The facts about Global Trade in Masks, Ventilators and Test Kits,' *The Interpreter, Lowy Institute*, 21 April 2020, available at https://www.lowyinstitute.org/the-interpreter/facts-about-global-trade-face-masks-ventilators-and-test-kits, accessed on 15 June 2020.
67. Xie Tao, ' How the West Failed the Rest in the COVID 19 Pandemic,' *The Diplomat*, 14 April 2020, available at https://thediplomat.com/2020/04/how-the-west-failed-the-rest-in-the-covid-19-pandemic/; accessed on 15 June 2020.
68. Pepe Escobar, ' China Rolls out the Health Silk Road,' *Asia Times*, 02 April 2020, available at https://asiatimes.com/2020/04/china-rolls-out-the-health-silk-road/; accessed on 15 June 2020.
69. 'Belt and Road to Boost China-Austria Closer Ties in all Areas,' *China Daily*, 26 April 2019, available at https://www.chinadaily.com.cn/cndy/2019-04/26/content_37462647.htm; accessed on 15 June 2020.
70. Escobar, 'China Rolls out the Health Silk Road,' n.68.
71. The State Council Information Office The People's Republic of China, Full Text: Fighting COVID 19: China in Action,' 7 June 2020, available at http://english.scio.gov.cn/whitepapers/2020-06/07/content_76135269.htm; accessed on 15 June 2020.
72. The State Council Information Office The People's Republic of China, Full Text: Fighting COVID 19: China in Action,' n.71.
73. Ibid.
74. Laurie Garett, 'How China's Incompetence Endangered the World,' *Foreign Policy*, 15 February 2020, available at https://foreignpolicy.com/2020/02/15/coronavirus-xi-jinping-chinas-incompetence-endangered-the-world/; accessed on 15 June 2020.
75. 'Li Wenliang: Coronavirus Death of Wuhan Doctor Sparks Anger,' *BBC*, 7 February 2020,

available at https://www.bbc.com/news/world-asia-china-51409801; accessed on 15 June 2020. Vivian Wang, 'China's Coronavirus Battle is Waning. Its propaganda Fight is Not,' *The New York Times*, 8 April 2020, available at https://www.nytimes.com/2020/04/08/world/asia/coronavirus-china-narrative.html; accessed on 15 June 2020.

76. 'U.S. Public Needs to Know the Truth of Chinese "Whistleblower": Yale Scholar,' *Xinhua*, 21 May 2020, available at http://www.xinhuanet.com/english/2020-05/21/c_139074845.htm; accessed on 15 June 2020.
77. The State Council Information Office The People's Republic of China, Full Text: Fighting COVID 19: China in Action,' n.71
78. Ibid.
79. 'COVID 19,' *The Wall Street Journal*, 13 March 2020, available at https://www.youtube.com/watch?v=DA18-ZXopyc, accessed on 15 June 2020.
80. Ibid.
81. Lisa Friedman and Brad Plumer, 'Trump's Response to Virus Reflects a Long Disregard for Science,' *The New York Times*, 28 April 2020, available at https://www.nytimes.com/2020/04/28/climate/trump-coronavirus-climate-science.html; accessed on 15 June 2020.
82. Huileng Tan, 'China' Owes Us': Growing Outrage over Beijing's Handling of the Coronavirus Pandemic,' CNBC, 24 April 2020, available at https://www.cnbc.com/2020/04/24/lawsuits-outrage-over-chinas-handling-of-the-coronavirus-pandemic.html, accessed on 15 June 2020.
83. Marc Thiessen, 'China Should be Legally Liable for the Pandemic damage it has Done,' *The Washington Post*, 09 April 2020, available at https://www.washingtonpost.com/opinions/2020/04/09/china-should-be-legally-liable-pandemic-damage-it-has-done/, accessed on 15 June 2020.
84. The State Council Information Office The People's Republic of China, Full Text: Fighting COVID-19: China in Action,' n.71
85. 'Xi Focus: Xi Emphasizes Strengthening National Defense, Armed Forces,' *Xinhua*, 26 May 2020, available at http://www.xinhuanet.com/english/2020-05/26/c_139089760.htm; accessed on 15 June 2020.
86. 'China Focus: "Be Ready to Win Wars," China's Xi Orders Reshaped PLA," *Xinhua*, 01 August 2017, available at http://www.xinhuanet.com//english/2017-08/01/c_136491455.htm; accessed on 15 June 2020.
87. 'China's Lavish Funds Lured U.S. Scientists. What did it get in Return?,' *The New York Times*, 02 June 2020, available at https://www.nytimes.com/2020/02/06/us/chinas-lavish-funds-lured-us-scientists-what-did-it-get-in-return.html; accessed on 15 June 2020; Smriti Mallapaty, ' China hides Identities of Top Scientific Recruits Amidst Growing US Scrutiny,' Nature Index, 22 October 2018, available at https://www.natureindex.com/news-blog/china-hides-identities-of-top-scientific-recruits-amidst-growing-us-scrutiny; accessed 15 June 2020.
88. The White House, 'President Donald J. Trump Is Protecting America From China's Efforts To Steal Technology And Intellectual Property,' 29 May 2020, available at https://www.whitehouse.gov/briefings-statements/president-donald-j-trump-protecting-america-chinas-efforts-steal-technology-intellectual-property/; accessed on 15 June 2020.
89. 'US Imposes New Rules on State-Owned Chinese Media Over Propaganda Concerns,' *ABC News*, 19 March 2020, available at https://www.abc.net.au/news/2020-02-19/us-new-rules-on-state-owned-chinese-media-propaganda-concerns/11979036; accessed on 15 June 2020.

21

COVID-19 and the Challenge of Global Governance

Manish

From the time China reported a novel coronavirus to the World Health Organization (WHO) on 31 December 2019, it took barely four months to become a pandemic, killing hundreds of thousands and growing daily. It is now clear that the novel severe acute respiratory syndrome coronavirus 2 (SARS-CoV-2) had been circulating in Wuhan, China, for some time before it was reported to the WHO. It is for sure that the Chinese authorities had hidden information. Given the totalitarian nature of the Chinese regime, it is certainly not surprising. China maintained that SARS-CoV-2 was not readily transmissible between humans.[1] With the number of reported COVID-19 infections now touching several million cases across 196 Westphalian entities at the time of writing, this pandemic is genuinely global in every sense of the word.[2]

Doubts have also been raised about the origin of the virus. *The Washington Post*, citing US diplomatic cables, indicated that the US officials were, earlier, worried about safety and management weaknesses at the Wuhan Institute of Virology (WIV). Since the place of origin of the current pandemic was Wuhan, suspicions were bound to be raised if a lab in Wuhan could have been the source of the virus. The US President Donald Trump and Secretary of State Mike Pompeo have both claimed that there is evidence about the pathogen coming from the lab in Wuhan. The WHO, however, has made it clear that Washington's claim was at best 'speculative,' and scientists believe that the coronavirus jumped from animals to humans, possibly at a wet market selling wild animals in Wuhan, China. This assertion also got support from the top US epidemiologist Anthony Fauci, who told the National Geographic, that all evidence so far 'strongly indicates' a natural origin.[3] Unfortunately, no independent investigation has until now been conducted to establish the source. Whatever be the origin of the outbreak, whether natural, accidental, or deliberate, by state or non-state actors, the bottom line is that societies need to be better prepared to prevent, mitigate or face the effects of epidemics and pandemics.[4]

Amongst the twentieth- century major crises, COVID-19 is different because it is truly universal. However, what is equally surprising is the failure of any global leadership to pre-empt or prevent the proliferation of COVID-19, and most significant in the case of China. Contrary to the assertions of timely response and containment of the virus in China made in a White Paper titled 'Fighting COVID-19: China in Action' released by China's State Council Information Office on 07 June 2020, the facts on the ground speak otherwise. China informed the WHO of several cases of atypical pneumonia in Wuhan on 31 December 2019, but it was already very late by then as a molecular dating estimate based on the SARS-CoV-2 genomic sequences indicates an origin in November 2019. ....". Several of the infections were linked to the Huanan Seafood Wholesale Market. But according to a study conducted at a Wuhan Hospital, the very first human case identified did not frequent this market. Not only that, the local government at Wuhan led by its Mayor Zhou Xianwang failed to control the early spread of the virus, but it also worked overtime to suppress the information.[5]

On the other hand, the WHO also fell short of its mandate of ensuring global health. As late as the 9th and 11th of January 2020, the WHO put out tweets either downplaying the situation or trying to undercut travel advisories that were anticipated. On 09 January 2020, the official Twitter handle of the WHO had this to say: "Novel coronavirus emerges periodically as we have seen. SARS emerged in 2002, and MERS emerged in 2012. Several known coronaviruses are currently circulating in animals that have not impacted humans". On 11 January 2020, they followed it up with a travel advisory stating: "WHO does not recommend any specific health measures for travellers to and from Wuhan China. It is generally considered that entry screening offers little benefit while requiring considerable resources". Even entry screening of passengers from Wuhan or China were discouraged.[6] It would be interesting to find out how many passengers moved to and from Wuhan before the city was finally locked down. The most notorious example came in the form of a single tweet from the WHO account on 14 January: "Preliminary investigations conducted by the Chinese authorities have found no clear evidence of human-to-human transmission of the novel coronavirus." That same day, the Wuhan Health Commission's public bulletin declared, "We have not found proof for human-to-human transmission." But by that point, even the Chinese government was offering caveats not included in the WHO tweet.[7] "The possibility of limited human-to-human transmission cannot be excluded," Further, the bulletin said, "but the risk of sustained transmission is low." It was only on the 20 and 21 January 2020 that the WHO conducted its first field visit to Wuhan.[8]

The full impact of the epidemic was not grasped even three weeks after China had notified the WHO.[9] It took another five weeks until, on 11 March 2020, that the Director-General of the WHO, Tedros Adhanom Ghebreyesus, declared COVID-19 as a pandemic. It also calls into question the WHOs failure to question China about the Whistle-blower doctor Li Wenliang, who in early December 2019 had privately warned his colleagues that a new SARS type illness had started manifesting – nearly a month before China grudgingly informed the WHO.[10]

The full economic and cyclical effects of China's belligerence and the under-reporting by the WHO of the incident are still in infancy – but the consequences certainly will be gigantic. The United Nations, too, was slow in coordinating a global response to the situation. With China vetoing a United Nations Security Council (UNSC) meeting on COVID-19, no further evidence is required of the failure of the UNSC at this critical moment in time. The United Nations was founded at the end of the Second World War "to save succeeding generations from the scourge of war, which twice in our lifetime has brought untold suffering to mankind" and "towards that end to unite our strength to maintain peace and security." But, seventy-five years later, we are being ravaged by another scourge of war – the COVID-19 pandemic – and we find ourselves ill-equipped as international comity of nations to win over it. It has shaken our national and international economic, social, and political order to its foundations. It has also exposed the weaknesses of the global health and biosecurity system, and above all, the weakness of our global governance system due to intransigence of Beijing and its policy of opacity, which has contributed significantly to the spread of the pandemic. The 'new' Cold War, which seems to be brewing for some time now between the United States and China, shows its true face under the harsh light of COVID-19. It will require our going back to the drawing board and reimagining the world as we did in 1945, for the survival of humankind.[11]

Tragically, biosecurity as a defense against biological warfare, bioterrorism, and pandemics has been underemphasized in national and international discourse. Not that the world was not aware of the impending pandemic threat. In a 2009

CIA Report, it was stated: "if a pandemic break, it should be in some markets in China, Southeast Asia, where people live close to livestock." And yet, it required a COVID-19, to awaken the world to the destructive potential of a pandemic, and- by extension- a vivid picture of what a biological war would look like. The COVID -19 pandemic thus has taught us many lessons which India and the world would do well to learn. Health issues have never raised a coordinated response globally or a sort of international mobilization, as we witness in case of a financial crisis or even an issue related to climate change.[12]

Fortunately for us, the conference of the Biological Weapons Convention (BWC) is scheduled for November 2021. It must, at the earliest, assess as to how the COVID-19 situation evolved from the biological weapons perspective. To recap, the BWC is a legally binding treaty that outlaws' biological arms. The BWC proscribes development, stockpiling, acquisition, retention, and production of biological agents and toxins "of types and in quantities that have no justification for prophylactic, protective or other peaceful purposes" and weapons, equipment, and delivery vehicles "designed to use such agents or toxins for hostile purposes or in armed conflict. The transfer of or assistance with acquiring the agents, toxins, weapons, equipment, and delivery vehicles are also proscribed. The Convention further requires states-parties to destroy or divert to peaceful purposes the "agents, toxins, weapons, equipment, and means of delivery" within nine months of the Convention's entry into force. However, the BWC does not ban the use of biological and toxin weapons but reaffirms the 1925 Geneva Protocol, which prohibits such use. It also does not ban biodefense programs. [13]

This chapter discusses the failures of global governance models. The first section argues that global governance institutions like the UN and the WHO have failed in disposing of their responsibilities. There is thus an urgent need for these institutions to be revisited and remodelled so that they have the ability, efficiency, and nimbleness to respond swiftly to global challenges. This will increasingly be defined in an integrated way to cover natural, accidental, and deliberately caused disease in humans, animals, and plants. As such, there are unconfirmed talks of the coronavirus having originated in a laboratory in Wuhan, with many theories about biological warfare programs and accidental release. Therefore, the second section of the chapter provides a spotlight on the inherent weaknesses of the BWC of 1975. The BWC is a disarmament treaty that does not prohibit the retention and use of biological agents, including coronaviruses, for prophylactic purposes which encompass medical research for diagnosis and immunization. It has no verification protocol to deal with any suspected use of biological agents. In the run-up to the ninth review conference of the BWC in 2021, India could engage in consultations with other powers to evolve a regime that can provide better oversight.[14] Given the consequences of COVID-19, there is an urgent need to strengthen the BWC. The final section deals with the way forward. The chapter argues that given the current and future global challenges, there is likely to be an increased demand for international cooperation in scenarios like COVID-19. International organizations, treaties, and conventions, therefore, need more flexibility, expertise, access, and proven ability to provide a rapid response, even if it means reforming these global institutions. Conventions like the BWC should also tighten the gaps within, deliberate upon having a new code of conduct like the Hague Ethical Guidelines agreed in 2015 for chemists under the Chemical Weapons Convention (CWC), which can well complement structural reforms in the UNSC and the WHO.

COVID-19 and the Global Response

The COVID-19 outbreak and the subsequent global response has placed all international institutions under scrutiny. The liberal world order and the idea of global governance now appear to be in shambles. The term global governance has loosely been defined as "the sum of the many ways individuals and institutions, public and private, manage their common affairs. It is a continuing process through which conflicting or diverse interests may be accommodated, and cooperative action may be taken. It includes formal…as well as informal arrangements that people and institutions have agreed to or perceive to be in their interest". The United Nations and its organs – the Security Council, WHO, G-20, international treaties, and the totality of institutions, regimes, and norms, procedures, taken together, constitute what is known as global governance.

In the COVID-19 era, critics have started to question global governance and associated multilateralism. No doubt, that functioning of multilateral institutions, like much else, requires reform today. As the COVID-19 crisis continues, any predictions or recommendations as to its further course can only be tentative. Its scale and duration can only be guessed at this point in time. But what is clear is that failures in protecting global health security will seriously affect the economy, politics, and the public sphere.[15] The pandemic seems to have exposed the liberal order and the international community as mirages, even as it demonstrates the terrible consequences of faltering global cooperation.[16]

Despite the damage to globalization caused by COVID-19 and keeping in mind that states will likely prioritize their immediate need to manage health and economic crises that local populations face, the question of the necessity of coordinating a global response to COVID-19 naturally surfaces. In that context, the benefits of international cooperation and information sharing are unlikely to recede along with the pandemic. The outbreak's aftershocks will leave shared global problems that are likely to linger: movement restrictions, high levels of unemployment, rising dissatisfaction with governing institutions, and open-ended measures adopted by authoritarian regimes to suppress civil liberties, assume more power and insert loyalists into sensitive positions under the fog of COVID-19.[17]

Notably, the pandemic has given a powerful impetus to confrontation in relations between the United States and China. Each has been quick to blame the other for creating a threat to all humankind. This confrontation directly threatens economic globalization and hinders efforts to improve institutions of global governance. All these elements make it even more challenging to reform institutions, which have not been able to adequately meet the task of organizing a collective response to current challenges. On the other hand, the daunting threats, both present, and future are now more evident than before.[18]

The dismal multilateral response to the pandemic reflects, in part, the decisions of specific leaders, especially Chinese President Xi Jinping and US President Donald Trump. Their behavior helps explain why the WHO struggled in the initial stages of the outbreak and why forums for multilateral coordination, such as the G-7, the G-20, and the UN Security Council, failed to rise to the occasion.[19]

The Failure of the UN System?

Although the ability of the UN Security Council to effectively produce resolutions on issues related to pandemics has been limited in the past, it has been worse during the COVID-19. There are at least two instances from the past, wherein states have shown exemplary cooperation in dealing with the disease. First, the Security Council's success in global health is exemplified in the passing of Resolution 1308 in 2000 on HIV/AIDS – when the United States was at the helm of a unipolar international system – and, second, Resolution 2177 in 2014 on the Ebola crisis in West Africa. Both resolutions were aimed towards a coordinated international response to the pandemic. Unfortunately, the spread of COVID-19 appears to have furthered the power dynamics between the United States and China. The world witnessed the US referring to COVID-19 as the 'Wuhan' or 'Chinese' virus followed by the Chinese propaganda that the United States was responsible for spreading the virus.[20] Perhaps, this US-China politics sabotaged efforts to reach a resolution on COVID-19 at the Security Council. China, which held the rotating presidency of the Security Council in March, blocked it from considering any resolution about the pandemic, arguing that public health matters fell outside the Council's 'geopolitical' ambit. This, however, was plainly untrue as the Resolution 2177 passed in 2014 shows, it designated the West African Ebola epidemic a "threat to international peace and security."[21]

On 25 March, UN Secretary-General António Guterres launched a humanitarian response plan to mitigate the effects of the coronavirus on fragile and war-torn states, which are home to approximately a billion people and a majority of the world's poor, as well as most of its 70 million refugees and internally displaced people. Yet with a budget of just 2 billion USD in UN funds, this plan had funding that was less than one-thousandth of what the United States had dedicated to its domestic response by early May. Significantly, within the multipolar setting of 2020, the spread of COVID-19 has exacerbated already strained US-China relations as well as relations between the United States and its long-standing allies, as demonstrated by President Trump's announcement – without prior coordination with the European Union – of a European travel ban.[22]

The Inept World Health Organisation

COVID-19 has also brought into the spotlight the WHO, which has a mandate that exceeds its capabilities. Member states have assigned it more and more tasks while limiting its independence and resources, setting the organization up for failure. The pandemic has revealed both the limits of the existing multilateral system and the costs of the system's failure.

Since 2000, the WHO has risen markedly in importance, as various new and re-emerging infectious diseases have threatened global health and security. The agency managed the global responses to the SARS epidemic in 2003, the H1N1 flu pandemic in 2009, the Ebola epidemic in 2014–16, and the Zika epidemic in 2015–16. In the wake of SARS, the World Health Assembly, the WHO's governing body, strengthened the International Health Regulations (IHR), the core legal prescriptions governing the state's conduct concerning infectious disease. The new IHR gave the WHO's director-general the authority to declare a "public health emergency of international concern" and required member states to increase their pandemic-response capacities. Meanwhile, an entire multilateral ecosystem of global public health arrangements blossomed alongside the WHO and its IHR, including the Global Alliance for Vaccines and Immunization (now called GAVI, the Vaccine Alliance), the Global Health Security Agenda, the World Bank's Pandemic Emergency Financing Facility, and the Africa Centres for Disease Control and

Prevention. The result is a global health infrastructure beyond the wildest dreams of the national leaders who confronted the 1918 influenza pandemic alone.[23]

The absence of cooperation in the COVID-19 crisis is, therefore, somewhat puzzling. Countries should be working together. The United States and the Soviet Union found it within their interests to cooperate (and even outdo each other) on smallpox eradication during the Cold War. More recently, the US and China cooperated on a range of issues in the Obama era from the financial crisis to climate change to the Ebola outbreak.[24]

In the health space, the best example of this in recent years is the leadership of the United States on combating HIV/AIDS that began during the presidency of George W. Bush. Though the WHO is playing a prominent role in leading the international response to the COVID-19 pandemic, yet its performance has been marred by its pandering to China.[25]

In China, the initial epicenter of the COVID-19 pandemic, the Xi government was slow to report the outbreak to the WHO, and it resisted full transparency after that. China was also slow to share transmission data and biological samples with the WHO. Outside China, many countries responded to the novel coronavirus by implementing international travel restrictions. On 31 January, Trump ordered the United States closed to foreigners who had recently travelled to China. On 11 March, without consulting US allies, it abruptly suspended air travel from Europe to the United States. Brazil, India, Israel, and Russia also implemented pandemic-related border restrictions that month. Other countries, such as France and Germany, either banned or imposed limits on the export of protective medical equipment. At the same time, WHO extolled Chinese President Xi Jinping's "very rare leadership" and China's "transparency." The bias has been so pronounced that Japanese Deputy Prime Minister Taro also asserted that, for many, the WHO is looking more like the "CHO" – the Chinese Health Organization.[26]

However, this time it was to do with WHO's leadership. Tedros, who became the agency's first non-physician chief in 2017 with China's support, was accused of covering up to three cholera outbreaks while serving as Ethiopia's health minister. Nonetheless, few would have imagined that, as WHO chief, the microbiologist and malaria researcher would be complicit in China's deadly deception. As the costs of the mismanagement continue to mount, a reckoning is becoming all but inevitable. An online petition calling for Tedros to resign garnered almost a million signatures. More consequential, President Donald Trump's administration has suspended the WHO's US funding, which accounts for 9.2% of its budget.[27]

The world needs the WHO. But if the agency is to spearhead international health policy and respond to disease outbreaks effectively, it must pursue deep reforms aimed at broadening its jurisdiction and authority. That won't happen unless and until the WHO rebuilds its credibility, beginning with new leadership.[28] The latter undoubtedly harmed global preparedness in the early days of the outbreak by failing to convey the seriousness of the virus and the situation. It is, therefore, essential to consider how to manage better international cooperation in a world that will continue to be deeply interconnected, but whose current international institutions are underperforming, which may render them increasingly irrelevant.[29]

The US response to all this – announcing the halting of funds to WHO – is the opposite of much-needed action-oriented and effective international leadership. The world is in the midst of an unfolding crisis. No wonder, another wave of the epidemic outbreak cannot be ruled out. There is no substitute for a structured, coordinated global response in which international organizations have to play an active role. International power vacuums are likely to be filled by disruptive actors. If the United States has claims against China's rising influence over international bodies, it is unlikely to remedy those complaints – in this case, a failure to convey accurate information on the gravity of the pandemic – by abandoning those organizations and perhaps even seeking to create parallel institutions. Current and future global challenges demand far better international cooperation and significantly more decisive action to avoid worst-case scenarios. Given the lack of action by important and relevant international political bodies in dealing with COVID-19, efforts and resources ought to be channeled to more flexible, technocratic international organizations that have the knowledge, access, and proven ability to provide rapid response to unfolding events. Considering that such organizations are not hermetically sealed off from the political environments in which they exist and operate, reforms should be articulated toward improving transparency and mechanisms to demand accountability on critical decisions. Although great-power competition is likely to be a feature of global dynamics for the foreseeable future, such steps would contribute to minimizing the risks of the dysfunction embodied and reinforced by the current international response to COVID-19.[30]

Is the Multilateral BWC Regime Effective?

The COVID-19 pandemic has once again given an opportune moment to turn the spotlight on global non-proliferation norms and the use of biological pathogens to attack populations, whether by state actors or in the hands of non-state actors, amorphous entities or a rogue microbiologist. The anthrax attacks of 2001 were not just one single incident. There may have been ample potential warnings of such imminent attacks in the past. One is still not sure if the 2009 H1N1 Influenza or the Ebola or even the COVID-19 are naturally occurring threats or an orchestrated bio-attacks. But clearly, it has demonstrated global and national shortcomings in our biodefense. Global efforts to prevent the deliberate use of biological pathogens appears to be now drifting. Fortunately for us, the Ninth Review Conference of the Biological Weapons Convention (BWC), to be held in 2021, could be an opportunity for reinvigorating the treaty.[31]

The Convention on the Prohibition of the Development, Production and Stockpiling of Bacteriological (Biological) and Toxin Weapons and on their Destruction usually referred to as the Biological Weapons Convention (BWC), or Biological and Toxin Weapons Convention (BTWC) was the first multilateral disarmament treaty banning the production of an entire category of weapons, entering into force in 1975.[32]

This Convention itself was the result of prolonged international negotiations to supplement the 1925 Geneva Protocol, which prohibited the use, but not possession or development of chemical and biological weapons. Fortunately, this treaty prohibits the "development, stockpiling, acquisition, retention, and production of biological agents and toxins of types and in quantities that have no justification for prophylactic, protective or other peaceful purposes." Ironically, the pace of biotechnology has expanded exponentially. New genome-editing tools have been developed which are dual-use, thereby posing the challenge for a robust prevention and response framework.[33] The BWC also does not have a verification protocol to deal with any suspected use of biological agents.[34] The issues which need immediate attention in the forthcoming Ninth Review Conference, in 2021 are as follows:

First, there has been a growing recognition of the challenges faced by BWC. After a careful introspection of the BWC, the scope of the BWC is somewhat ambiguous. The question is: what is to be banned, and what is to be exempted? This question becomes important today since the scientific and technological advances have lowered the barriers to acquiring and using a biological weapon. The debates about new developments-including gain-of-function experiments, potential pandemic pathogens, CRISPR and other genome editing technologies, gene drives, and synthetic biology- make the BWC a weak instrument.[35] But as we can see, the spirit behind the scope of the BWC and related activity is promoting biosafety or protecting people from germs and advancing biosecurity. As the BWC seeks to promote biosafety and biosecurity on a global scale, we have seen biosafety diplomacy emerge on the international scene.[36]

Equally true is the fact that the efforts to prevent biological terrorism. Possible use of microorganisms as a biological weapon by terrorists is a real concern now. India has earlier, in 2002, brought a resolution at the UN General Assembly, titled "Measures to prevent terrorists from acquiring the weapons of mass destruction."

Of late, the spread of bioweapons debate is starting to shift away from the BWC towards the UN Security Council Resolution 1540. This resolution was first approved in 2004 and imposes an obligation on all UN members to improve their legal authorities and bureaucratic capacities to prevent non-state actors from acquiring, developing, or using nuclear, biological, and chemical weapons. While the bioweapons treaty provides one of the foundations for UNSC Resolution 1540's mandate, the resolution appears to be becoming the preferred international vehicle for enhancing biosafety, biosecurity, export controls, and the criminalization of biological weapons.[37] Indeed, the UNSC can investigate complaints in this regard, but the veto power enjoyed by the permanent members, including China, makes it near impossible. In the run-up to the Ninth Review Conference of the BWC in 2021, India could engage in consultations with other powers to evolve a regime that can provide better oversight.[38]

Second, while most states, so far 183, have joined and ratified the BWC, still, there are many off the hook. Bringing them on board is one of the major challenges. Today the prohibition of the use of biological weapons is a rule of customary international humanitarian law, binding on all parties to all armed conflicts, including non-state armed groups.[39]

Third, equally problematic is the compliance of the BWC by member-states. This lack of an enforcement mechanism has undermined the effectiveness of the BWC, as it is unable to prevent systematic violations by the Soviet Union/Russia and others.[40] The verification of compliance of the treaty by BWC states requires implementation at the national level only. As we now know, most disarmament treaties have a very elaborate international monitoring regime. Although there is a lack of data to substantiate this point, it is widely believed that the implementation of BWC has been sloppy, and there have been violations in the past by the member states even after the entry into force of the BWC. For instance, during the 1970s, the Soviet Union expanded its existing offensive bio-weapons program. A research conglomerate of over 30 institutions produced and weaponized large quantities of bio-agents, including smallpox and the Marburg virus. These were reportedly tested under real-world conditions on an island in the Aral Sea. After the demise of the

Soviet Union, a trilateral process was initiated between the three BWC depositary powers – the US, the UK, and Russia – to investigate this matter. However, the inquiry was terminated in the mid-1990s without tangible results, having ultimately failed to shed full light on the Soviet bioweapons program.[41]

Under Saddam's regime, Iraq is thought to have produced pathogens and toxins for military purposes. More recently, it has been transpired that Syria also produced the toxin ricin. Terrorists, too, have been involved with biological agents. The Japanese-cult Aum Shinrikyo is known to have experimented with anthrax and botulinum toxin. In September and October 2001, letters containing anthrax spores were sent to two US senators and several US journalists. These letters resulted in 22 anthrax infections and five deaths, but the case was never officially solved.[42] China also seems to be having a robust bio-weapons program. The Wuhan Institute of Virology (WIV) of the Chinese Academy of Sciences (CAS) is one of 20 separate biomedical research institutes in CAS, but it is the only institute specializing in virology, viral pathology, and virus technology. It contains five research centers, including the Centre for Emerging Infectious Disease, Chinese Virus Resources and Bioinformatics Centre, Centre of Applied and Environmental Microbiology, and the Department of Analytical Biochemistry and Biotechnology. Recently, it also became China's first, and only, biosafety level 4 (BSL-4) laboratory.[43]

Fourth, the critical challenge to BWC is the so-called "response gap": i.e., how should the state parties react and respond in case of a biological attack. By extension, this would also mean how they would coordinate amongst themselves, with international organizations including the UN and the WHO, and between health and security sectors. The BWC has been discussing this issue under the assistance and cooperation, capacity-building for detecting, reporting, and responding to outbreaks of infectious disease or biological weapons attacks, including in the areas of preparedness, response, and crisis management and mitigation. Over a period, states have discussed the need to promote interagency coordination and multi-sectoral cooperation to prepare for, detect, and respond to infectious disease outbreaks, whether natural, accidental, or deliberate in nature. Also, states have realized the importance of supporting states in building defenses against new and emerging diseases and developing national capacity for responding to biological threats through detection, containment, and decontamination.[44] No country is likely to have all the resources at its immediate disposal to respond to a severe biological attack, and there is widespread recognition that there are many improvements that can be made in this area. Article VII of the BWC recognizes a need for means to enable prompt assistance under Article VII. Article VII states:

"States Parties to assist States which have been exposed to danger as a result of a violation of the Convention." To date, these provisions have not been invoked. [45]

Fifth, there is a greater need today to promote Confidence Building Measures (CBMs) – activities to be undertaken by States Parties to enhance transparency and reduce ambiguity about each other's implementation of the treaty.[46] This required annual reporting about activities at high biosafety level laboratories (BSL-3 and BSL-4), the exchange of information on biodefense programs, documentation on national legislation for the implementation of the BWC, and reporting of human vaccine production facilities. Since these CBMs have not been legally binding, more than half the state parties do not participate in them at all.[47]

In January 1995, the BWC signatory states began negotiations on a legally binding additional protocol to strengthen the BWC verification process. In March 2001, a draft protocol was tabled requiring verification of compliance with the BWC based on annual national reports about biodefense programs, vaccine production facilities, BSL-3 and BSL-4 laboratories, and installations with high production capabilities by way of voluntary visits, transparency visits, and clarification visits, under the auspices of an international BWC organization. The US opposed this draft, claiming that the BWC was unverifiable and that too much transparency could give rise to espionage against its pharmaceutical industry. Russia and China, also, were uncomfortable with the additional protocol.[48]

To avoid a complete termination of the multilateral process to strengthen the BWC, European and other Western countries advocated a substitute program that would consider the US interests. On the occasion of the Fifth Review Conference in November 2002, the states agreed to hold annual expert and states parties meetings on the following topics: National measures to implement the BWC, including national legislation; national measures to enhance safety in handling pathogenic microorganisms and toxins; improvements to international response capabilities in case of intentional deployment of biological weapons and outbreaks of diseases; strengthening of national and international efforts to identify and combat infectious diseases; and codes of conduct for scientists. Since 2003, these meetings have been held in the framework of the "Intersessional Process." In the meantime, the scope of topics has been expanded to include issues related to biosafety and biosecurity, assistance in case of an attack using bioweapons, and improvements of CBM.[49]

Sixth, the Sixth Review Conference, held in 2006, resolved to continue this successful practice and called for the establishment of a three-person BWC Implementation Support Unit (ISU) within the UN Office in Geneva to provide much-needed administrative and technical assistance to States Parties and other support activities for the BWC regime.[50] However, what we see is that the ISU is poorly staffed to meet the emerging trends and growing expectations of the member-states, and the financing of the BWC is also inadequate.[51]

Beyond COVID-19: The Way Forward

The BWC, to this day, remains the pillar of international biological weapons control. It has undoubtedly contributed to international peace and security. However, in response to a perceived violation, states under the BWC only have the choice of consulting with one another or of lodging a complaint with the United Nations Security Council (UNSC) in the hope of securing an enforceable UNSC Resolution with the consensus of all five permanent members of the Council. A state can also appeal to the International Court of Justice (ICJ), but not all states are legally bound by the BWC, nor have they necessarily all accepted the compulsory jurisdiction of the ICJ in all legal disputes. In short, the present international regime is inadequate for handling a biological weapons crisis and addressing its humanitarian and legal consequences.[52] The 2021 BWC conference will be of importance due to the COVID-19 pandemic. The developments in science and technology have brought many benefits to areas such as health, environment, and agriculture. However, we should also be conscious of the fact that unchecked and unregulated developments in science and technology, in some cases, might bring about unintentional catastrophes. In this regard, there is a need for a regular review of science and technology.[53] The upcoming review conference provides an excellent opportunity for discussing all these developments and exploring ways to strengthen the BWC.

At first glance, it can be said that the BWC does not have any direct correlation with pandemics such as the COVID-19. However, it is still not possible for scientists and experts to assess the reasons for the sudden occurrence of the COVID-19 outbreak. Whatever the real reason for this pandemic, it is necessary to underline that there is an urgent need to strengthen the Biological Weapons Convention with transparency and verification provisions for humanity to have a safer future.

Against the backdrop of the current pandemic, it is now inevitable to make a radical change in our mindsets related to the implementation of the BWC. In the current conditions, the BWC is more than a convention on WMDs. Negligence in its implementation might have a bearing on worldwide public health and international order. The COVID-19 pandemic has shown everyone around the world that microscopic pathogens indiscriminately infecting people can have just as many disruptive effects as wars waged with large armed forces and expensive military hardware. The 2021 BWC Review should, in the absence of a standing international body to oversee implementation of the BWC, deliberate upon placing the biological weapons under the jurisdiction of the existing Hague-based Organisation for the Prohibition of Chemical Weapons (OPCW). There are already instances, such as the 1925 Protocol, the Australia Group, the UNSCOM (United Nations Special Commission) and UNMOVIC (United Nations Monitoring, Verification and Inspection Commission) Commissions dealing with weapons of mass destruction in Iraq, and UNSC Resolution 1540, in which biological and chemical weapons are or have been dealt with jointly. The 2016 BWC Review Conference noted "the increasing convergence of biology and chemistry and its possible challenges and opportunities for the implementation of the Conventions".[54]

The BWC helped strengthen the norm against bioweapons, but it is dangerously inadequate today. The BWC's lack of a verification mechanism renders it useless against states secretly pursuing bioweapons. The Convention is also presently struggling for funds to fulfill basic needs and has far too few resources at hand. For example, the Chemical Weapons Convention (CWC) has about 500 employees, while the BWC's Implementation Support Unit has just three. More fundamentally, the Convention was also born in a time before gene editing, unmanned vehicles, and mass-casualty terrorism and is therefore ill-equipped to deal with the perils that arise from them.

In short, the BWC needs to be overhauled – and if that does not work, we need a new treaty. Aspiring international rule-makers like India should take the lead in shaping a new legal and administrative regime for the problem of bioweapons. The BWC (or its successor) needs to be supported by a scientific board of doctors and scientists from member states as well as representatives from the WHO and the Global Health Security Agenda. The BWC should work with other international organisations like the WHO to deal with outbreaks when they do happen. Coordinated global responses to such attacks would not only reduce the incentives for perpetrators; they would also help deal with natural outbreaks.

NOTES

1. Lawrence O. Gostin, 'COVID-19 Reveals Urgent Need to Strengthen the World Health Organization', *The JAMA Forum*, vol. 323, no. 23, 2020, p. 2361–62.
2. Manish Tewari, 'COVID-19 Is This Century's Global Inflection Point,' *Deccan Chronicle*, 27 June 2020, available at https://www.deccanchronicle.com/opinion/columnists/310320/covid-19-is-this-centurys-global-inflection-point.html, accessed 25 June 2020.
3. 'Pompeo Says "Enormous Evidence" Coronavirus Came from Wuhan Lab', *Deccan Herald*, 3

May 2020, available at https://www.deccanherald.com/international/world-news-politics/pompeo-says-enormous-evidence-coronavirus-came-from-wuhan-lab-833122.html, accessed on 25 June 2020.

4. Josh Rogin, 'Senators Demand Answers from Pompeo on Wuhan Lab Cables,' *Washington Post*, 29 April 2020, available at https://www.washingtonpost.com/opinions/2020/04/28/senators-demand-answers-pompeo-wuhan-lab-cables/, accessed on 25 June 2020.
5. Fu Yu, 'Wuhan Coronavirus and the Tacitus Trap,' *The Diplomat*, 31 January 2020, available at https://thediplomat.com/2020/01/wuhan-coronavirus-and-the-tacitus-trap/, accessed on 25 June 2020.
6. Manish Tewari, 'Does China Have a Case to Answer for Coronavirus Outbreak?' *The Asian Age*, 26 April 2020, available at https://www.asianage.com/opinion/columnists/260420/does-china-have-a-case-to-answer-for-coronavirus-outbreak.html, accessed on 24 June 2020.
7. Kathy Gilsinan, 'What's Wrong With the World Health Organization,' *The Atlantic*, 12 April 2020, available at https://www.theatlantic.com/politics/archive/2020/04/world-health-organization-blame-pandemic-coronavirus/609820/, accessed on 25 June 2020.
8. See note 2.
9. See note 2.
10. See note 8.
11. Lakshmi Puri, 'Biological Weapons and Biosecurity: Lessons from the COVID-19 War,' *Observer Research Foundation*, 9 May 2020, available at https://www.orfonline.org/expert-speak/biological-weapons-biosecurity-lessons-covid19-war-65893/, accessed on 26 June 2020.
12. Ibid.
13. Manish Tewari, 'The Post COVID-19 World,' *Observer Research Foundation*, 29 March 2020, available at https://www.orfonline.org/expert-speak/the-post-covid-19-world-63829/, accessed on 25 June 2020.
14. Sujan R. Chinoy, 'India Can Absorb Shocks of Pandemic, Take the Lead in Reshaping Global Order,' *The Indian Express*, 4 May 2020, available at https://indianexpress.com/article/opinion/columns/covid-19-pandemic-unsc-china-coronavirus-global-cases-india-lockdowm-sujan-r-chinoy-6392238/, accessed on 25 June 2020.
15. Igor Yurgens and Sergey Kulik, 'COVID-19 and Rebalancing the Global Agenda,' *Council on Foreign Relations*, 2020, available at https://www.cfr.org/sites/default/files/pdf/COVID-19%20and%20Rebalancing%20the%20Global%20Agenda.pdf, accessed on 22 June 2020.
16. Syed Akbaruddin, 'Multilateralism Post COVID-19,' *The Hindu*, 18 June 2020, available at https://www.thehindu.com/opinion/op-ed/multilateralism-post-covid-19/article31854731.ece, accessed on 22 June 2020.
17. Michal Hatuel-Radoshitzky and Ari Heistein, 'Global Governance and COVID-19: Why International Cooperation Still Matters,' *Council on Foreign Relations*, 2020, available at https://www.cfr.org/sites/default/files/pdf/Global%20Governance%20and%20COVID-19%2C%20Why%20International%20Cooperation%20Still%20Matters.pdf, accessed on 22 June 2020.
18. See note 15.
19. Huang Yukon and Jeremy Smith, 'Pandemic Response Reflects Unlearned Lessons of U.S.-China Trade War,' *Carnegie Endowment for International Peace*, 27 April 2020, available at https://carnegieendowment.org/2020/04/27/pandemic-response-reflects-unlearned-lessons-of-u.s.-china-trade-war-pub-81651, accessed on 25 June 2020.
20. See note 17.

21. Stewart M. Patrick, 'As COVID-19 Runs Rampant, the U.N. Security Council Must Act,' *World Politics Review*, 30 March 2020, available at https://www.worldpoliticsreview.com/articles/28640/as-covid-19-runs-rampant-the-u-n-security-council-must-act, accessed on 20 June 2020.
22. See note 17.
23. Tom Bernes, Lars Brozus and et al, 'Challenges of Global Governance Amid the COVID-19 Pandemic,' *Council on Foreign Relations*, May 2020, available at https://cdn.cfr.org/sites/default/files/report_pdf/challenges-of-global-governance-amid-the-covid-19-pandemic.pdf, accessed on 24 June 2020.
24. Joshua Busby, 'What International Relations Tells Us about COVID-19,' *E-International Relations*, 26 April 2020, available at https://www.e-ir.info/2020/04/26/what-international-relations-tells-us-about-covid-19/, accessed on 24 June 2020.
25. Ibid.
26. Bill Chappell, 'Coronavirus: Chaos Follows Trump's European Travel Ban; EU Says It Wasn't Warned,' *NPR*, 12 March 2020, available at https://www.npr.org/sections/goatsandsoda/2020/03/12/814876173/coronavirus-trump-speech-creates-chaos-eu-says-it-wasnt-warned-of-travel-ban, accessed on 25 June 2020.
27. Brahma Chellaney, 'The World Health Organization Must Stop Covering up China's Mistakes,' 23 April 2020, available at https://www.marketwatch.com/story/the-who-has-a-big-china-problem-2020-04-22, accessed on 22 June 2020.
28. Ibid.
29. See note 17.
30. See note 17.
31. Manish, 'The BWC Review: Issues and Challenges,' *Manohar Parrikar Institute for Defence Studies and Analyses*, July-December 2016, available at https://idsa.in/cbwmagazine/bwc-review-issues-and-challenges, accessed on 25 June 2020.
32. Ibid.
33. See note 31.
34. See note 14.
35. Filippa Lentzos and Gregory D. Koblentz, 'It's Time to Modernize the Bioweapons Convention,' *Bulletin of the Atomic Scientists*, 4 November 2016, available at https://thebulletin.org/2016/11/its-time-to-modernize-the-bioweapons-convention/, accessed on 20 June 2020.
36. Jesus S. Domingo, 'The Biological Weapons Convention (BWC) and Biosafety Diplomacy,' *Applied Biosafety*, vol. 13 no. 2, 2008, pp. 86–88.
37. See note 35.
38. See note 34.
39. 'Customary IHL - Rule 73. Biological Weapons,' *ICRC*, available at https://ihl-databases.icrc.org/customary-ihl/eng/docs/v1_rul_rule73, accessed on 25 June 2020.
40. Jonathan Tucker, 'Biological Weapons Convention (BWC) Compliance Protocol,' *NTI*, 1 August 2001, available at https://www.nti.org/analysis/articles/biological-weapons-convention-bwc/, accessed on 25 June 2020.
41. See note 31.
42. See note 31.
43. Corey Pfluke, 'Biohazard: A Look at China's Biological Capabilities and the Recent Coronavirus Outbreak,' *Air University (AU)*, 2 March 2020, available at https://www.airuniversity.af.edu/Wild-Blue-Yonder/Article-Display/Article/2094603/biohazard-a-look-at-chinas-biological-capabilities-and-the-recent-coronavirus-o/, accessed on 20 June 2020.

44. See note 31.
45. The 2017 Meeting of States Parties: Setting the Scene, *MSP Report 1*, available at http://www.bwpp.org/documents/Dailyreports/MSP17-01.pdf, accessed on 22 June 2020.
46. See note 36.
47. See note 31.
48. See note 31.
49. See note 31.
50. See note 36.
51. See note 31.
52. Carlo Trezza, 'COVID-19 Shows That the Biological Weapons Convention Must Be Strengthened,' 27 April 2020, available at https://www.europeanleadershipnetwork.org/commentary/covid-19-shows-that-the-biological-weapons-convention-must-be-strengthened/, accessed on 25 June 2020.
53. Teoman Ertuðrul Tulun, 'Urgent Need to Strengthen he Effective Implementation of The Biological Weapons Convention,' 2020, available at https://avim.org.tr/en/Yorum/URGENT-NEED-TO-STRENGTHEN-THE-EFFECTIVE-IMPLEMENTATION-OF-THE-BIOLOGICAL-WEAPONS-CONVENTION, accessed on 25 June 2020.
54. See note 52.

22

Coronavirus as God's Soldier: Assessing the Divine Retribution Narrative of Jihadi Organisations

Animesh Roul

The SARS-CoV-2 (Coronavirus) that causes COVID-19 has engulfed the whole world within weeks of its outbreak in the Chinese city of Wuhan in late December 2019. Within six months of its advent, over 8.24 million people have been infected with over four lakh deaths (as of mid-June 2020) and an ongoing major global disruption. The deadly Coronavirus pandemic has occupied centre stage in the international security discourse at present. Amid this unprecedented global crisis and healthcare chaos, evil intentions of ever opportunistic Islamist jihadi forces have come to light. While the nation states struggle to cope with the pandemic, the violent non-state actors, especially the militant Islamists and jihadists around the world, are found to be celebrating the deaths and destruction due to the spread of the disease. Surprisingly, some of the violent groups have adopted or are adhering to health guidelines issued by the World Health Organization (WHO) or The Centers for Disease Control and Prevention (CDC), even as they continue intense criticisms against these organizations by targeting the very foundations of these global health superstructures based on western science and knowledge. For example, the Taliban issued health advisories in accordance with WHO and CDC norms on Coronavirus in early March 2020 when a surge in suspected COVID-19 cases surfaced in Afghanistan, terming the pandemic as a divine test.[1]

For the Islamic extremists, the virus is a divine punishment unleashed by God (Allah) due to widespread disobedience and increasing human transgression against supreme law. They also claimed that the disease and deaths would soon bring the

'Day of Judgement.[2]' Certainly, the ongoing COVID-19 pandemic and the resultant global disruption provided a unique opportunity to transnational jihadi terrorist groups and their ideologues to justify God's law and Islamic way of life by despising Western values, culture and lifestyle. Heavily prejudiced, radical Islamic clerics blamed people's indifference towards Islam for the spread of the pandemic and argued that only Islamic teachings can save people from COVID-19. They have even urged people to join and follow Islam to be free from the wrath of Coronavirus. A section of Islamists exulted the disease spread in China as a 'punishment from Allah' for the alleged persecution of the Muslim Uighur population.[3] Even Islamist propaganda machinery worked overtime to criticise Iran and the Shia regime for the spread of the disease in Qom city, affected by the Coronavirus outbreak. The Islamic State group primarily accused Shia Iran of hypocrisy in believing in God at the time of distress and their polytheistic practices. In another seemingly weird analogy taking a dig at western societies, especially sluggish response to the COVID-19, jihadist cleric Abu Qatada al-Filistini criticised the UK (United Kingdom) government's response to the pandemic by stating that it aimed at eliminating pensioners to rid the government of their financial burden.[4]

Jihadists of all hues largely considered the COVID-19 pandemic as a God-sent force to punish the infidels and to help the believers like Jihadists of the world. Subsequently, the narrative shifted to portray COVID-19 as God's 'soldier' to teach lessons for everybody including Muslims to return to 'Allah'. This chapter examines major transnational Jihadist movements, Al Qaeda and Islamic State's responses towards the COVID-19 pandemic and how these major groups and their regional affiliates attempt to exploit the prevailing pandemic situation by spreading propaganda and inciting violence.

The Islamic State and COVID-19

Among the violent non-state groups, the first to issue advisory on Coronavirus was the Islamic State (IS). Its central leadership issued advisories for COVID-19 and dedicated a regular section on its weekly Arabic language magazine Al Naba for pandemic coverage starting late February 2020. But unlike the Taliban, it has based the guidelines on the teachings of Prophet Muhammad and the Quran. Through Al-Naba, the group has advised its members, followers and sympathisers across the world on how to protect oneself against disease and epidemics. With an infographic, it urged fellow members to put their trust in God and seek refuge in him from diseases and also mentioned that the spread of the disease is happening with God's command.

Much before the guidelines, the IS lauded the corona outbreak in China. In January, IS mentioned about the rising Coronavirus in *Al-Naba*, terming it as a punishment from 'God Almighty' for China's abuse of Uyghurs.[5] On 12 March 2020, the IS issued religious directives on how to protect oneself against the epidemic. The infographic did not mention 'Coronavirus', or 'COVID-19' as such, but suggested few usual preventive measures, e.g., to stay away from infected or sick persons, avoiding travel to the affected region (e.g. China and Iran), covering one's mouth when coughing, and handwashing etiquettes.[6]

Again, on 19 March issue of *Al Naba*, the IS urged its followers to take maximum advantage of the way this pandemic has engulfed and engaged the powerful countries of the world. In its editorial titled, "The Crusaders' worst nightmare", it has directed its foot soldiers to take advantage of world governments' preoccupation with the COVID-19 pandemic to step up their jihadist attacks, including in the West.[7] The initial IS directives which termed the disease simply as a deadly illness, also urged its supporters to keep their faith in Allah (God) and seek refuge in him stressing that diseases spread with 'His' command only. It has criticized Muslims who believe in the notion that the US or China was behind the spread of COVID-19 with the ulterior motive of global economic and security dominance. In response, the IS underscored that COVID-19 is not man-made or human-driven scourge, rather it is affecting mankind by Allah's order. However, it stressed several times in its media releases that COVID-19 could very well affect Muslims in China and elsewhere, irrespective of their faith.

Subsequently, the IS published views on the Coronavirus spread and how it has been disrupting global security. It urged violent attacks and incited its followers to take advantage of the widespread disruption and ongoing preoccupation of countries in the Middle East and Europe with the disease containment. It gloated in the late March 2020 edition of Al-Naba about the coalition force withdrawal from the al-Qaim base in western Iraq's Al Anbar province due to the COVID-19 pandemic. The IS weekly also rejoiced with media reports at that time about how the US may soon become the next epicentre of the pandemic.

The Islamic State's regional branches too came out with a similar narrative. One of its youngest branches, the Kashmir and India focused group Ansar ul Khilafa-e Hind (IS-India) urged its followers and fellow Muslims ("believers" in India and beyond) in one of its monthly magazines (Swat al-Hind or Voice of India, 25 March 2020) to take advantage of governments and security forces' preoccupation with COVID-19. It incited them to strike the infidels but to show mercy for Muslims. In an article titled 'Coronavirus', it said, "Know that sickness and healings are only by Allah's command [...] the ever increasing rate of COVID-19 that we are witnessing is a torment for the disbelievers and has brought the glad tidings for the believers." It further added, "Allah has made this disease a source of chaos amongst the nations of disbelief, and their militaries and police have been deployed in their streets and alleys, thus making them an easy target [...]. Use this opportunity to strike them with a sword or a knife or even a rope is enough to stop their breath, fill the streets with their blood."[8]

Besides the IS and affiliated groups, several IS sympathisers taking to social media (e.g RocketChat, Hoop and Telegram) have urged violent strikes against the West amid the pandemic. In early April, IS sympathisers and groups (e.g. the Greenb1rds group or AbuDujana07) shared a poster featuring London's iconic Tower Bridge and the US city of Chicago. The posters titled O Muwahhideen [true believers]! Hit them when they least expect it". The Greenb1rd group, which intermittently calls for "lone wolf" attacks against the West, hailed the Coronavirus outbreak as 'divine bio-weapon', describing the pandemic as "a soldier of Allah".[9]

Similarly, pro-IS groups circulated a statement titled "today, where are the titans? West & United States have lost the battle Coronavirus (COVID-19)" through RocketChat channel on 30 March 2020. The message made fun of western military and economic might. It said "by the divine command of Allah, all the Las Vegas hotels, gambling clubs have closed; the streets of prostitution in Amsterdam are closed, and by the command of Allah today, all countries of the world have closed down nudist clubs, gays, nightclubs, bars and many restaurants. By the command of Allah, today the largest number of planes during history is on the ground knocks down." It further added that "the whole world is searching for deliverance [...] where are the people who thought they were capable of it. Where are the titans?"[10]

On 28 May, an official audio statement from Islamic State spokesman Shaykh Abu Hamza al-Qurashi reiterated the Jihadist sentiments terming the COVID-19 as divine retribution. The 39-minute audio broadcast titled, "And the Disbelievers Will Know who Gets the Good End" (al Furqan Media) was circulated in several languages and on different platforms. "We rejoice today with the great torment of God that befell you", he said in his message adding that "God sent the weakest of his creatures – a creature that cannot be seen with the naked eye", obviously pointing towards the Coronavirus. Hamza al-Qurashi again gloated talking about the COVID-19 crisis by saying in these words: "O Crusaders, you have been afflicted because of the divine retribution for your evil deeds. You have fought the religion of Allah and His worshipers, and conspired against the Islamic State."[11] This message transcript was circulated in at least 10 languages through pro-IS social media outlets subsequently.

Al Qaeda and COVID-19

Unlike the Taliban or Islamic State, Al Qaeda entered late into the COVID-19 and jihad propaganda. Its first comment on the pandemic surfaced as late as 31 March, when Al Qaeda central coaxed Western nations and non-Muslims to join Islam, telling them "we want to share heaven with you just as we share this earth". In a six-page release titled 'The Way Forward', the Al Qaeda central command urged people of other faiths to take advantage of time in quarantine to read and learn about Islam. It chided the western and advanced nations by saying that the very "technological advancement and globalisation that Man took immense pride has become hid undoing [...] If someone sneezes in China, those in New York suffer from its consequences." It further reiterated that this pandemic is a 'punishment from the Lord of the Worlds for the injustice and oppression committed against Muslims' specifically and mankind in general by the Western powers.[12] Taking pride by saying 'Islam is a hygiene-oriented Religion', the same message took a dig at China and its unhealthy practices too with following words: "Let us not forget that COVID-19 emerged from one of the filthiest places on earth, the markets of Wuhan, where all known norms of decent and humane dietary practices were trampled upon. From insects to rodents and reptiles, in short everything unsafe for human consumption, or the consumption of which is prohibited in all revealed religions, was sold and consumed there."[13]

The group again condemned Western countries, particularly the UK and the US, for implementing COVID-19 policies that were allegedly designed to get rid of the weak and elderly. In its second issue of English-language magazine 'One Ummah', the Al Qaeda central blamed the Western philosophy for considering COVID-19 pandemic as a "final solution" to get rid of the 'aged' who are considered a burden on the economy and that is 'the savage reality of western materialism'.[14] It gloated that the microscopic soldier of Allah' (the Coronavirus) has exposed the bitter truths about the western countries. In its editorial, it rejoiced at the myriad problems grappling the US at present and said "Corona, internal divisions, racism, shambled economy and terrorist attacks would comprise five corners of America's 'pentagonal coffin'."[15]

Al Qaeda's regional affiliates too stepped up their campaigns exploiting Coronavirus spread in their respective regions spanning from Syria to Bangladesh. Syria based Hayat Tahrir al-Sham (HTS), one of the powerful pro-Al Qaeda jihadi groups in Syria, issued instructions to its fighters and followers to stay focussed and not to get distracted by the COVID-19. It urged its fighters to continue their anti-Shiites campaigns. The HTS leaders such as Abu Mariya al Qahtani called Coronavirus a temporary epidemic, but for him, Shiites are a permanent problem that has corrupted Islam and its people.[16]

HTS's Ebaa newsletter published an infographic in mid-March 2020 terming the Coronavirus a God-sent force that is here to kill those who are instrumental in killing Muslims all over the world. However, realising the power of the disease, it urged its followers to stay isolated, avoid gatherings and shaking hands with each other.[17] Similar to HTS, Al Qaeda's African affiliate al-Shabaab released an audio message about the Coronavirus pandemic on 29 April 2020. This audio message by its leader Sheikh Ali Mahmoud Ragi blamed the apostate' countries for the origin and spread of the Coronavirus to the Muslim nations. It further added that pandemics are a 'punishment from God to his servants to remind them of their sins and injustices and also to remind them that there is a harsher punishment awaiting them.' He reiterated the usual jihadi narrative against China i.e. God is avenging the crimes against the Uighur Muslims. It also took a dig at western powers (crusaders) presently under the grip of COVID-19 who have 'killed Muslims in Afghanistan, Iraq, Syria, Yemen, Somalia, and the Maghreb'.[18]

The Ansar-al Islam-Bangladesh (AAI), a regional affiliate of Al Qaeda in the Indian Subcontinent (AQIS) too has engaged in virtual campaign amid this ongoing pandemic situation in the country. While terming the COVID-19 as 'A curse from Allah', extremist leaders are highlighting the government's failure to tackle the virus spread and to find a cure and how it has brought back poverty upon the people.[19]

Disease as a Weapon?

A cursory look at various Jihadist ideologies suggests that Salafis and Takfiris are not averse to use disease as a weapon against their perceived enemy, i.e. western countries and people from other religions or faiths. Past records, jihadi literature, and intelligence inputs have proven that jihadi groups such as Al Qaeda and the Islamic States have both the capability and intention to use disease as a weapon. In the past, Al Qaeda's effort to acquire disease pathogens for the subversive purpose indicated its evil intention and motivations. Many efforts, though largely unsuccessful, have gone into these kinds of insidious projects, for example, "Yogurt Project" or 'Project al-Zabadi (Arabic') to develop chemical and biological weapons in the past.[20] Al Qaeda's Encyclopaedia of Jihad (vol. 11) documented and offered guidance on how to disperse potentially lethal biological organisms and poisons, ranging from botulinum toxin, anthrax and ricin. This volume has elaborated tactics and targets such as water and food supplies and how to maximize panic and fear by poisoning. A similar manual titled 'A Course in Popular Poisons and Deadly Gases' by Abu Hadhifa al-Shami too shed light on the group's future designs of biowarfare.[21] Jihadist ideologues like Anwar al Awlaki, too rationalized the use of biological pathogens against civilians population, promoting mass killings of 'disbelievers' in a war.[22]

Through violent terrorist groups have not succeeded in achieving a capability to either develop or use biological pathogens, their undying intention to procure causes a global concern, especially at a time when the global healthcare system is struggling to cope with a novel deadly virus such as Coronavirus. Previously, both Al Qaeda and Islamic State groups have attempted to exploit similar viral disease outbreaks such as Ebola and Zika virus. During the 2014 Ebola outbreak in West African countries, there were discussions in Al Qaeda circles on how to weaponise this deadly strains of the virus against the United States and other western countries. Pro-Al Qaeda English language virtual forum such as Ansar al-Mujahideen had a discussion on using the Ebola virus to strike terror into the hearts of the West (the US). The idea was floated in the forum about an intentional spread of disease into the territory of the US. It was suggested that any Al Qaeda member playing a bio-martyr, can do this by visiting epidemic zones in West Africa first and then by traveling to the US. The plot did not materialise for Al Qaeda as the use of Ebola through a bio-martyr seemed untenable and highly ambitious task from a bio-violence perspective.[23] Similarly, the Islamic State group members were found mulling the idea to spread the deadly Zika virus through infected mosquito to spread terror against the US and the European countries after they found out about the lethality of the virus. The 2016 Zika outbreak caused a grave global concern but the lethality brought out the evil intentions of jihadi groups such as the IS to the fore.[24]

Irrespective of past interests in deadly disease pathogens, either Al Qaeda and IS groups have not yet considering or at least thinking to exploit the Coronavirus yet. However, even though the harvesting of pathogens is quite an uphill task for terrorist groups, the very discourse on its possible use is unsettling.

Conclusion

Undoubtedly, the COVID-19 pandemic is a challenging and uphill crisis the modern world is confronting since the Second World War. This pandemic has virtually pushed countries' preoccupation with military and counterterrorism priorities to the back burner. Fearing widespread social and political unrest across the world, the United Nation Secretary General Antonio Guterres has rightly underscored that this pandemic is a significant threat to the maintenance of international peace and security. He underscored that this pandemic has exposed the inherent weaknesses and the dearth of preparedness in global public health systems. While raising the issue of a possible 'bio-terrorist' threat amid this ongoing crisis, Guterres speculated that violent 'Non-State groups' could gain access to virulent strains that could pose similar devastation to societies across the world. [25]

Taking advantage of this global chaos, Jihadist groups are trying to spread disinformation against the government's failure in handling a 'divine soldier'. Whether it is Al Qaeda or Islamic State, each group is trying to exploit the prevalent situation, preparing for consolidation and resurgence against their perceived enemies. Peddling fear, these transnational jihadist groups are attempting to establish legitimacy as well as bring more recruits and followers to their respective folds. Not only have they stepped up their propaganda campaign, they have also called to unleash mindless violence against societies overwhelmed with this public health emergency.

NOTES

1. 'Coronavirus: Taliban tells WHO it will 'Cooperate and Coordinate' with Health Workers as Virus Spreads,' *The Independent*, 18 March 2020, available at https://www.independent.co.uk/news/world/coronavirus-spread-afghanistan-taliban-health-workers-world-health-organisation-a9409366.html, accessed on 25 June 2020.
2. The concept of Judgment Day is a fundamental tenet of Islam which marks the end of the present world. On this day human being will be resurrected and judged by their act of righteousness and sinfulness. Accordingly, they will be rewarded 'heaven' or 'hellfire'. See, Juan e Campo, Encyclopedia of Islam, Facts on File Inc, New York, 2009, pp.413-414.
3. 'Scholar of Iran Calling Coronavirus 'Divine Punishment' got Infected Himself,' *Global Village Space*, 11 March 2020, available at https://www.globalvillagespace.com/scholar-of-iran-calling-coronavirus-divine-punishment-got-infected-himself/, accessed on 22 June 2020.
4. Coronavirus: See wetin ISIS, Boko Haram and oda jihadist leaders dey tok about COVID-19, *BBC News Pidgin*, 24 May 2020, available at https://www.bbc.com/pidgin/tori-52782460, accessed on 22 June 2020.
5. Bridget Johnson, 'ISIS Lauds 'Death and Terror' of Coronavirus Outbreak,' *Homeland Security Today*, 27 January 2020, available at https://www.hstoday.us/subject-matter-areas/counterterrorism/isis-lauds-death-and-terror-of-coronavirus-oubreak/, accessed on 25 June 2020.
6. 'Islamic Guidance on Dealing with Epidemics,' *Al Naba*, no. 225, 12 March 2020.
7. 'The Crusader's Worst Nightmare,' *Al Naba*, no. 226, 19 March 2020.
8. 'Coronavirus,' *Voice of Hind*, no. 2, March 2020, p.7.
9. 'Green B1rds (Unofficial Islamic State): "O Muwahideen! Hit Them When They Least Expect

It,' *Terrorism Research & Analysis Consortium Beacham Publishing*, 03 April 2020, available at http://www.trackingterrorism.org/chatter/cgi-green-b1rds-unofficial-islamic-state-o-muwahideen-hit-them-when-they-least-expect-it-cor, accessed on 23 June 2020.

10. 'Islamic State Supporters Circulate: Today, Where Are the Titans?!' *TRAC Chatter*, 30 March 2020, available at https://www.trackingterrorism.org/chatter/statement-islamic-state-supporters-circulate-today-where-are-titans-30-march-2020-battle-cor, accessed on 24 June 2020.
11. The full transcript of Hamza al-Qurashi's audio statement, *Voice of Hind*, no. 5, June 2020, p.6.
12. 'The Way Forward: A Word of Advice on the Coronavirus Pandemic,' *Al-Sahab Foundation*, 31 March 2020.
13. Ibid.
14. Salama al Najdi, 'The Corona Pandemic: Treatment of the Elderly From the perspective of Islamic Sharia and Western Philosophy,' *One Ummah*, no. 2, June 2020, pp.25-26.
15. 'One Ummah,' no. 2, *Al-Sahab Foundation*, June 2020, p.4.
16. 'Jihadist Perspectives on Coronavirus Pandemic: Primary Sources,' Cited in Aymenn Jawad Al-Tamimi, 25 March 2020, available at http://www.aymennjawad.org/2020/03/jihadist-perspectives-on-coronavirus-pandemic,accessed on 22 June 2020.
17. Hayy'at Tahrir al-Sham, 'How to Protect Yourself Against Coronavirus COVID -19?' *Ebaa News Agency*, 17 March 2020, available at https://www.trackingterrorism.org/chatter/infographic-ebaa-news-agency-hayyat-tahrir-al-sham-hts-how-protect-yourself-against-coronavi, accessed on 23 June 2020.
18. 'It Is Natural That We Will Rejoice In The Destruction of The Infidels In This Epidemic,' *TRAC Chatter*, 29 April 2020, available at https://www.trackingterrorism.org/chatter/statement-al-shabaab-movements-first-comment-corona-spokesperson-al-shabaab-it-natural-we-wi, accessed on 24 June 2020.
19. Kamran Reza Chowdhury, 'Bangladeshi Militants Take Advantage of COVID-19 Pandemic,' *BenarNews*, 18 June 2020, available at https://www.benarnews.org/english/news/bengali/covid-militancy-06182020155559.html, accessed on 23 June 2020.
20. Dan Darling, 'Abu Khabab and Project al-Zabadi,' *Long War Journal*, 19 September 2005, available at https://www.longwarjournal.org/archives/2005/09/abu_khabab_and_1.php, accessed on 24 June 2020.
21. Abu Hadhifa al-Shami's, 'A Course in Popular Poisons and Deadly Gases,' *Islamic Media Center (unspecified Year)*, a summary at "Survey of Prevalent Al-Qa' ida Manuals", available at https://www.aclu.org/files/fbimappingfoia/20150309/ACLURM016597.pdf, accessed on 25 June 2020.
22. Anwar al Awalki, 'Targeting the Populations of Countries at War with Muslims,' *Inspire* (Al-Malahem Media), vol. 8, 2011, pp, 41-47.
23. 'Bio-Martyrs: A Very Real Threat at Unique Moment in Time,' *Homeland Security Today*, 28 August 2014, available at https://www.hstoday.us/channels/global/exclusive-bio-martyrs-a-very-real-threat-at-unique-moment-in-time/, accessed on 28 June 2020.
24. Ted Reynolds, 'Seeing COVID-19 as an Opportunity,' *Cairo Review of Global Affairs*, 03 May 2020, available at https://www.thecairoreview.com/essays/seeing-covid-19-as-an-opportunity/, accessed on 25 June 2020.
25. "COVID-19 threatening global peace and security, UN chief warns", *UN News*, 10 April 2020, available at https://news.un.org/en/story/2020/04/1061502, accessed on 25 June 2020.

SECTION V

BIOLOGICAL SECURITY

23

After COVID-19: Time to Agree a Biosecurity Code of Conduct Under the Biological and Toxin Weapons Convention

Simon Whitby, Cheng Tang, Lijun Shang and Malcolm Dando

Largely out of sight of most people, States Parties to the Biological and Toxin Weapons Convention (BTWC) have been meeting at the United Nations in Geneva over the last two decades trying to find ways to strengthen the Convention following the failure to agree on a Protocol during the 1990s. Given the application of developments in science in the major offensive military biological warfare programmes of the Twentieth Century, where viruses, toxins, bacteria and fungi had been weaponised[1], one major concern for the States has been the impact of rapid advances in the life sciences on the potential ease with which novel and very dangerous biological and toxin weapons could be developed by States, Non-State Actors, or even individuals.[2] The devastating COVID-19 disease outbreak in early 2020 is likely to cause a major rethink about the dangers of natural, accidental and deliberate disease outbreaks in humans, animals and plants when the outbreak is eventually brought under control[3]. As part of that rethink, it should be possible now, 45 years after the Convention entered into force[4], to bring the protracted discussions on a Code of Conduct under the Convention to a successful conclusion at the 2021 9th Five-Year Review Conference of the BTWC. This would make a major contribution to the prevention of further such outbreaks by engaging life scientists effectively for the first time in support of the prohibition of biological weapons that are embodied in the BTWC.

The problem that concerns States Parties to the BTWC was set out at the turn of the century in 2000 by Matthew Meselson, Professor of Molecular Biology at Harvard University when he questioned whether, as all previous scientific and technological revolutions had been applied in major ways to hostile purposes, it was probable that the same would happen to the revolution in civil biotechnology unless we found ways to prevent that happening. He also thought that this would be a long drawn out struggle, stating that:[5]

> "...During the century ahead, as our ability to modify fundamental life processes continues its rapid advance, we will be able not only to devise additional ways to destroy life but will also become able to manipulate it – including the processes of cognition, development, reproduction and inheritance....Therein could lie unprecedented opportunities for violence, coercion, repression, or subjugation..."

And he pointed out that dangerous capabilities could be available to a much wider range of actors than were available in relation to nuclear weapons:

> "...Unlike the technologies of conventional or even nuclear weapons, biotechnology has the potential to place mass destructive capabilities in a multitude of hands and, in coming decades, to reach deeply into what we are and how we regard ourselves. It should be evident that any intensive exploitation of biotechnology for hostile purposes could take humanity down a particularly undesirable path."

In the following two decades these concerns were illustrated by a series of publications of experiments by civil scientists that caused increasing consternation amongst the security analysts about the possibility of their facilitating the development of novel biological weapons, and this led to a series of major meetings and reports about this *problem of dual use* – the fact that benignly-intended civil research might later be used by others for hostile purposes. It became clear during these two decades that a range of different means applied at various levels in a "Web of Prevention"[6] would be required in order to minimize the potential for the biotechnology revolution to be misapplied for hostile purposes.[7] This paper examines the evolution of the idea of a Code of Conduct under the Convention being a useful part of that web in meetings of the States Parties to the Biological and Toxin Weapons Convention (BTWC) during the past two decades.

Following the failure to bring the decade-long efforts to strengthen the Convention to a successful conclusion at the 2001 5th Review Conference the UK, as one of the three Depositary States for the Convention, produced a summary (a Green Paper) of the available options for developing the Convention in the run up to the recommencement of the meeting in late 2002. A review of this paper[8] noted that one option was "codes of conduct for professional bodies" but also noted that "[W]hile there would be benefits from such an international code of ethics, the Green Paper says nothing as to how such a code might be developed or implemented." Nevertheless, at the meeting in Geneva States Parties to the BTWC agreed that as part of the new Intersessional Process of annual meetings at Expert (MX) level (in the summer) and State Parties (MSP) level (later in the year) the content, promulgation, and adoption of codes of conduct for scientists would be the subject for the meetings in 2005.[9] These annual meetings in 2003, 2004 and 2005 would be used to discuss, and promote common understanding and effective actions to support the Convention.

The Initial Meeting on Codes of Conduct in 2005

By the time of the 2005 Meeting of Experts, the difficulties encountered in the later stages of the attempt to negotiate a verification system during the 1990s had reduced and there was certainly an attempt to deal seriously with the issue of codes of conduct with large numbers of papers being produced for the meetings in 2005 (Table 1).

Table 1: Papers produced for the 2005 Meeting on Codes of Conduct*

Background Papers
Four Papers by the Secretariat
One Presentation by the United States
State Working Papers (Total 35)
Argentina 1, Canada 7, UK 4, Germany 6, Russia 2, China 1, Japan 2, India 1, Indonesia 1, South Africa 1, Iran 1, Australia 4, Cuba 2, Korea 1, Italy 1
Additional Working Papers at the MSP
India 1, Russia 1

*Data from the UN website in Geneva under Biological Weapons Convention/Meetings and Documents.

The papers[10] by the Secretariat covered codes that referred to the BTWC, codes relevant to the life sciences that did not refer to the BTWC, elements of codes from other fields and relevant organisation, associations, professional bodies and institutions which could serve as sources of guidance in the formulation of codes of conduct. The presentation by the United States was a wide-ranging review of relevant codes in the United States.[11] It began by asking some basic questions about codes of conduct (Table 2).

Table 2: Some Basic Questions about Codes of Conduct*

What is a "Code of Conduct"?
- Formal statement of values and professional practices of a group of individuals with a common focus, either an occupation, academic field, or social doctrine.
- Defines the expectations and directs the actions of a group.

Examples of Codes of Conduct for the Life Science
- The Nuremberg Code
- The Belmont Report
- American Society of Microbiology (ASM) Code of Conduct
- Code of Ethics for the Life Sciences

Why a Code of Conduct for Dual Use Research?
- Government cannot oversee all scientists and experiments across the nation.
- Offers greatest opportunity for improving security of research at the level of individual scientists:
- Increases understanding of biosecurity;
- Persistent reminder of moral and ethical responsibilities:
- Creates a "culture of responsibility and accountability".
- Sets professional standards that may have legal implications.

*From BWC/MSP/2005/MX/MISC.4.

Canada similarly submitted a series of papers on common elements codes used in government, professional associations, academia and biodefence together with separate papers on the overlap between codes of conduct and legislation and on the functions of codes of conduct. However, the paper on the functions of codes also considered their possible weaknesses noting, for example, that:[12]

> "False or unrealistic expectations can damn the best of ideas. The creation of code of conduct that will make for a safer, happier, more productive work environment is a lofty goal, but one that will be doomed to failure if the code is ignored.... In addition, an ambitious code of conduct can be derailed by individuals who decide that they do not wish to follow its provisions, with no perceptible consequences to them. This is a key problem with virtually all codes of conduct that lack the power of applying sanctions to violators. Even a code that may have the backing of a financial, professional or legislative sanction may succumb to the pitfalls of disillusionment if not properly constructed."

A related point of particular interest here was raised by Australia in its Working Paper 29.[13] This stated that:

> "1. Amongst the Australian scientific community, there is a low level of awareness of the risk of misuse of the biological sciences to assist in the development of biological or chemical weapons. Many scientists working in 'dual-use' areas simply do not consider the possibility that their work could

> inadvertently assist in a biological or chemical weapons programme. *For most of these researchers, biological weapons issues may seem irrelevant and therefore strong advocacy is required to overcome natural resistance or ignorance...*" (emphasis added)

The paper therefore continued by reasoning it followed that"

> "... Introducing Codes of Conduct that highlight these issues is an important step in raising awareness. *However, it is not enough simply to put such Codes in place. Without effective measures to educate scientists about the existence and importance of such Codes, attitudes and awareness will remain largely unchanged.*" (emphasis added).

Brian Rappert and Malcolm Dando had reported just before the Meeting of Experts on the results of a series of seminars that they had conducted at life science departments in universities in the UK. They concluded that:[14]

> "There was little evidence from our seminars that participants:
>
> (a) Regarded bioterrorism or bioweapons as a substantial threat;
> (b) Considered that developments in the life sciences research contributed to biothreats;
> (c) Were aware of the current debates and concerns about dual-use research; or
> (d) Were familiar with the BTWC." (original emphasis).

These authors were therefore in agreement with the Australian position. Moreover, in a further paper before the Sixth Review Conference in 2006, they reported very similar findings from seminars in five other countries.[15] The need for education of life scientists was reiterated by the Russian Federation in a paper for the Meeting of States Parties later in 2005.[16] Russia supported the idea of a code and gave it as the first core element that scientists should "[B]e well informed of, and apply in their practice, international and national regulatory legal instruments on the prohibition of biological and toxin weapons." So even in 2005 just introducing a code of conduct was not seen to be sufficient to deal with the problem of the potential misuse of research by some of the States Parties.

The Meeting on Codes of Conduct in 2008

Given this level of interest it was unsurprising that the 6th Review Conference in 2006 decided that in 2008 during the Second Intersessional Process States Parties would focus on two topics, the second of which being:[17]

> "...Oversight, education, awareness raising, and adoption and/or

> development of codes of conduct with the aim of preventing misuse in the context of advances in bio-science and bio-technology research with the potential of use for purposes prohibited by the Convention."

Again in 2008, there were two contributions by the Implementation Support Unit on Codes of Conduct, Education and Awareness-Raising and a further eight Working Papers by States Parties, including by China,[18] on these topics. The most significant contribution was by the Netherlands. Their Working Paper stated that:[19]

> "A code is a set of principles and instructions that are binding on members of a particular group in a profession or industry.…Moreover, *codes can be classified into different types. Brian Rappert developed this typology…"* (emphasis added).

Brian Rappert, as a Sociologist, had suggested the typology that the Working Paper then set out. This typology can be summarised as follows:

- Aspirational Codes (Set Standards);
- Advisory Codes (Provide Guidelines); and
- Enforceable Codes (Make Legal Requirements).

Today, a decade and a half after Rappert's original 2004 paper, it is well worth reading, particularly his summary of the state of the discussions about codes of conduct at that stage:[20]

> "There is a renewed interest in codes to apply to the scientific and industrial life sciences community. Despite the extent and varied interest in a code or codes, there is a lack of detailed proposals about just what such a code or codes would entail. A close reading of the initial proposals shows that there are different concepts about who should devise codes; whether they should be voluntary or enforceable; what purpose they might serve (e.g., raise awareness, proscribe specific actions); what issues they should cover; by what mechanisms they could be agreed; whether a new code is necessary or existing ones should be augmented; and whether there should be a single universal code or various local ones…"

Rappert also argued that it could be very confusing if different people were discussing different types of codes. It has become clear that the discussions in Geneva are best related to an *Aspirational Code* that could be agreed at this international level and then implemented in a variety of codes to fit the different requirements in various countries.

What it is important to understand is that in 2008 it was widely thought that developing a code could be a means to raise awareness of the problem of dual use amongst scientists. This idea was in direct contradiction to the view put forward in 2005 by Australia. As was quite clearly stated in the Netherlands paper as *"[T]he main aim of the Dutch Code of Conduct on Biosecurity is to be seen as a contribution to awareness raising."* The code developed by the Netherlands was widely circulated for example by the InterAcademy Panel, but while the need for education was noted in the code there was no requirement for it to be in place to support the code. The impact of the lack of education was illustrated by the account given by Koos van der Bruggen of the surprise, among the young researchers in the Netherlands who researched on the airborne transmission of highly pathogenic avian influenza in 2011, at the consternation caused by the submission of their work for publication. According to this account, one of the researchers said that:[21]

> "...he never imagined that the paper would get a red light from the NSABB [National Science Advisory Board for Biosecurity in the United States] and become the focus of a heated international debate about the limits of academic freedom. Watching the flood of news coverage, 'it was strange to think that we had created all of that in our lab'..."

That in regard to an experiment that many security analysts would see as raising very obvious dual-use concerns.

Nevertheless, progress was being made in the development of educational material linked to the BTWC for life scientists. For example, at the 2008 Meeting of Experts Professor Norihiko Yamada made a Statement in the Non-Government Organisations section on a joint Japan/UK project on the development of an Educational Module for Life Scientists. The module is still available on the website of the Federation of American Scientists and consists of lecture slides, references and question topics for 21 lectures in five sections: Introduction; The Threat of Biological Warfare, Biological Terrorism and the International Prohibition Regime; The Dual-Use Dilemma and the Responsibilities of Scientists; National Implementation of the BTWC; and Building an Effective Web of Prevention to Ensure Benign Development.

Developing Ideas on Education in Support of Codes of Conduct

This lack of education about dual use was again brought to the attention of States Parties in a contribution by Japan in a joint Working Paper titled *Possible approaches to education and awareness-raising among life scientists* by Australia, Canada, Japan, New Zealand, Republic of Korea, Switzerland, Kenya, Sweden, Ukraine, United Kingdom and the United States at the Seventh Review Conference in 2011. Japan's contribution stated that:[22]

> "...the National Defense Medical College (NDMC) in Japan and the University of Bradford in the UK conducted collaborative research to analyse the current state of biosecurity education in Japan. The research found that there was a lack of educational topics on biosecurity despite a certain level of presence of dual-use references, mainly due to an absence of space in the existing curricula, an absence of time and resources to develop new curricula, an absence of expertise as well as doubt about the need for biosecurity education..."

The paper also noted that "[P]arallel to this survey, the NDMC and the University of Bradford also jointly developed an online learning module in applied dual-use biosecurity education." Moreover, given that level of interest in the topic amongst States Parties it was not surprising that the Review Conference decided that, under the Standing Agenda on developments in the field of science and technology related to the Convention, the Third Intersessional Process would consider:[23]

(d) voluntary codes of conduct and other measures to encourage responsible conduct by scientists, academia and industry;
(e) education and awareness-raising about risks and benefits of life sciences and biotechnology..."

Thus, the Meeting of States Parties in 2015 concluded that:[24]

> "To further address education and awareness-raising about risks and benefits of life sciences and biotechnology, States Parties recognized that the continuous and accelerating rate of progress in scientific knowledge requires the necessity of deepening a culture of responsible use of this knowledge, which takes into account the object and purpose of the Convention without undermining peaceful uses. In order to further efforts on education and awareness-raising about risks and benefits of life sciences and biotechnology, States Parties discussed the need to share information and knowledge on these developments, including dual-use research of concern."

Then in 2016 at the Preparatory Committee for the Seventh Review Conference, China and Pakistan put forward a significant proposal for the development of a template for a code of conduct. Their Working Paper stated that:[25]

> "With the aim to prevent abuse and misuse of bioscience and technology, fulfil the aims and objectives of the Convention and strengthen global biosecurity governance, China has proposed the development of a template of biological scientist code of conduct within the framework of the Convention in December 2015..."

The paper went on to point out that many States had indicated support for the idea and provided suggestions. The elements of the proposed code are set out in

Table 3A. The Working Paper proposed that States Parties should "[F]ully exchange views on the issue 'the development of the template of biological scientist code of conduct under the framework of the BWC' under relevant agenda of the Eighth Review Conference."

Table 3A: Elements of the 2015 China/Pakistan Draft Model Code of Conduct for Biological Scientists*

1. Ethical Benchmark
2. Legal Restraint
3. Research Integrity
4. Respect for the Object of Research
5. Applying Science Research and its Relevant Process
6. Constraint on the Spread of Research
7. Popularizing Science and Technology
8. Organisation's Role
9. International Exchange

* From BWC/CONF.VIII/WP.30

At the Review Conference itself Ukraine and the UK, reflecting on their joint studies and research, pressed the case for serious attention to be given to the education of scientists given the current lack of awareness of the Convention and its implications. Their joint Working Paper argued that:[26]

> "18. The Conference should therefore adopt the following language in the Final Declaration text for Article IV:
>
> > The Conference stresses the critical importance of biosecurity education and awareness-raising in achieving effective implementation of the Convention, which should be put into effect through national implementation measures, as appropriate, in accordance with the constitutional process and practices of each State Party.
>
> 19. The Conference notes that such measures could include…
>
> > (c) promoting the development and implementation of training and education programmes as well as training guides, handbooks and course materials, including raising awareness of the implications of dual use research and technology, for those granted access to biological agents and toxins relevant to the Convention, and especially for those with the knowledge or capacity to modify such agents and toxins…"

Ukraine, Japan and the UK again pressed the case for serious attention to be given to education at the 2017 Meeting of States Parties in a Working Paper on *Recent Developments in Education*. The joint paper suggested that:[27]

"19. There are a number of key points that States Parties might draw from these experiences, taking into account what is most appropriate given their own national structures and organisations:

The need to reach out and engage with stakeholders over a period, obtain their interest and support, and build networks; it is especially important to engage with staff who will deliver the teaching, and students who will study the materials, to ensure that learning will be effective.

The need to develop appropriate teaching materials, adapting what is already available for their own national circumstances and developing complementary material where necessary.

The benefits of international collaboration and shared experience and expertise.

The benefits of using websites and online techniques to facilitate communication and learning.

The importance of continuing efforts to ensure sustainability."

Finally, China and Pakistan made a clear-cut proposal for bringing this long period of development to a conclusion at the Ninth Review Conference in 2021. At the 2018 Meeting of Experts, they presented a Working Paper that included a draft *Model Code of Conduct for Biological Scientists* (Table 3B).

Table 3B: Elements of the 2018 China Draft Model Code of Conduct for Biological Scientists*

1. Ethical Standard
2. Research Integrity
3. Respect for the Object of Research
4. Process Management for Science Research
5. Constraint on the Spread of Research Outcome
6. Popularisation of Science and Technology
7. Institution's Role
8. Education and Training
9. Awareness and Engagement
10. International Exchanges

*From reference 24

Crucially, China's Working Paper stated:[28]

"9. Hereby, we propose to:

Continue in-depth discussion on the topic of 'development of a model code of conduct for biological scientists', with a view to reaching consensus on the content of the model code of conduct.

Facilitate the approval of the model code of conduct for biological scientists by the Ninth Review Conference, as well as the authorization by the Review

> Conference to work on implementation and promotion of the model code of conduct in the future inter-sessional process."

The presentation at the Meeting of Experts had been preceded by an international conference in Tianjin, China on *Building a Global Community of Shared Future for Biosecurity: Development of a Code of Conduct for Biological Scientists* at which China's ideas for the code were discussed in detail by a range of 28 experts from 14 different countries, 6 experts from international organisations and a large host delegation from China itself. The elements of the Code as set out in Table 3B.

It will be noted that there was a significant change in the elements of the code after the Tianjin meeting. As emphasised in Table 3B the elements 8 and 9 were added to the previous version of the code shown in Table 3A. The envisaged code of conduct now clearly had a key element (8) concerned with emplacement of an effective system of education for scientists which stated that:

> "8. (*Education and training*) Scientific community and professional associations should play an active role in education and training. Increase public awareness of the Convention, and *establish a safety education and training system for all parties involved in biotechnology research.* Biological scientists should be encouraged to engage in dialogue and cooperation with social scientists, philosophers and anthropologists, so as to have a better understanding of the possible ethical and social implication of relevant biological research and its outcome." (emphasis added)

It also had element 9 devoted to awareness-raising and engagement of scientists that stated:

> "9. (*Awareness and engagement*) *Biological scientists should be fully aware of the potential threats of dual-use research to human society, ecological environment and economic security.* It is advocated to promote the peaceful application of biological research achievements, to prevent the abuse and misuse of biological products, scientific knowledge, technology and equipment, and to consciously resist any unethical scientific conducts that are harmful to human society." (emphases added)

The new version of the code retained element 10 on the kind of international cooperation that will be needed for example to deal with threats of the kind illustrated by the present COVID-19 outbreak.

Then in his report of the meeting, the Chair of the MX2 Session on science and technology concluded that such a code of conduct would be one of the elements that had the most chance of being agreed at the Ninth Review Conference:[29]

> "...It is the Chair's view that...activities of the ISP should focus on issues that achieved greater commonality of approaches among delegations. In this regard, two areas could be explored: (i) risk assessment and management, and (ii) a voluntary code of conduct for biological scientists and relevant personnel."
>
> "The Chair sees the two topics above as those that could lead to a meaningful discussion during the remaining meetings of the ISP, in 2019 and 2020. They seem to present the best prospect for an agreed outcome on S&T [Science and Technology] issues in the 2021 Review Conference of the BWC..."

How this plays out will depend on how well meetings of the BTWC succeed in 2020 and 2021 in the lead up to the decision making 9th Review Conference. However, China's attitude to the misuse of biotechnology became very clear at the end of 2019 when the scientist who used CRISPR/Cas technology to edit the genomes of three human babies was sentenced to 3 years in jail and a large fine by a court in Shenzhen for illegal medical practice.[30]

International Comparisons

Of course, biological weapons are just one of the three types of generally acknowledged weapons of mass destruction and it is therefore not surprising that similar discussions have taken place in regard to chemical and nuclear weapons. The Organisation for the Prohibition of Chemical Weapons (OPCW) that implements the Chemical Weapons Convention (CWC) produced the *Hague Ethical Guidelines*, essentially an Aspirational Code of Conduct, in applying the norms of the practice of chemistry to support the CWC in 2015 (Table 4). There clearly exist differences between the code proposed by China for the BTWC (Table 3B) from that agreed for the CWC (Table 4). For example, the biological code necessarily has more emphasis on respect for the subjects of research as much more of the experimentation involves living organisms, but the clear prominence given to education and awareness-raising is obvious in both.

Table 4: Core Elements of The Hague Ethical Guidelines*

1. Sustainability
2. Education
3. Awareness and Engagement
4. Ethics
5. Safety and Security
6. Accountability
7. Oversight
8. Exchange of Information

* From the OPCW Website.

The newly established Advisory Board for Education and Outreach (ABEO) of the OPCW produced a major report in 2018 that emphasised the importance of active learning in engaging practicing scientists in maintaining and developing the prohibition to prevent the re-emergence of chemical weapons. The report stated that:[31]

> "One of the most important implications of this research is that 'active learning' methods, as opposed to traditional, lecture-based instruction in which students are passive recipients, produce better and longer lasting results. The results hold for factual information and for more fundamental concepts. The methods can be applied in many settings, including the classroom, the laboratory, or the field."

These developments related to the CWC have been reported by the OPCW in detail to meetings of the BTWC States Parties in recent years.[32] It is to be expected that the OPCW will over the coming years pursue a robust programme of education in support of the *Hague Ethical Guidelines*. Similarly, major developments have taken place in relation to nuclear security education. In 2012 it was already clear that significant efforts were being made to improve the security education of scientists (and others) connected with the nuclear industry. A Briefing Paper titled *Biosecurity Education for the Life Sciences: Nuclear Security Education Experience as a Model* stated that:[33]

> "The INSEN [International Nuclear Security Education Network] is a partnership between the IAEA and educational and research institutions, and competent authorities. Its mission is '*to enhance global nuclear security by developing, sharing and promoting excellence in nuclear security education*'. In order to achieve its main objective, namely to foster and support the implementation of nuclear security education, the Network has identified a set of key areas and activities for collaboration..." (original emphasis).

The text continued by setting out some of these key areas as follows:

- "Development of peer-reviewed textbooks, computer-based teaching tools and instructional material, including exercises and materials for laboratory work;
- Faculty assignment and development in the different areas of nuclear security through mutual faculty exchanges and/or joint development and implementation of in-depth nuclear security training programmes or school....
- Quality assurance: consistency with IAEA defined terminology described in the IAEA Nuclear Security Glossary, the Fundamentals and the Recommendations documents...

- Performance of surveys on the effectiveness of nuclear security education among students and faculty."

Even in 2012, this was an endeavour of a different order to anything being envisaged in relation to the BTWC even today.

The importance of the INSEN model was emphasised in a major review of the literature on dual use and responsible conduct in 2018. The authors concluding that:[34]

> "...We found that while there were discussions in the literature about specific elements of culture (management systems, leadership and/or personnel behavior, beliefs and attitudes, or principles for guiding decisions and behaviors), there was a general lack of integration of these concepts, as well as limited information about specific indicators or metrics and the effectiveness of training or similar interventions. We concluded that life scientists seeking to foster a culture of biosafety and biosecurity should learn from the substantial literature in analogous areas such as nuclear safety and security culture, high-reliability organizations, and the responsible conduct of research, among others."

Then in a follow-up effort to find means of assessing the Culture of Biosafety, Biosecurity, and Responsible Conduct in the Life Sciences an attempt has been made to modify the nuclear security approach for the life sciences. The working draft titled *Culture of Biosafety, Biosecurity, and Responsible Conduct in the Life Sciences: (Self) Assessment Framework* stated that:[35]

> "This tool intends to provide a measure of the organizational culture of biosafety, biosecurity, and responsible conduct to aid in the process of enhancing such culture at the local level through baseline and periodic assessments."

And it pointedly drew upon the nuclear security programme adding that:

> "While this is an attempt to adapt the nuclear safety and security culture model to the biological domain, future efforts to holistically integrate characteristics and indicators of an organizational culture across chemical, biological, and radiological/nuclear (CBRN) domains may help establish a framework for holistically assessing the CBRN safety and security culture in laboratories and other related organizations working with such hazardous materials. Such efforts will not be possible without the leadership of major international organizations and the support of professional associations."

In this tool biosafety, biosecurity and responsible is defined as:[36]

> "An assembly of beliefs, attitudes, and patterns of behavior of individuals

> and organizations that can support, complement or enhance operating procedures, rules, and practices as well as professional standards and ethics designed to prevent the loss, theft, misuse, and diversion of biological agents, related materials, technology or equipment, and the unintentional or intentional exposure to (or release of) biological agents."

Then, for a particular laboratory, assessments are made of the management systems in place; the behaviour of the leadership and personnel; the principles for guiding decisions and behaviours; and the beliefs, opinions and attitudes of those involved. For example, in regard to beliefs, opinions and attitudes people carrying out the self-assessment are asked to state the extent that they agree with a series of questions such as those set out in Table 5.

Table 5: Questions about Beliefs, Attitudes and Opinions*

1.	There is a risk of bioterrorism or an attack with a biological weapon.
5.	Biosafety and/or biosecurity deficiencies or vulnerabilities are corrected with a sense of urgency.
10.	I am aware that there are ethical, legal, and societal issues and consequences attached to my research.
13.	My organization has a culture that supports and encourages trust, collaboration, consultation, and communication with regard to biosafety and biosecurity.
14.	National policy and legislation relevant to the life sciences aim to provide protection against the misuse of science.
17.	I have received adequate training on the procedures necessary to conduct my work without compromising safety and security.
19.	Scientists have an obligation to do no harm.
20.	I do/would/will report my concerns to the appropriate people, authorities, and/or agencies if I become aware of activities that violate the Biological and Toxin Convention, United Nations Security Council resolution 1540, or international customary law.

From reference 31.

Answers to these questions can then be summarized in a colour chart to give a picture of the state of the organization in regard to biosafety, biosecurity and responsible conduct and from that picture suggestions can be made as to how the organization can be improved.

Conclusions

When the COVID-19 outbreak is over there will undoubtedly be many investigations about what happened and what should be done to prevent any further outbreaks – natural, accidental or deliberate – in the future. There will be many proposals put forward of various importance and difficulty of implementation. We would suggest that one important proposal should be the agreement of an *Aspirational Code of Conduct* under the BTWC as proposed by China with mandatory education in order to effectively engage life scientists in protecting their work from misuse. After almost 20 years of discussion, the proposal is well understood by many States Parties and could be agreed as a set of principles like the *Hague Ethical Guidelines* and then implemented in national codes of various kinds as fits different national circumstances.

In relation to awareness-raising and education initiatives of the kind that would be needed to underscore understanding of the relevance of such codes, important contributions in this connection have already resulted from the state – academic collaboration with the production by the University of Bradford of a Guide to Biological Security[37] that is accompanied by a Team-Based-Learning Handbook[38]. The chief objective of the latter is to supplement the former by combining teaching material in biological security with an active learning training approach – Team-Based Learning (TBL) - so as to empower educators, students and practitioners as they begin to engage with biological security. Further to this, the use by Bradford[39] of such techniques in proof of concept continuing professional development training has been undertaken under the auspices of the European Union's Human Brain Project where, in 2017 and 2018, evidence-based training of neuroscience professionals and practitioners at the Karolinska Institutet, Stockholm, demonstrated improvement in the knowledge and understanding of participants through engagement in discussions concerning the ethical, legal and social aspects of biological security.

The world is in the midst of a century of unprecedented change, and the 45-year-old Biological and Toxin Weapons Convention stands on a new starting line. It is to be hoped that the international community will take the commemoration of the 45th anniversary of the entry into force of the Convention as an opportunity to keep pace with the times, comprehensively advance the aims and objectives of the Convention, deepen international cooperation on biosecurity, and actively promote the establishment of a community of biological security for the destiny of mankind.

* * *

A presentation based on an earlier version of this paper was given at a meeting in St Petersburg in December 2019. M. R Dando, and S. Whitby, (2019) Towards Mandatory Education in Support of Biosecurity Codes of Conduct. Presentation at the Third Workshop of the Academic Network for European Security Studies, St Petersburg State University, 16–17 December.

This essay was published with the same title in CBW Magazine Vol. 13, No. 1, Jan-June 2020.

NOTES

1. Mark Wheelis, (ed.), *Deadly Cultures: Biological Weapons Since 1945*, Cambridge: Harvard University Press, 2006.
2. Malcolm R. Dando, *The New Biological Weapons: Threat, Proliferation, and Control*, Colorado: Lynne Rienner Pub, Boulder, 2001.
3. John Allen, Nicholas Burns, Laurie Garrett and et al, 'How the World Will Look After the Coronavirus Pandemic,' *Foreign Policy*, March 2020, available at https://foreignpolicy.com/2020/03/20/world-order-after-coroanvirus-pandemic/, accessed on 20 April 2020.
4. Jun Kong, 'Comprehensive Strengthening of the Biological Weapons Convention Mechanism: Promoting the Building of a Biosecurity Community of Human Destiny,' 2020, available at http://world.people.com.cn/n1/2020/0326/c1002-31648530.html?from=singlemessage&isappinstalled=0, accessed on 20 April 2020 (In Chinese).
5. Matthew Meselson, 'Averting the Hostile Exploitation of Biotechnology,' *The Chemical and Biological Weapons Conventions Bulletin*, 48, 2000, p. 16.
6. The concept of the 'Web of Prevention' was first proposed in the early 1990s by Graham S. Pearson (1993). Graham S. Pearson, 'Prospects for Chemical and Biological Arms Control: The Web of Deterrence,' *Washington Quarterly*, vol. 16, no. 2, January 2010, Pp. 145-162.
7. B. Rappert and C. McLeish (Eds.), 'A Web of Prevention: Biological Weapons,' *Life Sciences and the Governance of Research*, London: Earthscan, 2007.
8. G.S. Pearson, 'Return to Geneva: The United Kingdom Green Paper,' *Review Conference Paper No. 6*, University of Bradford, UK, 2002.
9. *Final Report of the Fifth Review Conference of the States Parties to the Convention on the Prohibition of the Development, Production and Stockpiling of Bacteriological (Biological) and Toxin Weapons and on their Destruction*, 2002, BWC/CONF.V/17, United Nations, Geneva.
10. United Nations, BWC/MSP/2005/MX/INF1 – INF.4., 2005, United Nations, Geneva.
11. *Presentations Submitted by the United States*, BWC/MSP/2005/MX/MISC.4, 2005, United Nations, Geneva.
12. *Thoughts on the Functions of Codes of Conduct: Potential Weaknesses and Solutions.* BWC/MSP/2005/MX/WP.6, Canada (2005), United Nations, Geneva,
13. Australia (2005) *Raising Awareness: Approaches and Opportunities for Outreach.* BWC/MSP/MX/WP.29. United Nations, Geneva, 13-27 April.
14. Malcolm R. Dando, and B. Rappert, *Codes of Conduct for the Life Sciences: Some Insights from UK Academia.* Briefing Paper No. 16 (Second Series), 2005, University of Bradford, May.
15. B. Rappert, M.I. Chevrier, and Malcolm R. Dando, *In-Depth Implementation of the BTWC: Education and Outreach.* Review Conference Paper No. 18, 2006, University of Bradford, November.
16. Russian Federation, *Basic Principles (Core Elements) of the Codes of Conduct of Scientists Majoring in Biosciences*, BWC/MSP/2005/WP.2, United Nations, Geneva, 2005.
17. *Final Report of the Sixth Review Conference of the States Parties to the Convention on the Prohibition of the Development, Production and Stockpiling of Bacteriological (Biological) and Toxin Weapons and on their Destruction*, United Nations, 2006, BWC/CONF.VI/6, United Nations, Geneva.
18. China, *Oversight of Science, Education and Awareness Raising, Coders of Conduct.* BWC/MSP/2008/MX/WP.18, United Nations, Geneva, 2008.
19. Netherlands, *Development of a Code of Conduct on Biosecurity.* BWC/MSP/2008/MX/WP.8, United Nations, Geneva, 2008.

20. Brian Rappert, 'Towards a Life Sciences Code: Countering the Threat from Biological Weapons,' Briefing Paper No. 13 (Second Series), University of Bradford, September 2004.
21. K. van der Bruggen, Gain-of-Function Experiments, *Chapter 2* (Box 2.3: Young scientists who did the job) in S. Whitby *et al* (Eds) *Preventing Biological Threats What You Can Do*, 2005, University of Bradford, UK. See also Schuurbiers, D. *et al* (2009) Implementing the Netherlands code of conduct for scientific practice – a cased study. *Sci Eng Ethics*, vol. 15, no. 2, pp. 213 - 231.
22. Australia *et al*, *Possible Approaches to Education and Awareness-Raising Among Life Scientists*. BWC/CONF/VII/WP.20/Rev.1, United Nations, Geneva, 2011.
23. United Nations, *Final Report of the Seventh Review Conference of the States Parties to the Convention on the Prohibition of the Development, Production and Stockpiling of Bacteriological (Biological) and Toxin Weapons and on their Destruction*. BWC/CONF.VII/7/ Corr.1, United Nations, Geneva, 2011.
24. United Nations, *Report of the Meeting of States Parties*. BWC/MSP/2015/6, United Nations, Geneva, 2015.
25. China and Pakistan, *Proposal for the Development of the Template of Biological Scientist Code of Conduct under the Framework of Biological Weapons Convention*. BWC/CONF.VIII/PC/WP.31, United Nations, Geneva, 2016.
26. Ukraine and UK, *Awareness-raising, Education, Outreach: An Example of Best Practice*. BWC/CONF.VIII/WP.10, United Nations, Geneva, 2016.
27. Ukraine, Japan and the UK, *Awareness-Raising, Education and Outreach: Recent Developments*. BWC/MSP/2017/WP.22, United Nations, Geneva, 2017.
28. China and Pakistan, *Proposal for the Development of a Model Code of Conduct for Biological Scientists under the Biological Weapons Convention*. BWC/MSP/2018/MX.2/WP.9, United Nations Geneva, 2018.
29. United Nations, *Chair's Report on MX2*. BWC/MSP/2018/CRP.3, United Nations, Geneva, 2018.
30. I. Sample, 'Chinese Scientist who Edited Babies' Genes Jailed for Three Years,' *The Guardian*, London, 31 December 2019.
31. Advisory Board on Education and Outreach, *Report on the Role of Education and Outreach in Preventing the Re-Emergence of Chemical Weapons*. AEBO-5/1. OPCW, The Hague, 12 February 2018.
32. C. Tang, and J.E. Foreman, *Development of the Hague Ethical Guidelines*, OPCW Presentation at the MX2 Experts Meeting, 9 August 2018, United Nations, Geneva; C. Tang, (2019) *Update on The Hague Ethical Guidelines*, Presentation by the Chair of the OPCW Scientific Advisory Board to the MX2 Experts Meeting, August. United Nations, Geneva.
33. T. Novossiolova, and G.S. Pearson, *Biosecurity Education for the Life Sciences: Nuclear Security Education Experience as a Model*, Briefing Paper No. 5 (Third Series), 2012, University of Bradford.
34. Dana Perkins, Kathleen Danskin and A. Elise Rowe and et al, 'The Culture of Biosafety, Biosecurity, and Responsible Conduct in the Life Sciences: A Comprehensive Literature Review,' *Applied Biosafety*, vol. 24, June 2018.
35. International Working Group on Strengthening the Culture of Biosafety, Biosecurity, and Responsible Conduct in the Life Sciences (2020) *Culture of Biosafety, Biosecurity, and Responsible Conduct in the Life Sciences: (Self) Assessment Framework*. January 2020 Working Draft.
36. *A Guide to Training and Information Resources on the Culture of Biosafety, Biosecurity, and Responsible*

Conduct in the Life Sciences, T*he International Working Group* on Strengthening the Culture of Biosafety, Biosecurity, and Responsible Conduct in the Life Sciences, 2019, available at https://absa.org/wp-content/uploads/2019/04/CULTURE_TRAINING_CATALOGUE.pdf, accessed on 28 April 2020.

37. S. Whitby, T. Novossiolova, G Walther and Malcolm R. Dando, 'Preventing Biological Threats: What You Can Do. A Guide to Biological Security Issues and How to Address Them,' *University of Bradford*, *Bradford Disarmament Research Centre*, 2015, p. 446, available at http://hdl.handle.net/10454/7821, accessed on 28 April 2020.
38. T. Novossiolova, 'Biological Security Education Handbook: The Power of Team-Based Learning,' *University of Bradford*, Bradford Disarmament Research Centre, 2016, p. 85, available at http://hdl.handle.net/10454/7822, accessed on 28 April 2020.
39. Shamin Patel, Linnaeus University, Sweden, Tutors: Malcolm Dando, and Simon Whitby, University of Bradford, UK. Team Based Learning Exerecise - Social, ethical and legal responsibilities of life sciences 1st HBP Curriculum Workshop Series - Research, ethics and Societal Impact. Karolinska Institutet, Stockholm, Sweden. 10-12 July 2017. Video recorded by the Human Brain Project Education Office - https://youtu.be/EFvraNKU1UE. And, Tutors: Malcolm Dando, Simon Whitby, Bradford University, UK Team-Based Learning Exercise - Social, ethical and legal responsibilities of life scientists. 2nd HBP Curriculum Workshop Series - Research, ethics and Societal Impact 15-17 November 2018. Karolinska Institutet, Stockholm, Sweden. Video recorded by the Human Brain Project Education Office - https://youtu.be/vQ_Dfm3jJp0 accessed on 29 April 2020.

24

Biological Security and Health in the Post-pandemic World: The Infectious Disease Community's 'Mushroom Cloud'?

David R Franz

Having served in the US Army at the interface of health and security for most of my career, I have often found myself on committees and boards in government where the topic was 'WMD' (Weapons of Mass Destruction). It was not unusual in those settings for there to be one or two 'biologists' to every ten nuclear physicists or arms control experts. When we got to infectious diseases or 'biodefense' portion of the agenda, some – not all – of the physicists would be ready for a 'break'. The biology was either too squishy for a brilliant engineering mind or just not that interesting. I might lean over to a friend – if I had one in the meeting – and whisper, "Too bad WE don't have a 'mushroom cloud.'"

The Cold War

During the Cold War and for ten years thereafter, the USA (United States of America) and other countries developed physical and medical countermeasures to protect their military forces from what we loosely called the "dirty dozen" biological agents previously weaponized by the Soviet Union (SU). Most of the threat agents for which we developed medical and physical countermeasures were similar to the weapons agents developed by the offensive programs of the US and its allies before 1972 when the biological weapons convention was signed.[1] Throughout this period, our defensive biological work was on a small scale, compared to our nuclear weapons programs, and probably little known or appreciated outside our service laboratories.

In the context of the COVID-19 pandemic,[2] some might find it interesting that the biological warfare agents developed by US and Soviet offensive programs were not highly contagious. For example, the list of characteristics sought by US weaponeers through the '60s read like this: pathogenic for humans or animals, causes disability or lethality, highly infectious but not contagious, medical countermeasures available, stable during logistical operations, stable in small particle aerosols, readily and rapidly producible, weaponized in munitions and delivery systems and produce desired effects on the target.[3] Through the 1990s, our own work focused on environmental detection, physical protection, vaccines and diagnostics. While we were attempting to protect our military force globally, we also 'practiced' by responding to emerging infectious diseases, mostly through collaborations with public health systems in Africa or South East Asia. The total science and technology budget for the US biodefense program was approximately 137 Million USD in 1997. The overall biodefense budget would jump to 14.5 Billion USD spent between 2001 and 2004 in response to the 'anthrax letters.'[4]

Post 9/11 and the 'Anthrax Letters'

After attacks on the World Trade Center and mailing of the 'anthrax letters' in September of 2001, the focus in biological defense turned toward protecting citizens from weapons produced by individuals or sub-state terrorist organizations. A self-proclaimed survival medicine expert – sounding like nature at its worst – listed the following as likely terrorist threat agent characteristics during that era: infectious and contagious, causing long-term debilitation or death, few available preventatives or therapies, easily deliverable to a target population and low likelihood of harming the perpetrators.[5] During this period, we quickly realized that it was significantly more difficult to protect citizens of any country than it had been to protect our hypothetical military force on a European battlefield. The threat agent list became more difficult to construct and the necessary medical countermeasures and defensive practices more difficult to define. Who should be vaccinated; against what agents; when? Furthermore, environmental detectors could not be placed everywhere, and ordinary citizens could not, or would not, carry a protective mask or would know when to don it. The problem became 'too hard' to solve with technical solutions. As Noble Laureate Joshua Lederberg told us, "There is no technical solution to the problem of biological weapons. It needs an ethical, human, and moral solution if it's going to happen at all. Don't ask me what the odds are for an ethical solution, but there is no other solution".[6]

Less than a decade into this phase we turned much of our biosecurity focus toward naturally occurring emerging infectious diseases. After all, we had seen essentially no more bioterrorism after the anthrax letters and the FBI's (Federal Bureau of Investigation) conclusion based on circumstantial evidence was that the letters were mailed by an 'insider' from one of our own labs.[7] So, we began a system of heavy-handed regulation and micromanagement of our domestic infectious disease laboratories where scientists worked with high-hazard pathogens.[8] We also soon turned our focus toward surprises that might come from nature rather than from nations, sub-national forces or even individuals.

Emerging Infectious Disease

That refocusing made sense, as the rate of occurrence of highly-pathogenic emerging infectious diseases was increasing: SARS (Severe Acute Respiratory Syndrome) in China, 2002; Chikungunya in numerous countries from 2007 to 2014; MERS (Middle East Respiratory Syndrome) in the Arabian Peninsula, 2012; Ebola in West Africa, 2014 and Zika in the Americas in 2015.[9] Almost in parallel with the Ebola outbreak in West Africa the Global Health Security Agenda[10] (GHSA) was endorsed by a group of, now more than 60, countries plus international organizations, NGOs (Non-Government Organisation) and private sector companies to help make the world safe and secure from infectious disease threats. The GHSA would evaluate preparedness and even support improvements in a supported nation's capability to respond to an outbreak or epidemic caused by an emerging infectious disease. Then, even as the West African Ebola epidemic spread, the financial condition of the GHSA worsened; the program may have disappeared but for an infusion of 'left-over Ebola money'.

By 2018, the US CDC (United States Centers for Disease Control and Prevention) was threatened with budget cuts to programs that conducted infectious disease research and support for other nations internationally.[11] That same year, the Trump administration made clear the low priority of pandemic preparedness and even the value of keeping a finger on the pulse of emerging diseases; it abolished the White House Office of Global Health Security and placed the responsibility for naturally emerging and intentional disease threats under the Weapons of Mass Destruction Directorate. [Note that the same office had been abolished by the second Bush administration as well as the Obama administration, only to be reinstated after the anthrax letter attacks and Ebola 2014 epidemic respectively.][12] Pandemic preparedness isn't easy when there is not a pandemic.

The Pandemic

And then in December of 2019, a handful of cases of SARS-like pneumonia were reported in a very large but little-known city in the middle of China: Wuhan. Almost overnight our world changed.[13] Now, we wish we had paid closer attention to medical epidemiologists and emerging disease experts who have been warning us for the last decade or more that a lethal pandemic was all but inevitable.[14,,15,,16] One organization in the US has described our situation during the COVID-19 pandemic as "forewarned but not forearmed".[17] Will we all learn from this global experience that we must make pandemic preparedness a priority going forward?

The World has Changed

As many of us sit in our homes, experiencing 'social distancing' for the first time, we often feel helpless, attempting to maintain working relationships and activities electronically while trying to fight the war on COVID-19 as best we can. Many watch, as their personal treasure and even livelihood, slip away and most of us watch as our nations' economies come sliding to a near halt. We are told that a vaccine will be the best answer, but there are still so many unknowns. We are hopeful. There are some promising drugs in the pipeline. Diagnostics must get better and faster, both for identification of virus-infected individuals and for serologic studies to see who is – possibly – protected by an antibody response. We could be doing better on contact tracing and isolation, but it is not easy in a democracy. What about herd immunity? We are sorting through a swirling mass of new and old science to find relevant public health information to aid in halting the pandemic.

It is too early to know how individuals, populations, nations and global organisations and their policies will change after the COVID-19 experience. It is likely that nations will reconsider their supply chains for critical medical devices, clothing, personal protective equipment, drugs and vaccines and maybe even for the basics like food and fuel. Just-in-time supply, while efficient for both producer and consumer may not be feasible when we are cut off from global supplies for many months. Access to enough medical materiel through the international shifting of inventories may work for a local or regional crisis but may not be logistically or politically possible in a crisis that impacts all of us globally. Modern medicine has allowed us to reduce hospital bed numbers *per capita*, but a number of countries in the COVID-19 crisis have had to improvise on the fly to house the massive number of humans needing intensive care. Will we change the way we build hospitals or even hotels and schools with the thought of quickly making them intensive care wards in a crisis? Will telemedicine or what some now call 'cyber care' becomes a larger component of healthcare delivery? So much has changed. Will infectious diseases be discussed more seriously as a national security issue in the future? How long will we remember?

Impact on Public Thinking

Will our citizens change the way they think about infectious diseases after this most traumatic experience? Will there be stronger public support for vaccines? Will we be more attuned to the principles of preventive medicine, public health and 'one health'?[18] Will we alter our lifestyles to reduce comorbidities such as obesity, diabetes, heart and pulmonary disease? Will our young people be drawn to careers in medicine and the biological sciences more strongly after this experience?

Nations and the International Community

Will we expect more from our governments, both local and national? Will we get more? In the US we have had a National Strategy for Pandemic Influenza (2005) and a Pandemic Influenza Plan (2017 Update); now, in the bright light of the COVID-19 pandemic, is the time to see what difference they made, and adjust as necessary.[19] Strategies and plans can be nothing more than a stack of papers on a shelf unless recommendations are kept up to date, implemented and practiced regularly. Will our political leaders take pandemic planning more seriously? We have been warned so many times but it is difficult to find support for a once-in-a-century event in a political world that measures time in two and four-year increments. Or is the once-in-a-century rule still valid for pandemics? A big piece of this pandemic planning must be driven by our domestic departments and ministries with initial coordination that can only happen at the top of our individual governments. It requires funding, of course, but even more importantly, sound and wise leadership. Much of this must occur within our own nations, but with transportation what it is today, we cannot afford to become isolationist in our thinking regarding infectious diseases. Remember, the 'bugs' know no borders. A highly contagious viral disease such as influenza or a coronavirus in my country today can literally be in your country tomorrow. We must work together.

Like never before in our lifetimes, we face a common enemy. This enemy doesn't respect the seal on the cover of our passports, political ideologies, economic power, military might, age or gender. Fortunately, to the degree that we had been working together internationally before the pandemic, we have been able to leverage relationships of friendship and trust between experts – scientists and clinicians – during the crisis. Global networks of scientific and clinical subject matter experts are powerful tools before, during and after a pandemic.[20] We must work together internationally.

A Role for Individuals

We have exceptional examples of science academies, academic centers, military-to-military programmes and even industrial partners working synergistically across international borders. When we look closely, however, it is often individuals within these systems and organizations who find a colleague with common technical interests anywhere in the world.[21] Common interests fuel more-open conversation and communication which leads to sharing what I have long called "good news and bad news". This kind of frank exchange over time results in trust between the two parties. Where trust exists, the relationships are often both sustained and supercharged. These nodes of friendship and trust between technical experts are empowered, in some cases, by connecting with other similar nodes to contribute to an even broader network of like-minded individuals. National leadership is, of course, central to domestic and global preparation for the next pandemic, but politics so often get in the way. However, through relationships of trust grounded in common technical interests, each of us as individuals can contribute our small piece to the 'fight', technically and through effective communication. Both enlightened leadership and excellent, networked subject matter experts are essential. And now, sadly, we biologists do have our very own 'mushroom cloud'. Let us learn from this global experience and respond wisely.

* * *

A shorter version of this essay was published with the same title in CBW Magazine, Vol. 13, No. 1, Jan-June 2020.

NOTES

1. The Biological Weapons Convention, available at https://www.un.org/disarmament/wmd/bio/ , accessed on 01 May 2020.
2. As I complete this manuscript, the United States has just passed the 100,000 mark in COVID-19 related deaths and is still averaging more than 1,000 deaths per day.
3. Personal Communication with William C. Patrick III, former US biological weapons expert, ca. 1997.
4. David R. Franz, 'The Dual Use Dilemma: Crying Out for Leadership,' *Saint Louis University Journal of Health Law & Policy*, Vol. 7, No. 1, Article 4, 2013, p. 8, available at https://scholarship.law.slu.edu/jhlp/vol7/iss1/4, accessed on 04 May 2020.
5. Alton, Joe, *Doom and Bloom*, 17 Oct. 2014, available at https://www.doomandbloom.net/, accessed on 05 May 2020.

Author's note: It is not clear how 'low likelihood of harming the perpetrators' is compatible with the other characteristics listed here.

6. Richard Preston, 'The Bioweaponeers,' *New Yorker*, March 9, 1998, pp 52-65.
7. National Research Council, Review of the Scientific Approaches Used During the FBI's Investigation of the 2001 Anthrax Letters, 2011, Washington, DC: The National Academies Press, available at https://www.nap.edu/catalog/13098/review-of-the-scientific-approaches-used-during-the-fbis-investigation-of-the-2001-anthrax-letters, accessed on 01 May 2020.
8. David R. Franz, 'Implementing the Select Agent Legislation: Perfect Record or Wrong Metric?' *Health Security*, pp. 290-294, August 2015, available at https://www.ncbi.nlm.nih.gov/pmc/articles/PMC4544819/, accessed on 01 May 2020.
9. Emerging Infectious Diseases, Baylor College of Medicine, available at https://www.bcm.edu/departments/molecular-virology-and-microbiology/emerging-infections-and-biodefense/emerging-infectious-diseases, accessed on 01 May 2020.
10. Global Health Security Agenda, available at https://ghsagenda.org/, accessed on 01 May 2020.
11. Ed Yong, 'The CDC Is About to Fall off a Funding Cliff,' *The Atlantic*, February 2, 2018, available at https://www.theatlantic.com/health/archive/2018/02/cdc-funding-pandemics/552224/ accessed on 08 May 2020.
12. Kenneth W. Bernard, 'The White House Signals that Bioterrorism and Disease Don't Matter – again,' *The Washington Post*, May 23, 2018, available at https://www.washingtonpost.com/opinions/the-white-house-signals-that-bioterrorism-and-disease-dont-matter--again/2018/05/22/5a5b0c0c-5dd1-11e8-b2b8-08a538d9dbd6_story.html, accessed on 10 May 2020.
13. Robin Muccari, Denise Chow and Joe Murphy, "Coronavirus Timeline: Tracking the Critical Moments of COVID-19," *NBC News*, May 11, 2020, available at https://www.nbcnews.com/health/health-news/coronavirus-timeline-tracking-critical-moments-covid-19-n1154341, accessed on 11 May 2020.
14. Michael T. Osterholm and Mark Olshaker, 'Deadliest Enemy: Our War against Killer Germs,' Boston/USA: Little, Brown and Company, 2017, available at https://wwwnc.cdc.gov/eid/article/24/1/17-1081_article, accessed on 12 May 2020.
15. Laurie Garrett, 'The Coming Plague,' New York: Tenth Printing, 1994 available at https://www.lauriegarrett.com/the-coming-plague, accessed on 12 May 2020.
16. Ali S. Khan and William Patrick, 'The Next Pandemic: On the Front Lines against Humankind's Gravest Dangers,' *EID Journal*, December 2017, v. 23, n.12, available at https://wwwnc.cdc.gov/eid/article/23/12/17-1137_article, accessed on 12 May 2020.
17. Blue Ribbon Study Panel on Biodefense is now the Bipartisan Commission on Biodefense, available at https://biodefensecommission.org/, accessed on 13 May 2020.
18. One Health Initiative will unite human and veterinary medicine, *One Health Initiative*, available at http://www.onehealthinitiative.com/, accessed on 14 May 2020.
19. National Pandemic Strategy, available at https://www.cdc.gov/flu/pandemic-resources/national-strategy/index.html, accessed on 14 May 2020.
20. Biological Threat Reduction Program, available at https://www.nap.edu/search/?term=bioloigal+threat+reduction+program, accessed on 15 May 2020.
21. Corrie Brown and David R Franz, 'Making Foreign Engagements Sustainable: it's personal,' *J Am Vet Med Assoc*, September 2016, vol. 249, no. 6, pp.576-577.

25

How Should South Asian States Respond to Global Biosecurity Concerns

Malinda Meegoda

Introduction

It is now virtually axiomatic to describe that certain pathogens such as viruses responsible for major global public health emergencies such as the 2002 SARS outbreak, and COVID-19 do not respect geographical boundaries irrespective of the origin of the viral strain. COVID-19, in particular, has exposed how ill-equipped the vast majority of countries remain in their capacity to contain global public health emergencies such as pandemics. The crisis has also sparked new discussions and re-opened debates on how states need to re-think, in the way they conceptualise national security and the list of priorities that come under the broad topic of national security.

With the understanding that ensuring proper biosecurity and biosafety requires a response that is global in nature, this paper will aim to highlight some of the major avenues that require urgent attention in terms of policy responses and international cooperation. The paper will also attempt to offer some policy suggestions regarding what countries and regional organisations based in South Asia could do to further enhance the web of prevention related to biosafety and biosecurity.

Biological Weapons and Non-State Actors

From a global health security and governance perspective, it is self-evident that bio-risk management is far removed from other analogous spheres of arms control. The most glaring distinction being that there are not any naturally occurring security risks present within nuclear, and other conventional weapons systems. With nuclear and conventional weapons human intent to weaponize the agent and the delivery device can eventually be traced to an actor even if the deployment of the delivery device is deemed inadvertent. Contrastingly, biosafety and biosecurity management is burdened with naturally occurring phenomena that stem from pathogens which include; bacterium, viruses, fungi, prions and toxins, in addition to the intentional weaponisation of some of these pathogens.[1]

The use of biological weapons on the battlefield has a long history going beyond modern warfare. For most of the twentieth century, several states such as the US, and the Soviet Union possessed active biological weapons programmes. During this period, evidence of open use of biological weapons in the battlefield, however, remains sparse with only a few of these having gained any traction such as the 'Yellow Rain' controversy in South East Asia.[2] However, even after the majority of states acceded to the Biological Weapons and Toxins Convention (BWC), thus eliminating their offensive programmes a few states were accused of continuing offensive biological weapons programmes.[3] While there hasn't been any documented use of biological weapons possessing the lethal virality of a weaponised smallpox virus in the 21st century, a few states have been accused of using toxins to carry out targeted assassinations.[4]

Currently, much of the concern of biological weapons is focused on the use and possession by non-state actors, and unauthorised access and misuse of dangerous pathogens by individuals working in laboratory settings. The three cases that are commonly cited to illustrate these two broad-ranging concerns include; the attempted failed attacks by the Aum Shinrikyo cult in 1990 and 1994, the poisoning of a salad bar in Portland, Oregon in the United States by members of the Rajneeshee religious cult in 1984, and the release of anthrax in Washington DC in 2001. The latter attributed to a scientist with a history of working with highly infectious diseases at the United States Army Medical Research Institute of Infectious Diseases (USAMRIID).[5]

Despite these frequently cited case studies, the reason why not many non-state actors have actively pursued biological weapons in greater quantity may have to do with two factors. The first being that weaponizing biological weapons requires a high degree of technical expertise and resources.[6] The Aum Shinrikyo cult was an outlier in many respects among non-state terror outfits. It was able to recruit many individuals possessing technical expertise working in lab settings and ties to professional institutions that the organization was able to recruit.[7] It also had access to financial and material resources through its member networks as evidenced by the scale of its biological weapons programme where the group produced several hundred metric tons containing the botulinum toxin. In addition to the technical hurdles, the other reason that perhaps non-state actors have refrained from using biological weapons may have to do with the effects of using biological weapons with its unpredictable nature. However, recent developments in the life sciences and associated technologies, some of the technical barriers that have historically prevented non-state actors from using biological weapons may wane. Furthermore given that a major motivation for actors involved in terrorism is to create a general sense of panic and fear coupled with the need to stay ahead of the developments in state-led counter-terrorism initiatives, it is quite plausible that attempts by non-state actors to utilise bioweapons may become more prevalent.

An important lesson to be learnt regarding non-state actors and their capabilities to develop Weapons of Mass Destruction (WMD) programmes is that very much like the state counterparts they need time to develop WMD programmes through a process of trial and error. This is often a luxury that these groups do not possess as possible surveillance by state intelligence and other law enforcement authorities would often force them to change tactics and methods which can disrupt the development cycle in their WMD programmes. A report compiled by the Centre for a New American Security (CNS) posthumously on Aum Shinrikyo's chemical and biological weapons programme arrived at a similar conclusion where the report states, "Insofar as this experience indicates, it is a story of evolution. Terrorists need time; time will be used for trial and error (tacit knowledge acquisition); trial and error entail risk and, in this case, provoked disruption".[8] However, other groups in the future if inclined could study these cases, and adapt more workable solutions with their programmes. States should heed the cautionary note offered in the previously mentioned CNS report which urges relevant authorities to look past the failures of these groups by stating that "Groups such as Aum expose us to risks uncomfortably analogous to playing Russian roulette. Many chambers in the gun prove to be harmless, but some chambers are loaded."[9]

Although, there have only been a handful of successful attacks conducted by non-state actors using biological weapons, the current evolution of biotechnology merits careful consideration of whether the advances in technologies such as gene editing will empower and enable more individuals or groups to consider it as a weapon of choice. With the ever-increasing role of the private sector in the life sciences and greater commodification of this knowledge base a depreciation of the cost of relevant equipment, questions should be asked if there be an increasing desire by terror outfits such to use a virus or bacteria acquired through a third party. Although bioweapons are commonly perceived as a way to infect populations with deadly diseases, groups could use it as a form of economic sabotage through actions aimed at crop destruction. For example, in the 1980s, way before the Liberation Tigers of Tamil Eelam (LTTE) had reached its zenith as a fighting force, there is evidence to suggest that the group had threatened to use biological agents to destroy crops that belonged to Sinhala communities.[10] Countries, especially in South Asia with large populations where food security challenges continue to be a persistent challenge, acts of agroterrorism using biological agents, could create widespread challenges to stability and security.

Bio-risk management and Research Activities

Even though the use of biological weapons has been sparse in recent times, what some are calling the 'democratisation of biology', through innovations in fields such as 'synthetic biology' could shorten the development cycle of biological weapons in the future.[11] Advances in synthetic biology most famously associated with tools, such as CRISPR (clustered regularly interspaced short palindromic repeats) are currently being fuelled by a complex and interactive web of political, economic, and social drivers. Many governments across the world including ones in South Asia are increasingly focusing on ways to utilise biotechnology for a myriad of reasons including; to maximise agricultural output, eradicate disease, and to increase the quality and scope of their knowledge-based economies. India's Department of Biotechnology (DBT) received a 17% increase in 2020 from the previous year in government allocated spending.[12] The resulting increased pace of innovation currently found in the life sciences, therefore, merit greater attention in managing the potential risks associated with such activity.

Bio-risk management in the lab is a multi-sectoral effort and should not simply be viewed as focusing narrowly on securing the physical properties of a designated facility. It should be viewed as an increasingly expansive approach that delves into the arenas of bioethics particularly with the dual-use nature of much of the life sciences. It requires the cooperation of states, industry and individual researchers to develop an appropriate methodological framework that can balance security and research objectives. Apart from the overall concern of dual-use, the other main point of concern when it comes to research activities in the life sciences remains the area known as gain-of-function research. Gain-of-function research refers to the effect of adding new functions in the form of new biological properties to an existing pathogen with the expectation that it may offer insights into other aspects of a pathogen like the nature of the transmission process of a particular viral strain. The effect of this type of research is that it leaves the door open for researchers to create potentially more dangerous pathogens with greater virality.

One of the most illustrative cases where significant concern was generated regarding gain-of-function research occurred in 2011 regarding research into the H5N1 virus, commonly known as avian bird flu. Two scientists Yoshihiro Kawaoka from the University of Wisconsin, Madison and Ron Fouchier of Erasmus Medical Center, in the Netherlands were able to create a new strain of the virus that appears to demonstrate that is possible to increase the virality of H5N1 without reducing any of its lethality.[13] The main concern was that by publishing the results the particular research was essentially giving the blueprint for malicious actors looking to create a pandemic pathogen. In the end following a review of the case by convened by the World Health Organisation (WHO) determined that on balance the research benefits outweighed all other concerns regarding accidental, or intentional misuse of the research findings.[14] The US National Science Advisory Board for Biosecurity (NSABB) which had earlier called for a redacted publication ultimately agreed with the conclusions of the WHO review mentioned earlier. However, what should be noted is that NSABB's later re-evaluation of the H5N1 study should not be taken as an endorsement that all future research similar to the H5N1 study would not merit greater scrutiny before publication. The NSABB rightly assessed that "research findings will likely emerge in the very near future that should not be widely disseminated because of a high risk of misuse."[15]

It is perhaps an appropriate time to consider whether a code of conduct can be developed among research scientists working in the life sciences when it comes to gain-of-function research activities. As a prerequisite to enabling a common code of conduct, more constructive efforts need to be made to increase the field of bioethics. A code of conduct should ideally prioritise three areas; risk analysis of individual research studies, an ability to demonstrate the greater good of a particular research undertaking and increase the quality and scope of the discussions between researchers and other key stakeholders to better inform the risks and benefits of dual-use research. Bioethics as a field of study is relatively new and is even more nascent in its development stage in developing countries situates in South Asia like Sri Lanka. One of the few institutions that are tasked with addressing these challenges in Sri Lanka like the Institute for Research and Development faces a lot of common resource constraints which is a common issue for institutes in other developing countries as well. In this regard, more assistance could be sought from bodies such as the Indian Council of Medical Research (ICMR) to uplift the collective knowledgebase regarding bioethics in South Asian countries such as Bangladesh, Nepal and Sri Lanka.

Increasing Regional Cooperation on Biosecurity and National Security in South Asia

South Asia as a geographical entity has among its more discernible characteristics; the presence of highly porous borders, the largest concentration of the global human population, and a highly diverse ecosystem of flora and fauna. These particular characteristics make the risk factors of future pandemics from spreading in the region all the more acute. Managing these risks effectively will require greater investments in infrastructure, international and regional cooperation. Current security dialogues in the South Asian region, in particular, have been dominated on the conventional and nuclear fronts and little attention has been paid to the inter-related issues pertaining to biosecurity and biosafety. In most regional security forums topics such as climate change, marine conservation tends to be relegated to a subcategory often referred to as 'non-traditional security threats. Even under the rubric of 'non-traditional security threats', Biosafety and biosecurity are topics rarely tabled for discussion at many of these fora.

India is currently unrivalled in the region in terms of the resources and scientific knowledge base it has accrued. It has a well-established pharmaceutical industry and a rapidly expanding life sciences industry, particularly on agricultural research. India also remains the only country in South Asia to possess BSL-4 laboratory facilities that conduct research on extremely dangerous pathogens.[16] While India overall has a robust system of integrated health ministries and institutes to implement proper biosafety procedures, it does not appear to have a concrete national biosecurity strategy that is present among other global powers. In comparison, the Obama administration in the US implemented a biosecurity strategy in 2009 which aimed to reduce the risk of both naturally occurring and deliberate disease outbreaks.[17] The strategy was noteworthy in the way in which it attempted to align the objectives with the overall foreign policy of the Obama administration. It readily recognised the increasingly globalising nature of the pharmaceutical and biotechnology industries and the rapid rate of diffused knowledge taking place in the life sciences. India in this regard should take some inspiration from the Obama administration's security strategy on biosecurity by emulating some of the key tenets of the document to create a national security strategy on biosecurity. India could invest in a bio-threat intelligence platform that comes directly under the Ministry of Defence designed to gather and coordinate intelligence among various scientific health communities both in the public and private sectors. In addition to upgrading India's capacity to increase its bio-surveillance of important infrastructures such as ports, and airports, it would also be an opportunity to share data with cooperating intelligence services among India's neighbouring countries. As with Obama's security strategy, adequate importance should be placed on improving public health in India and its neighbouring countries. Given India's favourable track record in health-related investments in the region such as the '119 Ambulance Services project' in countries like Sri Lanka, this would be an opportunity to build on.[18] Such investments should be the key cornerstone of any 'web of prevention' system of layered biosafety and security measures.

Ideally, while some of the initiatives should be championed by regional organisations such as SAARC (The South Asian Association for Regional Cooperation), and BIMSTEC (The Bay of Bengal Initiative for Multi-Sectoral Technical and Economic Cooperation), ongoing political disputes between member states that belong to these organisations has resulted in comprehensive multilateral cooperation on these issues unlikely. However, there is much scope for states to engage bilaterally either in the form of technical cooperation, security dialogues, and capacity building. On the security front, Sri Lanka, for example, engages in a series of security exercises such as the SLINEX naval exercises, and the Mithra Shakthi exercises between the armies of Sri Lanka and India. It is plausible to envision a specialised security exercise either bilaterally between India, Sri Lanka and other select South Asian or BIMSTEC partners countries to conduct exercises aimed at countering biological threats. These exercises could use the 'red teaming' methodology which is often described as, "the deliberate adoption of an adversarial perspective to better understand and predict security threats".[19] This could be also an opportunity to simultaneously broaden the scope of cooperating institutions beyond the militaries of the respective countries, by inviting public and private institutes working in the life sciences. A biological threat exercise conducted using common red teaming techniques such as simulations, and vulnerability probes could be instrumental in developing a greater understanding of the biological threats from a developing country perspective. It is crucial, that the undertaking of biological threat assessment exercises is comprehensively analysed to meet current compliance standards consistent under the Biological and Toxic Weapons Convention (BWC). Other states such as the US that have conducted biological weapons threat assessment programmes have in the past elicited apprehensions of human error, and dual-use concerns. The most common category of projects that have been subjected to BWC compliance concerns are ones with a focus on 'vulnerability probes' which could entail the use of actual pathogens. For example, 'Project Jefferson', a programme that falls into the category of 'vulnerability probes' was undertaken by the US Defence Intelligence Agency to reproduce a genetically-modified strain of anthrax.[20] Therefore, given these security concerns, emphasis on regional initiatives in South Asia should be given to implementing exercises that are focused on scenario analysis using appropriate simulation environments. In addition, commissioning joint 'analysis of alternatives' (AoA) studies could aid each state to decide what further investments are necessary to combat potential threats regarding biological agents.

When it comes to the question of the current status of the global governance aspect of biosecurity, there are some notable gaps and limitations regarding the harmonisation of regulations present in the various sectors. Since distinct and separate organisations are involved in the regulatory frameworks concerning environmental protection, health and disease control, and arms control there can be gaps in the overlapping regulatory frameworks. This is perhaps an area that regional organisations such as BIMSTEC and SAARC could look to address from a regional perspective. It would be desirable to create a regional initiative that would take into account the health of animals, plants, environment, and humans to plug knowledge gaps that may exist regionally. Such an initiative could garner support from an organisation such as BIMSTEC given the fact that public health, environment, and technology are already part of the fourteen priority areas agreed upon by BIMSTEC member countries.[21] Additionally, BIMSTEC's priority area on 'people-to-people contact' could be invoked to increase links between research scientists working on biotechnology among member states. Furthermore, these groups could be encouraged to participate in global meetings such as the Convention on Biodiversity (CBD), and the Biological and Toxic Weapons Convention. Such initiatives could go a long way in improving the collective response needed to manage bio-risks in the region.

Conclusion

Although this paper earlier noted how biological weapons are markedly distinct from other weapons of mass destruction, there is a current common political thread that still binds all categories of WMDs. The thread being that existing norms against any of these weapons remain extremely fragile. There are still persistent debates as to what counts as defensive research when it comes to biological weapons.

During the COVID-19 outbreak allegations quickly surfaced alleging that the COVID-19 pandemic was deliberately engineered or that it was the result of a biosafety breach at the Wuhan Institute of Virology.[22] Such allegations unaccompanied by robust evidence can have long-lasting destabilising impacts on regional and international stability. Under the current security backdrop where numerous arms control agreements such as the Intermediate Nuclear Forces (INF) treaty have been either revoked or are in serious jeopardy,[23] unqualified allegations during the time of a pandemic could not only disrupt current efforts to deal with the present crisis but could undermine the integrity and legitimacy of long-standing treaties such as the BWC and efforts to strengthen it. Given the unparalleled disruption COVID-19 has caused to the global economy, and public health there should be a renewed emphasis placed on reconstructing and reconfiguring foreign policy, security and health to adapt to these new and evolving challenges through greater international cooperation and convergence to act on these common existential threats.

NOTES

1. Thavaselvam, Duraipandian, and Rajagopalan Vijayaraghavan, 'Biological Warfare Agents,' *Journal of Pharmacy & Bioallied Sciences*, 2010, p.179-88.
2. J.B. Tucker, 'The Yellow Rain Controversy: Lessons for Arms Control Compliance,' *The Non-Proliferation Review*, 2001, available at https://www.nonproliferation.org/wp-content/uploads/npr/81tucker.pdf, accessed on 25 June 2020.
3. P. David, 'Biological Weapons: Soviet Union accused,' *Nature*, 1984.
4. Oliver Homes and Tom Phillips, 'Kim Jong-nam Killed by VX nerve Agent, say Malaysian Police,' *The Guardian*, 2017, available at https://www.theguardian.com/world/2017/feb/24/kim-jong-nam-north-korea-killed-chemical-weapon-nerve-agent-mass-destruction-malaysian-police, accessed on 25 June 2020.
5. US Department of Justice. Anthrax Investigation Summary, (n.d.), available at https://www.justice.gov/archive/amerithrax/docs/amx-investigative-summary2.pdf, accessed on 25 June 2020.
6. Ouagrham-Gormley and Sonia Ben, 'Barriers to Bioweapons: Intangible Obstacles to Proliferation,' *International Security*, vol. 36, no. 4, 2012, pp. 80–114.
7. Richard Danzig, Marc Sageman, Terrance Leighton and et al, 'Aum Shinrikyo Insights into How Terrorists Develop Biological and Chemical Weapons,' *Centre for a New American Security (CNS)*, 2012, available at https://s3.amazonaws.com/files.cnas.org/documents/CNAS_AumShinrikyo_SecondEdition_English.pdf?mtime=20160906080510, accessed on 26 June 2020.
8. Ibid.
9. See note 7.
10. Jeffrey Ryan and Jan Glarum, 'Biosecurity and Bioterrorism: Containing and Preventing Biological Threats,' *Butterworth-Heinemann*, 2011, p. 164.
11. I. Sample, 'Synthetic Biology Raises Risk of New Bioweapons, US Report Warns,' *The Guardian*,

2018. available at https://www.theguardian.com/science/2018/jun/19/urgent-need-to-prepare-for-manmade-virus-attacks-says-us-government-report, accessed on 26 June 2020.

12. J. Koshy, 'Budget 2020: Cheer for Science as Key Departments Get a Raise,' *The Hindu*, 2020, available at https://www.thehindu.com/business/budget/budget-2020-cheer-for-science-as-key-departments-get-a-raise/article30715689.ece#:~:text=The%20Department%20of%20Biotechnology%20(DBT,crore%20it%20spent%20last%20year, accessed on 28 June 2020.
13. M. Specter, 'The Deadliest Virus,' *The New Yorker*, 2012, available at https://www.newyorker.com/magazine/2012/03/12/the-deadliest-virus, accessed on 28 June 2020.
14. Guidance for adoption of appropriate risk control measures to conduct safe research on H5N1 transmission, World Health Organization, 2012, available at http://www.who.int/influenza/human_animal_interface/biosafety_summary/en/index.html, accessed on 25 June 2020.
15. Steven Kendall, Anne-Marie Mazza and Karin Matchett, 'Perspectives on Research with H5N1 Avian Influenza: Scientific Inquiry, Communication, Controversy,' *Summary of a Workshop, National Academies Press*, 2013.
16. Aarti Dhar, 'NIV Pune Lab gets BSL-4,' *The Hindu*, 29 July 2011, available at https://www.thehindu.com/news/national/niv-pune-lab-gets-bsl4/article2305614.ece, accessed on 28 June 2020.
17. G.D. Koblentz, 'From Biodefence to Biosecurity: The Obama Administration's Strategy for Countering Biological Threats,' *Int Affairs*, 2012, pp. 131-148.
18. '1990 Emergency Ambulance Service now Available Island-wide Under Indian Grant Assistance,' *The Daily Financial Times*, 24 June 2019, available at http://www.ft.lk/healthcare/1990-Emergency-Ambulance-Service-now-available-island-wide-under-Indian-grant-assistance/45-680517, accessed on 26 June 2020.
19. Lisa Zhang and Gigi Kwik Gronvall, 'Red Teaming the Biological Sciences for Deliberate Threats, Terrorism and Political Violence,' *Taylor and Francis Online*, 30 May 2018.
20. DIA Hopes to Grow Anthrax Variant to Test Vaccine, US Department of Defense, 2001, available at https://archive.defense.gov/news/newsarticle.aspx?id=44931, accessed on 25 June 2020.
21. The Bay of Bengal Initiative for Multi-Sectoral Technical and Economic Cooperation (BIMSTEC). BIMSTEC Priority Areas, available at https://bimstec.org/?page_id=199, accessed on 25 June 2020.
22. Matt Field and John Krzyzaniak, 'Why do Politicians Keep Breathing Life into the False Conspiracy Theory that the Coronavirus is a Bioweapon?, *Bulletin of Atomic Scientists*, 19 March 2020, available at https://thebulletin.org/2020/03/why-do-politicians-keep-breathing-life-into-the-false-conspiracy-theory-that-the-coronavirus-is-a-bioweapon/, accessed on 29 June 2020.
23. N. Götz, 'The Deep Crisis of Nuclear Arms Control and Disarmament: The State of Play and the Challenges,' *Journal for Peace and Nuclear Disarmament*, pp. 431-452.

26

The COVID Crisis: Implications and Lessons for United States – and Global – Biosecurity

Vikram Venkatram, Diane DiEuliis and James Giordano

COVID-19: Elucidation of Vulnerabilities in United States Biosecurity

The United States' (US) engagement of public health resources to meet the SARS-CoV-2 (COVID-19) crisis revealed vulnerabilities in testing and treatment components of biosecurity. The lack of tests made it difficult to track exactly how many people within each state, as well as the US at-large were and/or are affected, which has implications both for the extent of public health response and for consideration of approaches aimed at stabilizing and sustaining the national and international economy.

COVID-19 testing has utilized a polymerase chain reaction (PCR) method to analyze genetic material found within bodily fluids, to identify the presence of SARS-CoV-2 viral genetic material.[1] However, PCR testing has incurred a number of problems: there have been considerable delays in making test results available to healthcare professionals and patients; the test may provide false negative results if administered soon after initial infection;[2] and PCR methods only assess the presence of a current viral infection, but do not afford information about whether the test recipient has recovered from prior COVID-19 infection.

This latter issue is important. Following infection, the immune system produces antibodies that are specific to the virus, and which remain functional after recovery.[3] This antibody response also occurs in individuals who have been infected but do not develop signs or symptoms of disease.[4] Serological testing can assess the presence of viral-specific antibodies in a person's blood, and in this way detect the presence of an immune response (rather than the virus itself), thus identifying those individuals who will likely possess subsequent immunity – at least in the short-term.[5] This makes serological testing useful to enable evaluation of viral spread, how many individuals have been infected to date, and how many people remain vulnerable to infection. Such assessments would facilitate more accurate predictions about the trajectory of COVID-19, and could also be used to identify those individuals (that are most likely immune) who might provide the human resources necessary to stabilize and sustain the economy.[6]

Awareness and Preparedness: Crucial Factors in Biosecurity Response

To be sure, COVID-19 is a novel virus. However, coronaviruses and other viral species capable of producing rapid and broad epidemic, if not pandemic effects are well-known, and the risk and threat of such a viral pandemic to the US and global biosecurity were previously identified and communicated.[7] The lack of available treatments – coupled to initial insufficiency of critical care resources (e.g.-mechanical ventilators) - placed enormous pressure on healthcare systems and personnel, and prompted difficult decisions[8] about triage and prioritization of care[9] in public, military, and political domains.

An important step toward treating COVID-19 is the development and use of safe and effective antiviral agents. Antiviral therapy could be aimed at targeting different stages in viral infection, replication and dissemination processes. Another useful approach to COVID-19 therapeutics is antibody treatment that may take the form of drugs,[10] or the use of "convalescent plasma" taken from infected individuals who have recovered from COVID-19 and possess neutralizing antibodies.[11] Certainly, there are limitations that must be acknowledged and addressed when considering the use of antibody-based treatment methods. For example, at present, it remains uncertain if and to what extent such treatments are effective in practice, and even if shown to be efficacious and effective in real-world settings, it is likely that antibody-rich plasma will not be easily identifiable or copiously available, at least in the near-term. Still, such treatments are promising, if for nothing else than to serve as a stop-gap while time and resources are committed to developing antiviral therapeutics and/or a viable vaccine.

Yet here too, increased availability and accessibility of serological tests will be essential to reveal who has been infected, and therefore who may be potential plasma donors. Improving the ability to quickly produce these resources, and creating them with accessible supply will be vital to rectify the US' ability to effectively respond to pandemics – and other biological threats – at present and in the years to come. The COVID-19 pandemic has demonstrated that the US is currently ill-equipped in biosecurity preparedness and response. The rapid spread of the disease has forced citizens to drastically change their behavior,[12] dramatically impacted domestic and global dimensions of the national economy,[13] prompted concerns about[14] readiness of the military in times of crisis,[15] and in these ways, fostered genuine manifest risks to US national security.

Implications and Lessons to be Learned

There is no evidence to indicate or support that COVID-19 was an intentionally developed or delivered biological weapon.[16] It is a naturally occurring virus that spread zoonotically (from horseshoe bats to humans[17]) in pandemic proportion. Yet, the impact and effects that the COVID crisis has had upon the US is illustrative of inherent weaknesses, flaws, and vulnerabilities in domestic biosecurity that could be targeted and kinetically or non-kinetically leveraged by adversaries in the future. Therefore, it is clear that the US must improve its biosecurity preparedness and responsiveness in order to effectively and efficiently provide protection from both natural and man-made threats. We have previously stated, and re-iterate here that ongoing advancements in gene-editing,[18] the use of drones,[19] and increasing diversion[20] of information[21] all serve to force-multiply the risks to the US and the global biosafety and security. The current situation brings into stark relief that it is not an issue of absent or insufficient intelligence: pandemic risks and threats to US biosecurity were identified and noted.[22] Rather, the problem is a failure to (1) utilize and act upon accurate intelligence and forecasting, and (2) identify and rectify extant infrastructural and functional gaps and inadequacies in biosecurity systems, programs and their cooperativity and collaboration.

To remain apace with – or ahead of - the scope of current and near-term biosecurity threats it is vital to accept the fleeting nature of dominance, envision futures of contested or lost dominance, and prepare plans for rapid transformation of capabilities and deployment. Indeed, this pandemic has revealed gaps in national biosecurity entities and capabilities of surveillance, reliable information transfer, and coordination and mobilization of existing resources, goods, and services that are essential to both preparedness and prompt, effective, and sustained response. Thus, we call for an evolved view of the operational environment of the future. We contend that this environment will not be force-on-force in the traditional sense; nor will it require, or be defined by, kinetic power. Instead, the future operating environment will be one of disruption, not destruction (at least not proximately).[23]

Current technologies and those that are emerging with increasing rapidity on the global stage will dominate engagement spaces as weapons (i.e., means of contending against others) of choice. Novel non-kinetic approaches and both multi-domain and multi-dimensional applications have potential to incur longer-term, more strategically-latent, nonetheless, disruptive (and perhaps more profoundly influential) damage to nations, all while providing the initiator plausible deniability and depriving the recipient of means of recognizing and asserting claims of attribution and grounds for exerting justifiable retribution.

Thus, a lesson to be learned from the COVID crisis is that it is time to divest from sole concepts and commitments to physical warfare and to re-position. This expanded view requires acknowledgment, recognition, quantification of, and preparedness for disruptive threats and those that are could be predicted to be leveraged in the near future. This will take insight, integration of resources, organizations and services, and multi-disciplinary engagement and innovation.

An adage regarding science and technology advises that if something can be considered, there is a probability that it's already being worked upon (somewhere, and to some extent). The biosecurity community previously considered, and expressed concern, if not frank anxieties about the possibility – and manifest problems – of a pandemic. Many[24] of these[25] have been realized.[26] Surely, inadequacies in US biosecurity preparedness, and response capabilities – and the biological, psychological, socio-economic, and political effects that such gaps have incurred, have become evident to global tactical and strategic competitors, and potential adversaries. This prompts questions of "What might they work on?", and hence, and more urgently, "What will – or should – we work on?"

The Shield, Sword, and Ethical Balance of Biosecurity

Axiomatically, the goal of any biosecurity program is to shield individuals and the public from risks and threats to health and safety through systems of risk and threat analyses, and preparedness. Effective shielding must consider both the risk/threat as well as the agent(s) being threatened. The former requires assessment and surveillance of current and potential detriments and dangers to public safety and health. The latter necessitates the evaluation of individual and group vulnerabilities in and across a variety of levels. Too small a shield will not protect against the threats against which it is intended. Too large and/or broad a shield can require unsustainable effort and resources. As well, insufficient shielding will less than fully accord – and thereby leave accessible – the weaknesses of those it is designed to protect. While over-extensive shielding can be excessively burdensome, and in this way both impractical and inefficient.

There are times and circumstances, however, that shielding is insufficient, and when a proverbial sword must be developed and employed to thwart a threat. The "blade" of this sword is two-sided: To be of value it must be of substance and sharpness to meet the threat(s) against which it will be used. However, forging such an instrument requires (1) knowledge of that upon which the blade is to render effect, and (2) testing and evaluation of its mettle.

We contend that these requirements are reciprocal in their intention and effects, in that the elements of biosecurity must be assessed for usefulness against risks and threats posed by an adversary at present, and in light of realistic probabilities, possibilities, and/or potentialities in the near-, intermediate- and more distal future, respectively.[27] Thus arises a conundrum: How can – and should – the capabilities and limits of biosecurity functions be evaluated without (1) risking those doing the testing; and (2) implicitly or explicitly expanding and/or advancing what destructive forces are possible, if not probable, given tendencies toward both what has been called the "technologic imperative"[28] and the trends of brinkmanship?

Arguably, biosecurity serves a defined public good in its disciplinary and functional role in protecting the polis. As a public good, programmes of biosecurity must be authentic (i.e. - actually do what they claim), non-wasteful (i.e., not misuse resources) and uphold community trust in their focus, scope and practices.[29] But communities differ, and cultural histories, needs, values, philosophies and ethics that define various nations' identity, ideologies – and the relative "good(s)" that these instantiate, must be recognized, if not responsibly and respectfully addressed.

Therefore, it is meaningful to ask if and what lessons have been learned for strengthening the shield and sharpening the sword of biosecurity from both the COVID crisis, and acknowledgment of current and near-future ecological, scientific, technological, and geopolitical realities? To appraise and navigate this rapidly changing landscape, we have proposed an operational risk assessment and mitigation paradigm to inform the development and use of new biomedical techniques and technologies, inclusive of those that can be employed in/for biosecurity purposes.[30] Important to this approach is regard for cultural and circumstantial contexts of use, and we have opined the potential utility and value of cosmopolitan ethics from which to obtain or develop precepts that could be multi-nationally applicable, and from which more "locally contextual" principles may be taken for specific instances of particular inter-cultural engagements.[31]

To be sure, such a recipe and task is complex – and complicated – in its development and articulation, especially given the dual-usability of any proactive biosecurity efforts that identify and address naturally-occurring and/or man-made threats. Moreover, the possibilities for, and (we have posited) probabilities of (1) human use and/or modification of naturally-occurring threats; (2) *de novo* human-developed threats are increasing, given new and more facile methods in[32] gene-editing,[33] synthetic,[34] biology,[35] big data,[36] and artificial intelligence.

A realistic assessment of the dual-use validity and value of biosecurity preparedness, readiness, and response begs the question of which ethical system(s) would provide the most authentic consideration, and most effective guidance and governance of the relative benefits, burdens, risks and harms involved.[37] The ethical approach(es) used should recognize and seek to clarify – and balance – the often-fuzzy definitions and boundaries of various nations' and cultures' public health and safety, and international security and defense.[38] The ethical toolkits to guide and govern these decisions and actions may require revisiting. Certain existing positions, precepts, and postures may need revision, as might development of new views and methods of engaging multi-national issues, questions, and problems that can – and likely will – arise given the scientific, technological, and political capabilities at hand, as well as those[39] that are lacking.[40] We have called for a whole-of-nation approach to addressing emerging threats[41] to biosecurity.[42] But this alone will be ineffectual, as this is neither the time nor the circumstances for stances of nationalistic isolationism. Rather, any whole-of-nation engagement must be multi-nationally cooperative to enable effective surveillance, prompt notification, tactical flexibility of resource utilization and response, and fixity in strategic planning to ensure the success of outcomes. It is our hope that lessons learned from the current crisis can be leveraged to foster more capable, ethically sound biosecurity in the future.

* * *

Portions of this chapter have been adapted with permission from the authors' previous published works, "COVID-19: lessons to be learned for national biosecurity and future operational environments: appearing in the *Journal of Defense Research and Engineering*; and "The shield and sword of biosecurity: Balancing the ethics of public safety and global preparedness", appearing in the *American Journal of Bioethics*. This work was supported, in part, by funding from the Henry Jackson Foundation and Leadership Initiatives (JG).

NOTES

1. Australian Government Department of Health, 'How Testing Works for COVID-19,' *Therapeutic Goods Administration (TGA), Australian Government Department of Health*, 27 March 2020, available at https://www.tga.gov.au/how-testing-works-covid-19, accessed on 29 June 2020.

2. 'Testing for COVID-19.' *Centers for Disease Control and Prevention*, 15 April 2020, available at https://www.cdc.gov/coronavirus/2019-ncov/symptoms-testing/testing.html, accessed on 29 June 2020.
3. Scot E. Dowd, Marilyn J. Halonen, and Raina M. Maier, 'Chapter 12 - Immunological Methods,' *Environmental Microbiology* 2nd ed., 2009, pp. 225–41, available at https://doi.org/10.1016/B978-0-12-370519-8.00012-2
4. Adam Rogers. 'Blood From COVID-19 Survivors May Point the Way to a Cure,' *Wired, Conde Nast*, 24 March 2020, available at https://www.wired.com/story/an-old-source-for-potential-new-covid-19-drugs-blood-serum/, accessed on 29 June 2020.
5. Stephen M. Hahn, 'Coronavirus (COVID-19) Update: Serological Tests,' *U.S. Food and Drug Administration (FDA)*, 7 April 2020, available at https://www.fda.gov/news-events/press-announcements/coronavirus-covid-19-update-serological-tests, accessed on 29 June 2020.
6. Daniel M. Gerstein and James Giordano, 'How to Reopen America,' *CNN, Cable News Network*, 27 March 2020, available at https://www.cnn.com/2020/03/27/opinions/reopen-america-coronavirus-gerstein-giordano/index.html., accessed on 29 June 2020.
7. John Walcott, 'The Trump Administration Is Stalling an Intel Report That Warns the U.S. Isn't Ready for a Global Pandemic,' *Time USA*, 9 March 2020, available on https://time.com/5799765/intelligence-report-pandemic-dangers/ accessed 29 June 2020.
8. Ariana Eunjung Cha, and Laurie McGinley, 'Who Gets a Shot at Life If Hospitals Run Short of Ventilators?,' *The Washington Post (WP Company)*, 7 April 2020, available at https://www.washingtonpost.com/health/2020/04/07/ventilators-rationing-coronavirus-hospitals/, accessed on 29 June 2020.
9. Sheri Fink, 'The Hardest Questions Doctors May Face: Who Will Be Saved? Who Won't?,' *The New York Times Company*, 21 March 2020, available at https://www.nytimes.com/2020/03/21/us/coronavirus-medical-rationing.html, accessed on 29 June 2020.
10. Margaret Hynds, '4 Things to Know about Possible Antibody Treatments for COVID-19,' *CBS News CBS Interactive*, 7 April 2020, available on https://www.cbsnews.com/news/four-things-to-know-about-possible-antibody-treatments-for-covid-19/, accessed on 29 June 2020.
11. 'Recommendations for Investigational COVID-19 Convalescent Plasma,' *U.S. Food and Drug Administration (FDA)*, 13 April 2020, available on https://www.fda.gov/vaccines-blood-biologics/investigational-new-drug-ind-or-device-exemption-ide-process-cber/recommendations-investigational-covid-19-convalescent-plasma, accessed 29 June 2020.
12. Jenesse Miller, 'Bracing for Coronavirus, U.S. Residents Are Changing Their Behavior,' *University of Southern California News*, 13 March 2020, available at https://news.usc.edu/166834/coronavirus-survey-usc-behavior-changes-health-economic-fallout/, accessed 29 June 2020.
13. Brian Menickella, 'COVID-19 Worldwide: The Pandemic's Impact on the Economy and Markets,' *Forbes Magazine*, 8 April 2020, available at https://www.forbes.com/sites/brianmenickella/2020/04/08/covid-19-worldwide-the-pandemics-impact-on-the-economy-and-markets/#668ce0c428c3, accessed on 29 June 2020.
14. Mark Cancian, 'How Coronavirus Could Hurt U.S. Military Readiness,' *Forbes Magazine*, 11 March 2020, available at https://www.forbes.com/sites/markcancian/2020/03/11/will-covid-19-devastate-military-readiness/#1770cd0c1e10, accessed on 29 June 2020.
15. Diane DiEuliis and Laura Junor, 'Ready or Not: Regaining Military Readiness during COVID19,' *Strategic Insights, Institute for National Strategic Studies*, 10 April 2020, available at https://inss.ndu.edu/Media/News/Article/2145282/ready-or-not-regaining-military-readiness-during-covid19/, accessed on 29 June 2020.

16. Bruce Y. Lee, 'No, COVID-19 Coronavirus Was Not Bioengineered. Here's the Research That Debunks That Idea,' *Forbes Magazine*, 17 March 2020, available at https://www.forbes.com/sites/brucelee/2020/03/17/covid-19-coronavirus-did-not-come-from-a-lab-study-shows-natural-origins/#602176ef3728, accessed on 29 June 2020.
17. David M. Morens, Jeffery K. Taubenberger, and Peter Daszak, 'Escaping Pandora's Box - Another Novel Coronavirus: NEJM,' *New England Journal of Medicine*, 2 April 2020, available at https://www.nejm.org/doi/full/10.1056/NEJMp2002106?query=TOC, accessed on 29 June 2020.
18. Diane DiEuliis and James Giordano, 'Gene editing using CRISPR/Cas9: implications for dual-use and biosecurity,' *Protein Cell 9*, 2018, pp. 239–240, available at https://doi.org/10.1007/s13238-017-0493-4, accessed on 29 June 2020.
19. Joseph DeFranco, 'Dark Side of Delivery: The Growing Threat of Bioweapon Dissemination by Drones,' *Defence IQ*, 24 January 2020, available at https://www.defenceiq.com/cyber-defence-and-security/articles/the-dark-side-of-delivery-the-growing-threat-of-bioweapon-dissemination-by-drones, accessed on 29 June 2020.
20. Diane DiEuliis, Charles D. Lutes, and James Giordano, 'Biodata Risks and Synthetic Biology: A Critical Juncture,' *Journal of Bioterrorism & Biodefense*, 4 April 2018, available at https://inss.ndu.edu/Portals/97/Documents/Publications/Articles/biodata-risks-and-synthetic-biology-a-critical-juncture.pdf?ver=2018-04-04-100001-330, accessed on 29 June 2020.
21. James Giordano, 'Weaponizing the Brain: Neuroscience Advancements Spark Debate,' *National Defense Magazine, National Defense Industrial Association*, 11 May 2017, available at https://www.nationaldefensemagazine.org/articles/2017/5/11/weaponizing-the-brain-neuroscience-advancements-spark-debate, accessed on 29 June 2020.
22. John Walcott, 'The Trump Administration Is Stalling an Intel Report That Warns the U.S. Isn't Ready for a Global Pandemic,' *Time Magazine*, 9 March 2020, available at https://time.com/5799765/intelligence-report-pandemic-dangers/, accessed on 29 June 2020.
23. Joseph P. DeFranco, Diane DiEuliis, L.R. Bremseth, J.J. Snow, and James Giordano, 'Emerging technologies for disruptive effects in non-kinetic engagements,' *HDIAC Currents*, vol. 6, no. 2, 2019, pp. 49-54.
24. Rocco Casagrande, 'Assessing the Risks and Benefits of Conducting Research on Pathogens of Pandemic Potential,' *Gryphon Scientific*, 2015, available at https://www.gryphonscientific.com/resources/gain-of-function/#1545916149863-1000f696-4d32, accessed on 29 June 2020.
25. 'DNI Coats Opening Statement on the 2019 Worldwide Threat Assessment of the U.S. Intelligence Community,' 29 January 2020, available at https://www.dni.gov/index.php/newsroom/congressional-testimonies/item/1949-dni-coats-opening-statement-on-the-2019-worldwide-threat-assessment-of-the-us-intelligence-community, accessed on 29 June 2020.
26. David Sanger, Eric Lipton, Eileen Sullivan, and Michael Crowley, 'Before Virus Outbreak, a Cascade of Warnings Went Unheeded,' *The New York Times*, 19 March 2020, available at https://www.nytimes.com/2020/03/19/us/politics/trump-coronavirus-outbreak.html, accessed on 29 June 2020.
27. See note 23.
28. Hans Lenk, 'Technokratie als Ideologie: Sozialphilosophische Beitrage zu Einem Politischen Dilemma', *Stuttgart, Ger: Kohlhammer Press*, 1973.
29. W.F. May, 'Contending images of the healer in an era of turnstile medicine,' in JK Walter and EP Klein (eds.) *The Story of Bioethics: From Seminal Works to Contemporary Explorations*, Washington DC: Georgetown University Press.
30. James Giordano, 'Toward an Operational Neuroethical Risk Analysis and Mitigation Paradigm

for Emerging Neuroscience and Technology (neuroS/T),' *Exp Neurol*, vol. 287, no. 4, 2017, pp. 492-495.

31. John R. Shook and James Giordano, 'A principled, cosmopolitan neuroethics: Considerations for international relevance,' *Phil Ethics Humanities in Med*, vol. 9, no.1, 2014.
32. James Giordano, J.J. Snow, and Joseph P. DeFranco, 'Weaponized Prions: Much ado about Nothing, or Big Concerns about little Proteins?,' *DefenceIQ*, vol. 12, no. 42, 2019.
33. Diane DiEuliis and James Giordano, 'Why Gene Editors like CRISPR/Cas may be a game-changer for neuroweapons,' *Health Security*, vol. 15, no. 3, 2017, pp. 296-302.
34. J.J. Snow and James Giordano, 'Public safety and national security implications of the horsepox study,' *Health Security*, vol. 16, no. 2, 2018, pp. 1-3.
35. Diane DiEuliis, Charles D. Lutes, and James Giordano, 'Biodata risks and synthetic biology: A critical juncture,' *Journal of Bioterrorism and Biodefense*, vol. 9, no. 1, 2018, pp. 2-14.
36. Diane DiEuliis, James Giordano, 'Neurotechnological convergence and "big data": A force-multiplier toward advancing neuroscience,' in J Collmann and SA Matei (eds.), *Ethical Reasoning in Big Data: An Exploratory Analysis.* NY: Springer, 2016.
37. John R. Shook and James Giordano, 'Neuroethical engagement on interdisciplinary and international scales,' in E Racine and J Aspler (eds.), *Debates About Neuroethics*, NY: Springer, 2017.
38. M. Tennison, James Giordano, J. Moreno, 'Security threat versus aggregated truths: Ethical issues in the use of neuroscience and neurotechnology for national security,' in J. Illes and S. Hossein (eds.), *Neuroethics: Anticipating the Future.* Oxford: Oxford University Press, 2017, pp. 531-553.
39. James Giordano, E. Lanzilao, John R. Shook, and R. Benedikter, 'Guidare la neuroscienza e lo sviluppo della persona nel XXI secolo: Una prospettiva naturalistica e cosmopolita per la neuroetica,' *L'Arco di Giano*, vol. 80, 2015, pp. 147-164.
40. E. Lanzilao, John R. Shook, R. Benedikter, and James Giordano, 'Advancing neuroscience on the 21st century world stage: The need for – and proposed structure of – an internationally relevant neuroethics,' *Ethics Biol Engineer Med*, vol. 4, no. 3, 2013, pp. 211-229.
41. James Giordano, L.R. Bremseth, Joseph P. DeFranco, 'Dual- and non-kinetic use of Chinese brain science: Current activities and future implications,' in N. Petersen (ed.), *Chinese Strategic Intentions: A Deep Dive into China's Worldwide Activities*, Department of Defense, Strategic Multilayer Assessment Group- Joint Staff/J-3/Pentagon Strategic Studies Group, November 2019.
42. See note 23.

Editors' Musings

In the 1960s researchers of experimental psychology provided an opinion that holds ground even today. They had argued that normally when humans are presented with information, they tend to remember the first and last elements and are more likely to forget the middle ones. COVID-19 is an ongoing crisis with no end in-sight. The information and analysis presented in this work is probably at a time close to the midpoint of the crisis. It is expected that even the middle of this story is important to take note of. The nature of the coronavirus catastrophe is so overwhelming that even during the midpoint of the crisis there should be an interest to understand in which direction the world is moving. COVID-19 is a unique story where we know the location of the origin of the threat, however, still there is no clarity about how this threat has originated. The middle of this story is about an ongoing saga of the genuine attempts being made by many to overcome the crisis. The world had never witnessed anything like this before and hence some confusion about the nature of the response required continues. Presently, there are no indications about how this story would end. Also, it is very difficult to extrapolate the expiration. Still the story needs to be told because after all, it is a challenge to the existence of the human race on earth.

The world has been addressing the threat from pandemics since the earliest days of organized human activity. However, the nature and impact of COVID-19 is something not witnessed and experienced earlier. Till this date, the challenge is continuing, the infections are happening, and the risk of coronavirus spreading is far from over. The situation continues to remain grim and there are no immediate remedies in sight. The last couple of months demonstrate that the world everyday reaches a new and dreadful record. By the end of June 2020, there have been more than 500,000 deaths globally owing to this pandemic. Some countries are continuing to see a rapid increase in cases and deaths while some have effectively curbed transmission. However, at a few locations, the infections are re-occurring.

It is becoming obvious that transmission is increasing in the zones where the administration is allowing the reopening of normal activities.

The handling of this pandemic has been a unique experience for every country. The biggest causality of this pandemic (so far) has been the most developed state in the world, the United States of America (USA). This made the rest of the world realise that they need to think quickly and find answers to the challenges on their own. Apart from the US, many of the other developed states which are known to have a very sound health infrastructure are also facing a major crisis. There is a possibility that since the US and Europe got affected during the early phase of the pandemic, hence they were caught totally off-guard while the rest of the world had time to prepare themselves.

The entire world went under lockdown since February/March 2020 and started opening up around May 2020. Hence, broadly this volume is based on the experiences of both the lockdown phase and the post-lockdown phase. The first six months of 2020 could be viewed as a period of learning and experimentation for almost every state. By the end of February/early March, particularly after realising the enormity of this threat, the world started reacting with urgency. Various creative, innovative and out-of-box ideas were placed on the table. The imaginative use of various available technologies has been visible and some quick modifications in the existing technologies are being undertaken to suit the requirements. Particularly in the field of vaccine development, various collaborative efforts are visible. There is a realisation that technology alone can offer the world a way out of this major health disaster.

Presently, states are trying to realize a delicate balance between shielding their populations from the corona infection to minimizing the socio-political and economic damage. They were (are) forced to announce the lockdown to restrict the spread of the disease, but this has adversely impacted the livelihoods of the population. Job loss is the biggest problem, which the world needs to address in the immediate future. Today, the world is at the crossroads, where there is not much of a choice ahead of them. If they continue with the lockdown then there is a possibility that people could die of hunger, otherwise there could be deaths from the infection.

Along with health, the other biggest casualty is the economy. Within the first six months of the COVID-19 crisis itself, the economy has taken a major shock which almost all countries in the world are unable to resolve. The World Bank has already predicted negative growth for most countries. The real challenge for most economies is to co-exist with the COVID-19 (till the antidote is available) and prosper. Also, much would depend on the nature, extent and expanse of the second wave of COVID-19 (if it happens).

This pandemic has been an eye-opener for everyone from doctors to politicians and from students to scientists. There has been a new revelation for the industry, that a few industrial sectors can actually follow a successful model of work from home. Webinars have become the buzzword for many sectors. This medium has proved its utility beyond doubt. It has made people realise that how much local, regional and international travel was unnecessarily taking place for all these years. All in all, the world has successfully managed to migrate towards using various digital platforms for the conduct of various activities. However, there remains two prevalent challenge: that of cybersecurity and the disparity between digital haves and have-nots.

Social media has played an important role during this crisis. Initially, possibilities seemed endless, but over a period of time there is some realisation about the limits of social media too. Misinformation and fake news made many realise that in these times of crisis they should be careful about depending on these platforms. Globally, the entertainment industry and sports agencies are found using these platforms to their advantage and are ensuring that their relevance remains intact for their audiences.

Unfortunately, nation-states are still found continuing with their age-old rivalries and differences. Even during these times of crisis, a few states are found pushing for their geostrategic agenda. It appears that even during the extreme nature of the crisis, a few powers are not ready to look beyond the petty power politics. Probably, they are using the global health emergency to their advantage to pursue their strategic agenda. Also, many states appear to have identified the World Health Organization (WHO) as a scapegoat for the crisis. This appears to be more of a diversionary tactic so that they hide failures of their health sector which were not ready to address the possibility of pandemics.

Also, there is much talk that, 'a different world order is on the anvil in the post-COVID-19 era'. It looks a bit premature to make a definitive statement in this regard at this point in time. Even today, the major powers in the world are found to be relentlessly continuing with their military agenda. They are unlikely to give up the 'order' which they have created to suit their aspirations. Initially, states could make some changes with regard to established practices, methods of working and processes of development of norms and regulations in the post-COVID-19 era. Also, the world could slow down with regard to various global activities in the foreseeable future. However, at this stage, major systemic changes look difficult. Could there be a diminishing role for the US and Europe in the near future? It would be difficult to give a definitive answer, however, there is a possibility that important powers in the world would try to (mostly collectively) ensure that the world order is not dominated by China.

It could be a 'goldmine' for an agency or a country that invents the vaccine and/or a medicine first. They also would require a reasonable industry infrastructure to produce them to fulfil the global requirement. There is a likelihood that such a state could probably (mostly covertly) use this opportunity to further its geo-strategic and geo-economic agenda.

It is sad that for all these years the world has concentrated on how to reach the Moon and Mars, what destructive power an atom can produce and many other inventions. However, collectively the human community have failed to strengthen their healthcare systems with solutions ready to address the threat from possible pandemics. Today, the entire world is living on the hope that come January/February 2021 and we would have a vaccine in hand and then all would be fine. But, does the world have a plan B available?

APPENDIX

DRAFT Landscape of COVID-19 Candidate Vaccines – 29 June 2020

17 Candidate Vaccines in Clinical Evaluation

Platform	*Type of candidate vaccine*	*Developer*	*Coronavirus target*	*Current stage of clinical evaluation/regulatory status-Coronavirus candidate*	*Same platform for non-Coronavirus candidates*
Non-Replicating Viral Vector	ChAdOx1-S	University of Oxford/ AstraZeneca	SARS-CoV2	Phase 3 ISRCTN89951424 Phase2b/3 2020-001228-32 Phase 1/2 PACTR202006922165132 2020-001072-15	MERS, Influenza, TB, Chikungunya, Zika, MenB, Plague
Non-Replicating Viral Vector	Adenovirus Type 5 Vector	CanSino Biological Inc./ Beijing Institute of Biotechnology	SARS-CoV2	Phase 2 ChiCTR2000031781 Phase 1 ChiCTR2000030906	Ebola
RNA	LNP-encapsulated mRNA	Moderna/NIAID	SARS-CoV2	Phase 2 NCT04405076 Phase 1 NCT04283461	Multiple candidates
Inactivated	Inactivated	Wuhan Institute of Biological Products/Sinopharm	SARS-CoV2	Phase 1/2 ChiCTR2000031809	
Inactivated	Inactivated	Beijing Institute of Biological Products/Sinopharm	SARS-CoV2	Phase 1/2 ChiCTR2000032459	
Inactivated	Inactivated+alum	Sinovac	SARS-CoV2	Phase 1/2 NCT04383574 NCT04352608	SARS
Protein Subunit	Full length recombinant SARS CoV-2 glycoprotein nanoparticle vaccine adjuvanted with Matrix M	Novavax	SARS-CoV2	Phase 1/2 NCT04368988	RSV; CCHF, HPV, VZV, EBOV

RNA	3 LNP-mRNAs	BioNTech/Fosun Pharma/Pfizer	SARS-CoV2	Phase 1/2 2020-001038-36 NCT04368728	
Inactivated	Inactivated	Institute of Medical Biology, Chinese Academy of Medical Sciences	SARS-CoV2	Phase 1 NCT04412538	
DNA	DNA plasmid vaccine with electroporation	Inovio Pharmaceuticals	SARS-CoV2	Phase 1 NCT04336410	Multiple candidates
DNA	DNA Vaccine (GX-19)	Genexine Consortium	SARS-CoV2	Phase 1 NCT04445389	
Non-Replicating Viral Vector	Adeno-based	Gamaleya Research Institute	SARS-CoV2	Phase 1 NCT04436471 NCT04437875	
Protein Subunit	Native like Trimeric subunit Spike Protein vaccine	Clover Biopharmaceuticals Inc./ GSK/Dynavax	SARS-CoV2	Phase 1 NCT04405908	HIV, REV Influenza
Protein Subunit	Adjuvanted recombinant protein (RBD-Dimer)	Anhui Zhifei Longcom Biopharmaceutical/Institute of Microbiology, Chinese Academy of Sciences	SARS-CoV2	Phase 1 NCT04445194	MERS
RNA	LNP-nCoVsaRNA	Imperial College London	SARS-CoV2	Phase 1 ISRCTN17072692	EBOV; LASV, MARV, Inf (H7N9), RABV
RNA	mRNA	Curevac	SARS-CoV2	Phase 1 NCT04449276	RABV, LASV, YFV; MERS, InfA, ZIKV, DENV, NIPV
RNA	mRNA	People's Liberation Army (PLA) Academy of Military Sciences/ Walvax Biotech	SARS-CoV2	Phase 1 ChiCTR2000034112	

DISCLAIMER: These landscape documents have been prepared by the World Health Organization (WHO) for information purposes only concerning the 2019-2020 global of the novel coronavirus. Inclusion of any particular product or entity in any of these landscape documents does not constitute, and shall not be deemed or construed as, any approval or endorsement by WHO of such product or entity (or any of its businesses or activities). While WHO takes reasonable steps to verify the accuracy of the information presented in these landscape documents, WHO does not make any (and hereby disclaims all) representations and warranties regarding the accuracy, completeness, fitness for a particular purpose (including any of the aforementioned purposes), quality, safety, efficacy, merchantability and/or non-infringement of any information provided in these landscape documents and/or of any of the products referenced therein. WHO also disclaims any and all liability or responsibility whatsoever for any death, disability, injury, suffering, loss, damage or other prejudice of any kind that may arise from or in connection with the procurement, distribution or use of any product included in any of these landscape documents.

132 Candidate Vaccines in Preclinical Evaluation

Platform	*Type of candidate vaccine*	*Developer*	*Coronavirus target*	*Current stage of clinical evaluation/regulatory status-Coronavirus candidate*	*Same platform for non-Coronavirus candidates*
DNA	DNA plasmid vaccine S,S1,S2,RBD &N	National Research Centre, Egypt	SARS-CoV2	Pre-Clinical	
DNA	DNA with electroporation	Karolinska Institute/Cobra Biologics (OPENCORONA Project)	SARS-CoV2	Pre-Clinical	
DNA	DNA with electroporation	Chula Vaccine Research Center	SARS-CoV2	Pre-Clinical	
DNA	DNA plasmid vaccine	Osaka University/AnGes/ Takara Bio	SARS-CoV2	Pre-Clinical	
DNA	DNA	Takis/Applied DNA Sciences/ Evvivax	SARS-CoV2	Pre-Clinical	
DNA	Plasmid DNA, Needle-Free Delivery	Immunomic Therapeutics, Inc./ EpiVax, Inc./PharmaJet	SARS-CoV2	Pre-Clinical	SARS
DNA	DNA plasmid vaccine	Zydus Cadila	SARS-CoV2	Pre-Clinical	
DNA	DNA vaccine	BioNet Asia	SARS-CoV2	Pre-Clinical	
DNA	DNA vaccine	University of Waterloo	SARS-CoV2	Pre-Clinical	
DNA	DNA vaccine	Entos Pharmaceuticals	SARS-CoV2	Pre-Clinical	
DNA	bacTRL-Spike	Symvivo	SARS-CoV2	Pre-Clinical	
Inactivated	Inactivated whole virus	National Research Centre, Egypt	SARS-CoV2	Pre-Clinical	
Inactivated	Inactivated	Beijing Minhai Biotechnology Co., Ltd.	SARS-CoV2	Pre-Clinical	
Inactivated	TBD	Osaka University/BIKEN/ NIBIOHN	SARS-CoV2	Pre-Clinical	
Inactivated	Inactivated + CpG 1018	Sinovac/Dynavax	SARS-CoV2	Pre-Clinical	
Inactivated	Inactivated + CpG 1018	Valneva/Dynavax	SARS-CoV2	Pre-Clinical	
Inactivated	Inactivated	Research Institute for Biological Safety Problems, Rep of Kazakhstan	SARS-CoV2	Pre-Clinical	
Live Attenuated Virus	Codon deoptimized live attenuated vaccines	Codagenix/Serum Institute of India	SARS-CoV2	Pre-Clinical	HAV, InfA, ZIKV, FMD, SIV, RSV, DENV

Live Attenuated Virus	Codon deoptimized live attenuated vaccines	Indian Immunologicals Ltd/ Griffith University	SARS-CoV2	Pre-Clinical	
Non-Replicating Viral Vector	Adeno-associated virus vector (AAVCOVID)	Massachusetts Eye and Ear/ Massachusetts General Hospital/AveXis	SARS-CoV2	Pre-Clinical	
Non-Replicating Viral Vector	MVA encoded VLP	GeoVax/BravoVax	SARS-CoV2	Pre-Clinical	LASV, EBOV, MARV, HIV
Non-Replicating Viral Vector	Ad26	Janssen Pharmaceutical Companies	SARS-CoV2	Pre-Clinical	Ebola, HIV, RSV
Non-Replicating Viral Vector	Replication defective Simian Adenovirus (GRAd) encoding SARS-CoV-2 S	ReiThera/LEUKOCARE/ Univercells	SARS-CoV2	Pre-Clinical	
Non-replicating Viral Vector	MVA-S encoded	DZIF – German Center for Infection Research/ IDT Biologika GmbH	SARS-CoV2	Pre-clinical	Many
Non-replicating Viral Vector	MVA-S	IDIBAPS-Hospital Clinic, Spain	SARS-CoV2	Pre-clinical	
Non-Replicating Viral Vector	Adenovirus-based NasoVAX expressing SARS2-CoV spike protein	Altimmune	SARS-CoV2	Pre-Clinical	Influenza
Non-Replicating Viral Vector	[E1-, E2b-, E3-] hAd5-COVID19-Spike/ Nucleocapsid	ImmunityBio, Inc. & NantKwest, Inc.	SARS-CoV2	Pre-Clinical	flu, Chik, Zika, EBOV, LASV, HIV/SIV, Cancer
Non-Replicating Viral Vector	Ad5 S (GREVAX™ platform)	Greffex	SARS-CoV2	Pre-Clinical	MERS
Non-Replicating Viral Vector	Oral Ad5 S	Stabilitech Biopharma Ltd	SARS-CoV2	Pre-Clinical	Zika, VZV, HSV-2 and Norovirus
Non-Replicating Viral Vector	Adenovirus-based + HLA-matched peptides	Valo Therapeutics Ltd	Pan-Corona	Pre-Clinical	
Non-Replicating Viral Vector	Oral Vaccine platform	Vaxart	SARS-CoV2	Pre-Clinical	InfA, CHIKV, LASV, NORV; EBOV, RVF, HBV, VEE

(*Table Contd.*)

Platform	*Type of candidate vaccine*	*Developer*	*Coronavirus target*	*Current stage of clinical evaluation/regulatory status-Coronavirus candidate*	*Same platform for non-Coronavirus candidates*
Non-Replicating Viral Vector	MVA expressing structural proteins	Centro Nacional Biotecnología (CNB-CSIC), Spain	SARS-CoV2	Pre-Clinical	Multiple candidates
Non-Replicating Viral Vector	Dendritic cell-based vaccine	University of Manitoba	SARS-CoV2	Pre-Clinical	
Non-Replicating Viral Vector	Parainfluenza virus 5 (PIV5)-based vaccine expressing the spike protein	University of Georgia/ University of Iowa	SARS-CoV2	Pre-Clinical	MERS
Non-Replicating Viral Vector	Recombinant deactivated rabies virus containing S1	Bharat Biotech/Thomas Jefferson University	SARS-CoV2	Pre-Clinical	HeV, NiV, EBOV, LASSA, CCHFV, MERS
Non-Replicating Viral Vector	Influenza A H1N1 vector	National Research Centre, Egypt	SARS-CoV2	Pre-Clinical	
Non-Replicating Viral Vector	Inactivated Flu-based SARS-CoV2 vaccine + Adjuvant	National Center for Genetic Engineering and Biotechnology (BIOTEC) /GPO, Thailand	SARS-CoV2	Pre-Clinical	
Protein Subunit	Subunit	Helix Biogen Consult, Ogbomoso & Trinity Immonoefficient Laboratory, Ogbomoso, Oyo State, Nigeria.	SARS-CoV2	Pre-Clinical	
Protein Subunit	Protein Subunit S, N, M&S1 protein	National Research Centre, Egypt	SARS-CoV2	Pre-Clinical	
Protein Subunit	Protein Subunit	University of San Martin and CONICET, Argentina	SARS-CoV2	Pre-Clinical	
Protein Subunit	RBD protein fused with Fc of IgG + Adj.	Chulalongkorn University/ GPO, Thailand	SARS-CoV2	Pre-Clinical	
Protein Subunit	Capsid-like Particle	AdaptVac (PREVENT-nCoV consortium)	SARS-CoV2	Pre-Clinical	
Protein Subunit	Drosophila S2 insect cell expression system VLPs	ExpreS2ion	SARS-CoV2	Pre-Clinical	
Protein Subunit	Peptide antigens formulated in LNP	IMV Inc	SARS-CoV2	Pre-Clinical	

Protein Subunit	S protein	WRAIR/USAMRIID	SARS-CoV2	Pre-Clinical	
Protein Subunit	S protein +Adjuvant	National Institute of Infectious Disease, Japan	SARS-CoV2	Pre-Clinical	Influenza
Protein Subunit	VLP-recombinant protein + Adjuvant	Osaka University/BIKEN/ National Institutes of Biomedical Innovation, Japan	SARS-CoV2	Pre-Clinical	
Protein Subunit	Microneedle arrays S1 subunit	Univ. of Pittsburgh	SARS-CoV2	Pre-Clinical	MERS
Protein Subunit	Peptide	Vaxil Bio	SARS-CoV2	Pre-Clinical	
Protein Subunit	Adjuvanted protein subunit (RBD)	Biological E Ltd	SARS-CoV2	Pre-Clinical	
Protein Subunit	Peptide	Flow Pharma Inc	SARS-CoV2	Pre-Clinical	Ebola, Marburg, HIV, Zika, Influenza, HPV therapeutic vaccine, BreastCA vaccine
Protein Subunit	S protein	AJ Vaccines	SARS-CoV2	Pre-Clinical	
Protein Subunit	Ii-Key peptide	Generex/EpiVax	SARS-CoV2	Pre-Clinical	Influenza, HIV, SARS-CoV
Protein Subunit	S protein	EpiVax/Univ. of Georgia	SARS-CoV2	Pre-Clinical	H7N9
Protein Subunit	Protein Subunit EPV-CoV-19		EpiVax	SARS-CoV2	Pre-Clinical
Protein Subunit	S protein (baculovirus production)	Sanofi Pasteur/GSK	SARS-CoV2	Pre-Clinical	Influenza, SARS-CoV
Protein Subunit	gp-96 backbone	Heat Biologics/Univ. Of Miami	SARS-CoV2	Pre-Clinical	NSCLC, HIV, malaria, Zika
Protein Subunit	Molecular clamp stabilized Spike protein	University of Queensland/ GSK/Dynavax	SARS-CoV2	Pre-Clinical	Nipah, Influenza, Ebola, Lassa
Protein Subunit	Peptide vaccine	FBRI SRC VB VECTOR, Rospotrebnadzor, Koltsovo	SARS-CoV2	Pre-Clinical	Ebola
Protein Subunit	Subunit vaccine	FBRI SRC VB VECTOR, Rospotrebnadzor, Koltsovo	SARS-CoV2	Pre-Clinical	
Protein Subunit	S1 or RBD protein	Baylor College of Medicine	SARS-CoV2	Pre-Clinical	SARS
Protein Subunit	Subunit protein, plant produced	iBio/CC-Pharming	SARS-CoV2	Pre-Clinical	

(*Table Contd.*)

Platform	*Type of candidate vaccine*	*Developer*	*Coronavirus target*	*Current stage of clinical evaluation/regulatory status-Coronavirus candidate*	*Same platform for non-Coronavirus candidates*
Protein Subunit	Recombinant protein, nano-particles (based on S-protein and other epitopes)	Saint-Petersburg Scientific Research Institute of Vaccines and Serums	SARS-CoV2	Pre-Clinical	
Protein Subunit	COVID-19 XWG-03 truncated S (spike) proteins	Innovax/Xiamen Univ./GSK	SARS-CoV2	Pre-Clinical	HPV
Protein Subunit	Adjuvanted microsphere peptide	VIDO-InterVac, University of Saskatchewan	SARS-CoV2	Pre-Clinical	
Protein Subunit	Synthetic Long Peptide Vaccine candidate for S and M proteins	OncoGen	SARS-CoV2	Pre-Clinical	
Protein Subunit	Oral E. coli-based protein expression system of S and N proteins	MIGAL Galilee Research Institute	SARS-CoV2	Pre-Clinical	
Protein Subunit	Nanoparticle vaccine	LakePharma, Inc.	SARS-CoV2	Pre-Clinical	
Protein Subunit	Recombinant spike protein with Advax™ adjuvant	Vaxine Pty Ltd/Medytox	SARS-CoV2	Pre-Clinical	
Protein Subunit	Plant-based subunit (RBD-Fc + Adjuvant)	Baiya Phytopharm/ Chula Vaccine Research Center	SARS-CoV2	Pre-Clinical	
Protein Subunit	OMV-based vaccine	Quadram Institute Biosciences	SARS-CoV2	Pre-Clinical	Flu A, plague
Protein Subunit	OMV-based vaccine	BiOMViS Srl/Univ. of Trento	SARS-CoV2	Pre-Clinical	
Protein subunit	Structurally modified spherical particles of the Tobacco Mosaic Virus (TMV)	Lomonosov Moscow State University	SARS-CoV2	Pre-Clinical	Rubella, Rotavirus
Protein Subunit	Spike-based	University of Alberta	SARS-CoV2	Pre-Clinical	Hepatitis C
Protein Subunit	Recombinant S1-Fc fusion protein	AnyGo Technology	SARS-CoV2	Pre-Clinical	
Protein Subunit	Recombinant protein	Yisheng Biopharma	SARS-CoV2	Pre-Clinical	
Protein Subunit	Recombinant S protein in IC-BEVS	Vabiotech	SARS-CoV2	Pre-Clinical	

Protein Subunit	Orally delivered, heat stable subunit	Applied Biotechnology Institute, Inc.	SARS-CoV2	Pre-Clinical	
Protein Subunit	S-2P protein + CpG 1018	Medigen Vaccine Biologics Corporation/NIAID/Dynavax	SARS-CoV2	Pre-Clinical	
Protein Subunit	Peptides derived from Spike protein	Axon Neuroscience SE	SARS-CoV2	Pre-Clinical	
Protein Subunit	Protein Subunit	MOGAM Institute for Biomedical Research, GC Pharma	SARS-CoV2	Pre-Clinical	
Protein Subunit	RBD-based	Neovii/Tel Aviv University	SARS-CoV2	Pre-Clinical	
Protein Subunit	RBD-based	Kentucky Bioprocessing, Inc	SARS-CoV2	Pre-Clinical	
Protein Subunit	Outer Membrane Vesicle (OMV)-subunit	Intravacc/Epivax	SARS-CoV2	Pre-Clinical	
Protein Subunit	Outer Membrane Vesicle (OMV)-peptide	Intravacc/Epivax	SARS-CoV2	Pre-Clinical	
Protein Subunit	Spike-based (epitope screening)	ImmunoPrecise/LiteVax BV	SARS-CoV2	Pre-Clinical	
Replicating Viral Vector	YF17D Vector	KU Leuven	SARS-CoV2	Pre-Clinical	
Replicating Viral Vector	Measles Vector	Zydus Cadila	SARS-CoV2	Pre-Clinical	
Replicating Viral Vector	Measles Vector	Institute Pasteur/Themis/Univ. of Pittsburg Center for Vaccine Research/Merck	SARS-CoV2	Pre-Clinical	West Nile, Chik, Ebola, Lassa, Zika
Replicating Viral Vector	Measles Vector	FBRI SRC VB VECTOR, Rospotrebnadzor, Koltsovo	SARS-CoV2	Pre-Clinical	
Replicating Viral Vector	Measles Virus (S, N targets)	DZIF – German Center for Infection Research/CanVirex AG	SARS-CoV2	Pre-clinical	Zika, H7N9, CHIKV
Replicating Viral Vector	Horsepox vector expressing S protein	Tonix Pharma/Southern Research	SARS-CoV2	Pre-Clinical	Smallpox, Monkeypox
Replicating Viral Vector	Live viral vectored vaccine based on attenuated influenza virus backbone (intranasal)	BiOCAD and IEM	SARS-CoV2	Pre-Clinical	Influenza

(*Table Contd.*)

Platform	*Type of candidate vaccine*	*Developer*	*Coronavirus target*	*Current stage of clinical evaluation/regulatory status-Coronavirus candidate*	*Same platform for non-Coronavirus candidates*
Replicating Viral Vector	Recombinant vaccine based on Influenza A virus, for the prevention of COVID-19 (intranasal)	FBRI SRC VB VECTOR, Rospotrebnadzor, Koltsovo	SARS-CoV2	Pre-Clinical	Influenza
Replicating Viral Vector	Attenuated Influenza expressing an antigenic portion of the Spike protein	Fundação Oswaldo Cruz and Instituto Buntantan	SARS-CoV2	Pre-Clinical	Influenza
Replicating Viral Vector	Influenza vector expressing RBD	University of Hong Kong	SARS-CoV2	Pre-Clinical	
Replicating Viral Vector	Replication-competent VSV chimeric virus technology (VSVÄG) delivering the SARS CoV-2 Spike (S) glycoprotein	IAVI/Merck	SARS-CoV2	Pre-Clinical	Ebola, Marburg, Lassa
Replicating Viral Vector	VSV-S	University of Western Ontario	SARS-CoV2	Pre-Clinical	HIV, MERS
Replicating Viral Vector	VSV vector	FBRI SRC VB VECTOR, Rospotrebnadzor, Koltsovo	SARS-CoV2	Pre-Clinical	
Replicating Viral Vector	VSV-S	Israel Institute for Biological Research/ Weizmann Institute of Science	SARS-CoV2	Pre-Clinical	
Replicating Viral Vector	M2-deficient single replication (M2SR) influenza vector	UW–Madison/FluGen/ Bharat Biotech	SARS-CoV2	Pre-Clinical	Influenza
Replicating Viral Vector	Newcastle disease virus vector (NDV-SARS-CoV-2/Spike)	Intravacc/Wageningen Bioveterinary Research/Utrecht Univ.	SARS-CoV2	Pre-Clinical	
Replicating Viral Vector	Avian Paramyxovirus Vector (APMV)	The Lancaster University, UK	SARS-CoV2	Pre-Clinical	
RNA	LNP-mRNA	Translate Bio/Sanofi Pasteur	SARS-CoV2	Pre-Clinical	
RNA	LNP-mRNA	CanSino Biologics/Precision Nano Systems	SARS-CoV2	Pre-Clinical	
RNA	LNP-encapsulated mRNA cocktail encoding VLP	Fudan University/ Shanghai JiaoTong University/RNACure Biopharma	SARS-CoV2	Pre-Clinical	

RNA	LNP-encapsulated mRNA encoding RBD	Fudan University/ Shanghai JiaoTong University/RNACure Biopharma	SARS-CoV2	Pre-Clinical	
RNA	Replicating Defective SARS-CoV-2 derived RNAs	Centro Nacional Biotecnología (CNB-CSIC), Spain	SARS-CoV2	Pre-Clinical	
RNA	LNP-encapsulated mRNA	University of Tokyo/ Daiichi-Sankyo	SARS-CoV2	Pre-Clinical	MERS
RNA	Liposome-encapsulated mRNA	BIOCAD	SARS-CoV2	Pre-Clinical	
RNA	Several mRNA candidates	RNAimmune, Inc.	SARS-CoV2	Pre-Clinical	
RNA	mRNA	FBRI SRC VB VECTOR, Rospotrebnadzor, Koltsovo	SARS-CoV2	Pre-Clinical	
RNA	mRNA	China CDC/Tongji University/ Stermina	SARS-CoV2	Pre-Clinical	
RNA	mRNA	Arcturus/Duke-NUS	SARS-CoV2	Pre-Clinical	Multiple candidates
RNA	LNP-mRNA	Chula Vaccine Research Center/ University of Pennsylvania	SARS-CoV2	Pre-Clinical	
RNA	mRNA in an intranasal delivery system	eTheRNA	SARS-CoV2	Pre-Clinical	
RNA	mRNA	Greenlight Biosciences	SARS-CoV2	Pre-Clinical	
RNA	mRNA	IDIBAPS-Hospital Clinic, Spain	SARS-CoV2	Pre-Clinical	
VLP	Enveloped Virus-Like Particle (eVLP)	VBI Vaccines Inc.	SARS-CoV2	Pre-Clinical	
VLP	S protein integrated in HIV VLPs	IrsiCaixa AIDS Research/IRTA-CReSA/Barcelona Supercomputing Centre/Grifols	SARS-CoV2	Pre-Clinical	
VLP	VLP + Adjuvant	Mahidol University/ The Government Pharmaceutical Organization (GPO)/Siriraj Hospital	SARS-CoV2	Pre-Clinical	
VLP	Virus-like particles, lentivirus and baculovirus vehicles	Navarrabiomed, Oncoimmunology group	SARS-CoV2	Pre-Clinical	

(Table Contd.)

Platform	*Type of candidate vaccine*	*Developer*	*Coronavirus target*	*Current stage of clinical evaluation/regulatory status-Coronavirus candidate*	*Same platform for non-Coronavirus candidates*
VLP	Virus-like particle, based on RBD displayed on virus-like particles	Saiba GmbH	SARS-CoV2	Pre-Clinical	
VLP	Plant-derived VLP	Medicago Inc.	SARS-CoV2	Pre-Clinical	Flu, Rotavirus, Norovirus, West Nilevirus, Cancer
VLP	ADDomerTM multiepitope display	Imophoron Ltd and Bristol University's Max Planck Centre	SARS-CoV2	Pre-Clinical	
VLP	Unknown	Doherty Institute	SARS-CoV2	Pre-Clinical	
VLP	VLP	OSIVAX	SARS-CoV1 SARS-CoV2	Pre-Clinical	
VLP	eVLP	ARTES Biotechnology	SARS-CoV2	Pre-Clinical	Malaria
VLP	VLPs peptides/whole virus	Univ. of Sao Paulo	SARS-CoV2	Pre-Clinical	
Unknown	Unknown	Tulane University	SARS-CoV2	Pre-Clinical	
Unknown	Unknown	Université Laval	SARS-CoV2	Pre-Clinical	
Unknown	Unknown	Adeleke University	SARS-CoV2	Pre-Clinical	

DISCLAIMER: These landscape documents have been prepared by the World Health Organization (WHO) for information purposes only concerning the 2019-2020 global of the novel coronavirus. Inclusion of any particular product or entity in any of these landscape documents does not constitute, and shall not be deemed or construed as, any approval or endorsement by WHO of such product or entity (or any of its businesses or activities). While WHO takes reasonable steps to verify the accuracy of the information presented in these landscape documents, WHO does not make any (and hereby disclaims all) representations and warranties regarding the accuracy, completeness, fitness for a particular purpose (including any of the aforementioned purposes), quality, safety, efficacy, merchantability and/or non-infringement of any information provided in these landscape documents and/or of any of the products referenced therein. WHO also disclaims any and all liability or responsibility whatsoever for any death, disability, injury, suffering, loss, damage or other prejudice of any kind that may arise from or in connection with the procurement, distribution or use of any product included in any of these landscape documents.

Index